Drug Absorption Studies: In Situ, In Vitro and In Silico Models

Drug Absorption Studies: In Situ, In Vitro and In Silico Models

Editor

Im-Sook Song

MDPI • Basel • Beijing • Wuhan • Barcelona • Belgrade • Manchester • Tokyo • Cluj • Tianjin

Editor
Im-Sook Song
Department of Pharmaceutics
Kyungpook National University
Daegu
Korea

Editorial Office
MDPI
St. Alban-Anlage 66
4052 Basel, Switzerland

This is a reprint of articles from the Special Issue published online in the open access journal *Pharmaceutics* (ISSN 1999-4923) (available at: www.mdpi.com/journal/pharmaceutics/special_issues/Absorption).

For citation purposes, cite each article independently as indicated on the article page online and as indicated below:

LastName, A.A.; LastName, B.B.; LastName, C.C. Article Title. *Journal Name* **Year**, *Volume Number*, Page Range.

ISBN 978-3-0365-2461-0 (Hbk)
ISBN 978-3-0365-2460-3 (PDF)

Contents

About the Editor vii

Preface to "Drug Absorption Studies: In Situ, In Vitro and In Silico Models" ix

Marta Kus-Slowinska, Monika Wrzaskowska, Izabela Ibragimow, Piotr Igor Czaklosz, Anna Olejnik and Hanna Piotrowska-Kempisty
Solubility, Permeability, and Dissolution Rate of Naftidrofuryl Oxalate Based on BCS Criteria
Reprinted from: *Pharmaceutics* **2020**, *12*, 1238, doi:10.3390/pharmaceutics12121238 1

Kazuya Sugita, Noriyuki Takata and Etsuo Yonemochi
Dose-Dependent Solubility–Permeability Interplay for Poorly Soluble Drugs under Non-Sink Conditions
Reprinted from: *Pharmaceutics* **2021**, *13*, 323, doi:10.3390/pharmaceutics13030323 13

Lyubov Dyshlyuk, Stanislav Sukhikh, Svetlana Noskova, Svetlana Ivanova, Alexander Prosekov and Olga Babich
Study of the ¡span style="font-variant: small-caps"¿l¡/span¿-Phenylalanine Ammonia-Lyase Penetration Kinetics and the Efficacy of Phenylalanine Catabolism Correction Using In Vitro Model Systems
Reprinted from: *Pharmaceutics* **2021**, *13*, 383, doi:10.3390/pharmaceutics13030383 33

Mette Klitgaard, Anette Müllertz and Ragna Berthelsen
Estimating the Oral Absorption from Self-Nanoemulsifying Drug Delivery Systems Using an In Vitro Lipolysis-Permeation Method
Reprinted from: *Pharmaceutics* **2021**, *13*, 489, doi:10.3390/pharmaceutics13040489 47

Csilla Bartos, Patrícia Varga, Piroska Szabó-Révész and Rita Ambrus
Physico-Chemical and In Vitro Characterization of Chitosan-Based Microspheres Intended for Nasal Administration
Reprinted from: *Pharmaceutics* **2021**, *13*, 608, doi:10.3390/pharmaceutics13050608 61

Im-Sook Song, So-Jeong Nam, Ji-Hyeon Jeon, Soo-Jin Park and Min-Koo Choi
Enhanced Bioavailability and Efficacy of Silymarin Solid Dispersion in Rats with Acetaminophen-Induced Hepatotoxicity
Reprinted from: *Pharmaceutics* **2021**, *13*, 628, doi:10.3390/pharmaceutics13050628 73

Yusuke Kono, Iichiro Kawahara, Kohei Shinozaki, Ikuo Nomura, Honoka Marutani, Akira Yamamoto and Takuya Fujita
Characterization of P-Glycoprotein Inhibitors for Evaluating the Effect of P-Glycoprotein on the Intestinal Absorption of Drugs
Reprinted from: *Pharmaceutics* **2021**, *13*, 388, doi:10.3390/pharmaceutics13030388 89

Anallely López-Yerena, Maria Pérez, Anna Vallverdú-Queralt, Eleftherios Miliarakis, Rosa M. Lamuela-Raventós and Elvira Escribano-Ferrer
Oleacein Intestinal Permeation and Metabolism in Rats Using an In Situ Perfusion Technique
Reprinted from: *Pharmaceutics* **2021**, *13*, 719, doi:10.3390/pharmaceutics13050719 107

Ji-Min Kim, Seong-Wook Seo, Dong-Gyun Han, Hwayoung Yun and In-Soo Yoon
Assessment of Metabolic Interaction between Repaglinide and Quercetin via Mixed Inhibition in the Liver: In Vitro and In Vivo
Reprinted from: *Pharmaceutics* **2021**, *13*, 782, doi:10.3390/pharmaceutics13060782 123

Surendra Poudel and Dong Wuk Kim
Developing pH-Modulated Spray Dried Amorphous Solid Dispersion of Candesartan Cilexetil with Enhanced In Vitro and In Vivo Performance
Reprinted from: *Pharmaceutics* **2021**, *13*, 497, doi:10.3390/pharmaceutics13040497 . . . . **137**

Bo Tang, Yu Qian and Guihua Fang
Development of Lipid–Polymer Hybrid Nanoparticles for Improving Oral Absorption of Enoxaparin
Reprinted from: *Pharmaceutics* **2020**, *12*, 607, doi:10.3390/pharmaceutics12070607 . . . . **155**

Noriaki Nagai, Ryotaro Seiriki, Saori Deguchi, Hiroko Otake, Noriko Hiramatsu, Hiroshi Sasaki and Naoki Yamamoto
Hydrogel Formulations Incorporating Drug Nanocrystals Enhance the Therapeutic Effect of Rebamipide in a Hamster Model for Oral Mucositis
Reprinted from: *Pharmaceutics* **2020**, *12*, 532, doi:10.3390/pharmaceutics12060532 . . . . **167**

About the Editor

Im-Sook Song

Im-Sook Song received her undergraduate degree in Manufacturing Pharmacy, College of Pharmacy from Seoul National University in 1996 and her master's degree in Pharmaceutics, College of Pharmacy from Seoul National University in 1998. In 2001, she completed her Ph.D. degree in Biopharmaceutics, College of Pharmacy, Seoul National University. Then, she trained in the Department of Molecular Pathology, University of Texas MD Anderson Cancer Center, Houston, Texas as a postdoctoral fellow. She joined the Pharmacogenomics Research center, Inje University School of Medicine, Korea in 2006 as an Assistant professor. In 2012, she joined College of Pharmacy, Kyungpook National University, Korea as a Professor.

She has published more than 50 papers during recent five years in the area of Pharmacokinetics including drug transport, drug metabolism, and drug interaction and also in the area of pharmaceutical formulations to increase the bioavailability of drugs.

Preface to "Drug Absorption Studies: In Situ, In Vitro and In Silico Models"

Since the oral administration of drugs remains the route of choice for the treatment of numerous drugs, the intestinal permeability of orally administered drugs has been widely used to determine the rate and extent of the intestinal absorption of drugs. The solubility, dissolution, and gastrointestinal physiology including transit, pH condition, mechanisms for gut metabolism and transport could also affect the intestinal absorption of orally administered drugs. Several strategies have been developed to estimate the oral bioavailability of drugs and to understand or overcome the issues associated with low oral bioavailability. The implementation of in situ, in vitro, and in silico methods, followed by in vivo evaluation, can guide to obtain the acceptable oral bioavailability in the drug development and formulation process.

This Book serves to highlight the mechanisms related to the low intestinal drug absorption, the strategies to overcome the obstacles or intestinal drug absorption, and in situ, in vitro, and in silico methodologies to predict to intestinal drug absorption.

This Book presents a series of drug absorption studies and related technologies that predict intestinal permeation of drugs that govern the pharmacokinetic features of therapeutic drugs. It also contains the mechanistic understanding regarding the first-pass metabolism and intestinal efflux that modulate the pharmacokinetics of drug and suggest the formulation strategies to enhance the bioavailability of investigated drugs.

Im-Sook Song
Editor

pharmaceutics

Article

Solubility, Permeability, and Dissolution Rate of Naftidrofuryl Oxalate Based on BCS Criteria

Marta Kus-Slowinska [1,2], Monika Wrzaskowska [2], Izabela Ibragimow [2], Piotr Igor Czaklosz [2], Anna Olejnik [3,*] and Hanna Piotrowska-Kempisty [1,4,*]

1 Department of Toxicology, Poznan University of Medical Sciences, 30 Dojazd St., 60-631 Poznan, Poland; marta.kus-slowinska@ethifarm.pl
2 Research and Development Department of Ethifarm, Ethifarm Manufacturing Plant, 9 Stefana Zeromskiego St., 60-544 Poznan, Poland; monika.wrzaskowska@ethifarm.pl (M.W.); izabela.ibragimow@ethifarm.pl (I.I.); piotr.czaklosz@ethifarm.pl (P.I.C.)
3 Department of Biotechnology and Food Microbiology, Poznan University of Life Sciences, 48 Wojska Polskiego St., 60-627 Poznan, Poland
4 Department of Basic and Preclinical Sciences, Institute of Veterinary Medicine, Nicolaus Copernicus University in Toruń, 7 Gagarina St., 87-100 Torun, Poland
* Correspondence: anna.olejnik@up.poznan.pl (A.O.); hpiotrow@ump.edu.pl (H.P.-K.); Tel.: +48-618-466-008 (A.O.); +48-618-470-721 (H.P.-K.)

Received: 13 November 2020; Accepted: 17 December 2020; Published: 19 December 2020

Abstract: The Biopharmaceutics Classification System (BCS) was conceived to classify drug substances by their in vitro aqueous solubility and permeability properties. The essential activity of naftidrofuryl oxalate (NF) has been described as the inhibition of the serotonin receptors ($5\text{-}HT_2$), resulting in vasodilation and decreasing blood pressure. Since the early 1980s, NF has been used to treat several venous and cerebral diseases. There is no data available on the BCS classification of NF. However, based on its physical-chemical properties, NF might be considered to belong to the 1st or the 3rd BCS class. The present study aimed to provide data concerning the solubility and permeability of NF through Caco-2 monolayers and propose its preliminary classification into BCS. We showed that NF is a highly soluble and permeable drug substance; thus, it might be suggested to belong to BCS class I. Additionally, a high dissolution rate of the encapsulated NF based on Praxilene® 100 mg formulation was revealed. Hence, it might be considered as an immediate-release (IR).

Keywords: naftidrofuryl oxalate; solubility; permeability; dissolution profiles; pharmaceutical availability; BCS drug classification

1. Introduction

Pharmacokinetics characterizes the drug's behavior in the body from its administration to excretion. It describes five major physical and chemical properties: liberation, absorption, distribution, metabolism, and elimination (LADME). The first two stages of LADME are characterized by the Biopharmaceutical Classification System (BCS), introduced by Amidon et al. in 1995 [1]. BCS is a scientific framework for classifying drug substances based on their aqueous solubility and intestinal permeability, which largely allows the prediction of a given drug substance bioavailability (BA) in human blood plasma. The BA of drugs depends mainly on their physicochemical properties (solubility, dissociation, and lipophilicity), dosage form (influence of excipients on active pharmaceutical ingredients (API) properties), and the route of administration (oral—liver metabolism) [2,3].

Naftidrofuryl hydrogen oxalate (NF, $C_{24}H_{33}NO_3$, $C_2H_2O_4$; synonym: nafronyl oxalate), as a pharmacologically active drug compound, is a mixture of four stereoisomers [4]. NF is a white powder freely soluble in water and ethanol (with pKa 8.2 at 30 °C) [5,6]. It selectively inhibits 5-hydroxytryptamine type 2A (serotonin; type 5-HT_{2A}) receptors present in vascular smooth muscle cells, platelets, and endothelial cells (in vascular and cerebral tissues). In vascular cells, NF causes vascular vasodilation (by preventing smooth muscle contraction) and decreases blood pressure [7]. Furthermore, it inhibits serotonin-induced platelet aggregation and platelet- induced vasospasm [8]. NF has also been shown to increase the ATP level in fibroblast and endothelial cells by improving the aerobic metabolism in the blood vessel wall [4]. As a drug product, NF has been mainly used for the treatment of intermittent claudication (since 80th) [9], less often also for stroke [10] and dementia [11].

A literature review of NF pharmacokinetics properties is detailed in Table 1. The main NF capsules manufacturer states that the peak plasma concentration (C_{max}) occurs about 30 min after oral dosing [12]. The relative BA of 100 mg NF administered orally was estimated 121% (oral solution containing 100 mg of NF as a reference was used) [6]. Furthermore, based on the pharmacokinetic data presented by Brodie et al., the high relative BA of NF (approx 100% following oral administration of 100 mg tablets) can be suggested [13]. However, the results of several studies about BA of NF are controversial. Nishigaki et al. showed that the relative bioavailability of 100 mg NF after its oral administration was within the 20–23% range. The authors concluded that this was due to the large first-pass elimination metabolism (80%) [14]. Additionally, the pharmacokinetic analysis performed in the dogs has also demonstrated a low absolute BA of 250 mg NF in the range of 0.3–2.7% due to presystemic and/or first-pass metabolism [15].

After absorption, NF is distributed and stored predominantly in fatty tissue [16]. NF is primarily biotransformed in hepatocytes to three acidic metabolites, among which NF free acid (3-(1-naphthyl)-2 tetrahydrofurfuryl propionic acid) is the main one [17,18]. Less than 1% of absorbed NF is excreted in urine within 48 h of administration, while most of it appears to be eliminated with the bile [19].

Table 1. Summary of literature data on the NF pharmacokinetics.

Dosage Form	Dosage [mg]	No. of Patients	$T_{1/2}$ [h]	T_{max} [h]	C_{max} [ng/mL]	AUC [ng/mL*h]	BA [%]	Reference
oral	nd	nd	nd	nd	nd	nd	30	[20]
oral (gelatin capsules)	50	n/d	0.68	1.1	350	nd	76	[21]
oral (capsules)	100	2	1.2	0.5	203	nd	nd	[13]
intravenous	40	18	nd	nd	nd	nd	nd	[16]
oral (gelatin capsules)	300	12	1.79	0.94	922	2022	nd	[21]
oral (fasted)	100	12	1.3	0.8	238	500	19.7	[14]
oral (nonfasted)			1.6	2	181	583	23.0	
	100			1	209	630	121	
oral (tablets)	300	9	nd	0.9	590	1271	77	[6]
	300			1.2	645	1955	114	
oral (tablets)	200	30	3.41	2.75	279	1797	nd	[22]
oral (tablets)	200	12	4.4	1.3	174	1504	nd	[23]

nd = no data; $T_{1/2}$ = half life; T_{max} = the time taken to reach the maximum concentration; C_{max} = the peak plasma concentration; AUC = area under curve; BA = bioavailability.

NF drug products are widely distributed all over the world. The clinical dose of naftidrofuryl is 100 or 200 mg for all its dosage forms (capsules and tablets).

To the best of the authors' knowledge, there is no data concerning the permeability of NF or its BCS classification. Hence, to fulfill the literature gap, the present study aimed to provide data concerning aqueous solubility and permeability of NF through Caco-2 monolayers and propose its preliminary classification into BCS. We performed three experiments concerning the solubility, permeability, and dissolution of NF largely based on the BSC guidelines for the pharmaceutical industry [24,25]. However, industry guidelines are mainly focused and directed for biowaiver approach applicants.

Hence, in the present study, several issues in experimental design and data evaluation differ from the formal requirements.

2. Materials and Methods

2.1. Reagents and References

The acetonitrile (ACN; VWR Chemicals, Fontenay-sous-Bois, France) and water (H_2O; VWR Chemicals, Fontenay-sous-Bois, France) for the HPLC assay were of chromatographic grade. Other reagents were of analytical grade: hydrochloric acid (HCl, Chempur, Piekary Slaskie Poland), disodium hydrogen phosphate (Na_2HPO_4; Chempur, Piekary Slaskie, Poland), ammonium acetate ($CH_3CO_2NH_4$; Chempur, Piekary Slaskie, Poland), sodium acetate (CH_3COONa; Chempur, Piekary Slaskie, Poland), glacial acetic acid (CH_3COOH; Chempur, Piekary Slaskie, Poland), and orthophosphoric acid (85%; H_3PO_4; Chempur, Piekary Slaskie, Poland). The media solutions used for solubility and dissolution tests were prepared according to European Pharmacopoeia (EP) Chapter 4–Reagents.

A British Pharmacopoeia Certificated Reference Standard of Naftidrofuryl oxalate (BPCRS, Cat no. 362) was used for all the performed assays. Additionally, we used the Caffeine standard (CAF) (Sigma Aldrich–Merck Group, Darmstadt, Germany) for permeability tests as a reference. Praxilene® 100 mg Capsules (Merck Serono Ltd., Feltham, UK) was employed as a drug reference product. Each Praxilene capsule contained 100 mg of naftidrofuryl oxalate.

Naftidrofuryl oxalate (Sigma Aldrich–Merck Group, Darmstadt, Germany), magnesium stearate (Peter Greven Nederland C.V., Venlo, Netherland), and talc (C.H. Erbslöh, Krefeld, Germany) used for the in-house capsules were obtained from Ethifarm (Ethifarm, Poznan, Poland). Hard gelatin capsules, size 3 (Capsugel, Morristown, NJ, USA) used in the drug dosage manufacture were provided by Ethifarm (Ethifarm, Poznan, Poland).

2.2. Solubility Test

The solubility by equilibrium method was performed in three different media (0.1 M HCl, acetate buffer, and phosphate buffer), with a pH of 1.2, 4.5, and 6.8, respectively, based on European Medicines Agency (EMA) guideline [24]. Saturated solutions of NF in given media were prepared by adding an excessive amount of the drug until obtained a saturated solution (presence of visible precipitate on the tube). The samples were then incubated at 37 °C ± 0.5 (incubator chamber; Binder GmbH, Tuttlingen, Germany) for 24 h in an orbital agitation of 45 rpm (LLG-uniLOOPMIX 2 orbital shaker, LLG GmbH, Hamburg, Germany). After equilibration, the sample was filtered (0.45 µm) and diluted with the appropriate solution to the concentration within the linear calibration range. Drug concentration measurement was performed by a validated UV spectrophotometric method at $\lambda = 283$ nm with optical path 0.2 cm and spectrum recorded on 250–350 nm range (JASCO V-530 double-beam apparatus with Spectra Manager software, JASCO, Tokyo, Japan). The experiments were carried out in triplicate.

The dose number (D_0) for each pH buffer solution was calculated using the following equation:

$$D_0 = DOSE/V_0/S \quad (1)$$

where DOSE is the highest dose strength (mg), V_0 is the water volume (assumed to be 250 mL), and S is the aqueous solubility (mg/mL). Drug substances with $D_0 \leq 1$ are classified as high solubility drugs, while drugs with $D_0 \geq 1$ are assigned as low solubility drugs [26].

2.3. Cytotoxicity Analysis

The MTT (3-(4,5-dimethyl-2-thiazolyl)-2,5-diphenyl-2H-tetrazolium bromide) test (Sigma Aldrich–Merck Group, Darmstadt, Germany) was used to establish an appropriate concentration of analyzed substances NF and CAF in the Caco-2 cell line. To determine the effects of materials tested on cell viability, confluent stock cultures were detached using trypsin and seeded in 96-well plates at a density of 2×10^4 cells/well. They were allowed to attach overnight and then exposed for 2 h (time of transport across monolayer) for seven different NF/CAF concentrations in Hank's Balanced Salt Solution (HBSS, Sigma Aldrich–Merck Group, Darmstadt, Germany) pH 7.4 in the range of 0.0 mg/mL to 1.0 mg/mL. After NF/CAF discarding, the mixture of growth medium and MTT (5 mg/mL) was added. Cells were incubated for 3 h until intracellular purple formazan crystals were visible under a microscope, and then dimethyl sulfoxide (DMSO), (POCH-Avantor, Gliwice, Poland) was added to each well to dissolve purple crystals of formazan. The absorbance was measured using a spectrophotometric method (BioTek U.S., Winooski, VT, USA) at a wavelength of 540 nm.

2.4. The Culture of Caco-2 Colon Cancer Cells

The colon cancer Caco-2 cell line (ATCC® HTB-37™) was purchased from ATCC (American Type Culture Collection, Manassas, VA, USA) and used as the model of the epithelial intestinal permeability layer. Caco-2 cells were cultured in Dulbecco's Modified Eagle's Medium (DMEM, Merck Group, Darmstadt, Germany) supplemented with 1% nonessential amino acids mixture (MEM NON, Merck Group, Darmstadt, Germany), 20% fetal bovine serum (FBS, Merck Group, Darmstadt, Germany), and 2 mM L-glutamine, 100 U/mL penicillin and 0.1 mg/mL streptomycin solution (Merck Group, Darmstadt, Germany). For the transport monolayer preparation, the Caco-2 cells were seeded at $4 \times 10^5/cm^2$ into transparent membranes inserts with 0.4 μm pore size (Millipore–Merck Group, Darmstadt, Germany) in 6-wells plates (Corning-Life Science, Durham, NC, USA). The cells were cultured for 22 days at 37 °C in a humidified atmosphere containing 5% CO_2 and 95% air. The integrity of the Caco-2 monolayer was evaluated by measuring the Trans Epithelial Electrical Resistance (TEER) every 48 h. The cells were considered to be suitable for use in the permeability study if the average TEER value was >600 Ohm × cm^2 (Millicell ERS-2 Voltohmmeter, Millipore–Merck Group, Darmstadt, Germany).

2.5. Permeability Test

The permeability tests of NF and CAF solutions were performed in two directions: apical-to-basolateral (A–B) and basolateral-to-apical (B–A) in triplicate at 37 °C with shaking at 100 rpm for 2 h. For transport assay, drug substances (NF, CAF) were dissolved in the transport buffer solution (HBSS with 25 mM HEPES, pH 7.4) and applied in the apical or basolateral compartment in compliance with transport direction. At 15 min intervals, the sample from the acceptor compartment was taken during a 2-h transport experiment. Each sample volume (150 μL) was replaced with a fresh pre-heated (37 °C) transport buffer. The total solution volume in the apical and basolateral compartments was maintained at 2 mL and 4 mL, respectively. HPLC analysis was used to determine the concentration of the compound transported. Quantitative chromatographic analyses were performed using the reverse phase HPLC method and UV-VIS detector (Waters UPLC Acquity H-class apparatus with Empower 3.0 software, Waters Corporation, Milford, MA, USA). The analytical method of NF was based on British Pharmacopoeia monograph Naftydrofuryl capsules (with slight modifications) [27], while CAF was based on the European Pharmacopoeia monograph [5]. The chromatographic parameters for NF were set as follows: column (4.6 mm × 250 mm; 5 μm) filled with silica modified by phenyl groups (Spherisorb Phenyl columns, Waters Corporation, Milford, MA, USA). The liquid phase was a mixture of 55 volumes of ACN with 45 volumes of 0.05 M sodium acetate (pH 4.0 with 85% *v/v* orthophosphoric acid). The isocratic flow rate was set as 1 mL/min and the detection wavelength on $\lambda = 283$ nm. The retention time of Naftidrofuryl peak was about 10 min. Following the modifications, this chromatographic method was validated to be suitable for the assay. Transport data, including apparent permeability coefficient (P_{app}) that reflects the rate at which compounds pass the intestinal barrier, were calculated according to the protocols described by Tavelin et al. [28] and Hubatsch et al. [29].

2.6. *In-House NF Capsules Preparation*

In-house 100 mg capsules with Naftidrofuryl oxalate were prepared as a test product (laboratory scale) for the NF dissolution profile assay. The in-house NF capsules were made according to the Praxilene® 100 mg Capsules formulation, as presented in the Praxilene SPMC [12] in the proportions shown in Table 2.

Table 2. Composition of the developed in-house NF capsules.

Ingredients	Quantity (Per One Capsule)	Function
Naftidrofuryl oxalate	100 mg	active ingredient
Talc	rest of the unit filling weight	filler
Magnesium stearate	up to 0.5% of the unit filling weight	lubricant

2.7. *In Vitro Dissolution Test and Data Evaluation*

The release rate of NF (from in-house NF capsules vs. Praxilene® 100 mg Capsules) was determined by using automated dissolution apparatus (European Pharmacopoeia, Type II; Erweka DT 828/1000 LH; Erweka GmbH, Langen, Germany) with paddles operating at a rotation speed of 50 rpm in 37 °C (±0.5 °C). The parameters for the dissolution test: 900 mL of three different dissolution media (0.1 M HCl, acetate buffer, phosphate buffer) with pH of 1.2, 4.5, and 6.8 respectively were used. Twelve in-house NF capsules (and 12 Praxilene units) were tested in each dissolution medium. The concentration values of the released NF were recorded at the following time points: 5, 10, 15, 20, 30, and 45 min. Samples (10 mL) of the tested solutions were withdrawn, then filtered (0.2 μm nylon syringe filter), and subsequently subjected to quantitative assessment by validated spectrophotometric method (as described in Section 2.2—Solubility test). The dissolution data were statistically evaluated using the two factor (f_1, f_2) method, according to the United States Food and Drug Administration (FDA) guideline [25]. As the first step, the spectrophotometric results were qualitatively evaluated (% RSD—relative standard deviation percentage) to ensure that they are suitable for the two factors calculation stage and, subsequently, for the dissolution profiles comparison and evaluation. The aggregated % RSD was calculated based on all the three dissolution media timepoints results obtained. However, the % RSD not exceeding 20% of the results obtained in the early time points (up to 10 min) and 10% for the subsequent timepoints is mandatory in this approach. The difference factor (f_1) and similarity factor (f_2) were calculated according to the FDA guidelines [25,30]. The two curves are considered to be similar if the value for f_1 is not greater than 15% (0–15), while the value of f_2 is greater than 50% (50–100) [25,30].

3. Results

3.1. *Solubility Test*

The maximum dose strength for NF is 200 mg (according to data on https://www.drugs.com/international/naftidrofuryl.html). Using the equilibrium solubility method, we showed a high solubility of NF in all buffers pH range 1.2–6.8. The lowest value of solubility (about 169 mg/mL) was observed on acetic acid conditions (pH 4.5), and the highest value (about 290 mg/mL) was obtained in pH 6.8. Thus, the calculated minimum dose/solubility ratio (D/S) was lower than 250 mL, and the dose number (D_0) was less than 1 in each medium. The results of the equilibrium solubility are shown in Table 3.

Table 3. Solubility results of 200 mg NF in three different pH media at 37 °C. Results of the three replicates are presented as the mean ± SD.

Dose (D) (mg)	pH	Solubility (S) (mg/mL)	D/S Ratio (mL)	D_0
200	1.2	279.00 ± 15.69	0.69	0.003
	4.5	169.00 ± 6.79	1.19	0.005
	6.8	290.40 ± 19.83	0.67	0.003

3.2. Permeability Assay on Caco-2 Cell Line

To assess the permeability of NF across the Caco-2 monolayer, we selected CAF classified as the reference standard for highly permeable and BCS class I substances [24,25].

3.2.1. Effect of NF and CAF on Caco-2 Cells Viability

The concentrations of the drugs to be used for the permeability tests were established by using the MTT viability test. The highest concentration of the test compounds with no cytotoxic effect on Caco-2 cells was preferred. To evaluate the cytotoxic activity of NF and CAF, the Caco-2 cells were exposed for two hours to the concentration ranges of each compound from 0.0 mg/mL to 1.0 mg/mL. The MTT results (Figure 1) showed that NF caused a more cytotoxic effect, as compared to CAF since only the highest concentration of CAF (1.00 mg/mL) slightly decreased the viability of Caco-2 cells (~92%). In contrast, 0.250 mg/mL of NF concentration caused down-regulation of cell viability to ~67%. Hence, in the permeability study, we used 0.200 mg/mL and 0.125 mg/mL of NF concentrations as they were not cytotoxic in the Caco-2 cell line.

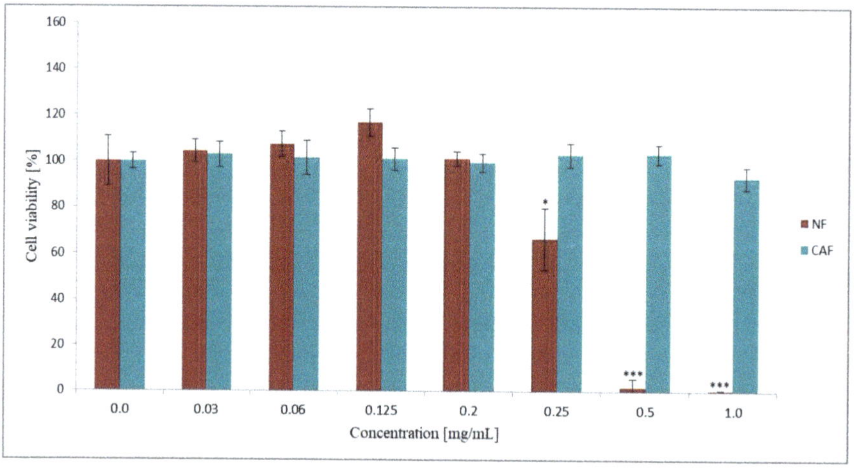

Figure 1. The effect of NF and CAF on Caco-2 cell viability. Results of the three independent replicates are presented as the mean ± SD. *** $p < 0.001$ and * $p < 0.05$.

3.2.2. Caco-2 Permeability Assay

The intestinal epithelial Caco-2 cell culture model was applied to determine the permeability of NF and CAF across the intestinal barrier. TEER value measurements monitored the integrity of the Caco-2 monolayers during 22-day cultivation. The TEER parameter stabilized at 614 ± 24 Ω cm^2 on the 7th day of culture. Only monolayers with TEER values beyond 600 Ω cm^2 were used in the transport experiments. Bidirectional transport was analysed at two NF concentrations (0.125 mg/mL and 0.200 mg/mL) to determine the drug dose permeability relationship. CAF, as a reference intestinal permeable compound, was transported across the Caco-2 barrier at a concentration of 0.500 mg/mL. No cytotoxicity of NF and CAF at the concentrations tested after 2-h transport was observed. The TEER measurement indicated the high integrity of Caco-2 cell monolayers before and after permeability experiments (data not shown).

Based on HPLC data, the NF and CAF transport kinetics and the apparent permeability coefficient (P_{app}) values were evaluated. The "weighted normalized cumulative amount of transported compound" for simplicity commonly named in the literature "cumulative fraction transported" (CFT) in the receiver compartment of the Caco-2 experimental model increased linearly with time, independently on transport direction (Figure 2). The time-course analysis of NF and CAF intestinal permeability showed that CFT was significantly higher in the absorptive direction (A-B transport) than in the secretory direction (B–A transport). This was also confirmed by the Papp values determined for NF and CAF transported in A–B and B–A direction (Table 4).

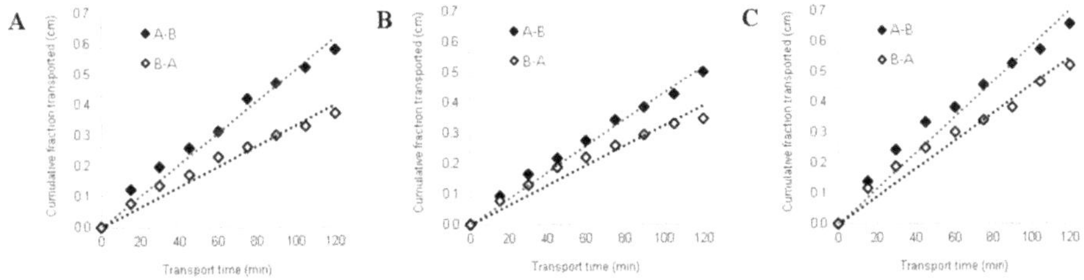

Figure 2. The experimentally (◊) and theoretically (········) determined "cumulative fraction transported" of naftidrofuryl oxalate (NF) and caffeine (CAF) versus time in bidirectional A–B and B–A transport across Caco-2 cell monolayer. NF concentrations in donor compartments were established at 0.125 mg/mL (**A**) and 0.200 mg/mL (**B**). CAF transport was analyzed at an initial concentration of 0.5 mg/mL (**C**).

Table 4. Apparent permeability coefficients (P_{app}) of naftidrofuryl oxalate (NF) and caffeine (CAF) determined in the Caco-2 intestinal barrier model (n = 3).

		$P_{app} \times 10^{-6}$ (cm/s)	
Drug Substance	**Concentration (mg/mL)**	**Apical-to-Basolaterial Transport**	**Basolaterial-to-Apical Transport**
NF	0.125	131.9 ± 34.8	84.1 ± 4.7
NF	0.200	100.8 ± 15.1	78.8 ± 1.0
CAF	0.500	161.3 ± 19.7	126.5 ± 2.4

The results obtained from transport experiments showed that in vitro permeability of NF across the Caco-2 intestinal barrier is relatively high. The P_{app} values estimated for A–B transport of NF at both concentrations were higher than 100 × 10^{-6} cm/s. Permeability coefficients for B–A transport were calculated at 84.1 × 10^{-6} cm/s and 78.8 × 10^{-6} cm/s for NF at concentrations of 0.125 mg/mL and 0.200 mg/mL, respectively (Table 4). The results obtained from transport studies confirmed high intestinal permeability of CAF in both transport directions.

3.3. Dissolution Profiles Comparison

The in vitro dissolution testing was performed based on EMA guideline [24]. NF was released from both products, Praxilene, and the in-house NF capsules, very rapidly > 85% in less than 15 min. The dissolution rate of NF capsules was independent of pH and buffer species of the dissolution media. We observed a slightly faster release NF from in-house NF capsules than a reference product (Praxilene). The results of dissolution profiles of NF from in-house NF capsules and Praxilene are shown in Figure 3.

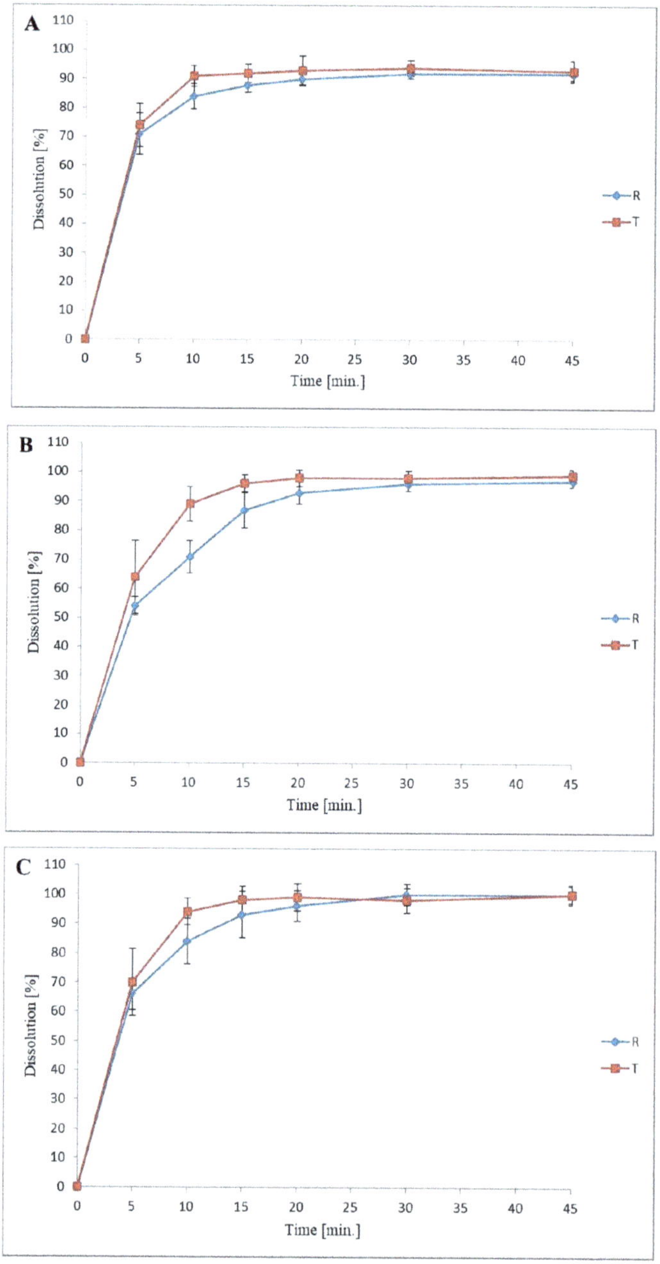

Figure 3. Comparative assessment of the in vitro release profiles of NF from in-house NF capsules (T, tested product) and Praxilene (R, reference product) in three different media 0.1 M HCl (**A**), acetate buffer (**B**), and phosphate buffer (**C**). Each time point on the curves shows the aggregated (n = 12) average percentage of NF release level from these products.

According to EMA, the confirmation of two curves (dissolution profiles) is not required for the IR product (≥85% in 15 min) [24]. Nevertheless, the mathematical estimation with standard statistical analysis was performed. The raw data (% RSD of the results in early dissolution time points, up to 10 min., of not more than 20%, and no more than of 10% in the subsequent time points) are consistent with the EMA guideline (Table 5) [24].

Table 5. The % RSD values for the in vitro release profiles of NF from in-house NF capsules (T, tested product) and Praxilene (R, reference product) in three different media 0.1 M HCl, acetate buffer, and phosphate buffer.

Time Point [min.]	0.1 M HCl pH 1.2 (%RSD)		Acetate Buffer pH 4.5 (%RSD)		Phosphate Buffer pH 6.8 (%RSD)	
	R	T	R	T	R	T
5	10.0	10.0	5.8	19.8	8.3	16.3
10	5.2	4.1	7.7	6.7	9.2	4.8
15	2.9	3.5	7.1	3.2	8.5	4.7
20	2.1	5.4	4.1	2.9	5.3	4.6
30	1.9	2.8	2.3	2.4	3.6	4.3
45	2.3	3.9	2.0	2.3	2.8	3.3

The statistical evaluation of the two profiles similarity was performed using the two factors (f_1, f_2) method. The summary of the results is presented in Table 6. Our results showed a mathematical similarity between the dissolution profiles of the test (in-house NF capsules) and the reference product (Praxilene) for each medium ($f_2 \geq 50$); the EMA guideline [24] was met. The release profiles showed the most significant similarity in pH 1.2 and 6.8 ($f_1 \leq 15$, $f_2 \geq 50$), while in pH 4.5, they were on the border of the accepted criteria ($f_2 = 51$, $f_1 = 11$).

Table 6. Summary of f_1 and f_2 values for dissolution profiles curves in three different media.

Requirement	0.1 M HCl pH = 1.2	Acetate Buffer pH = 4.5	Phosphate Buffer pH = 6.8
Difference factor f_1 (profiles are similar when $f_1 \leq 15$)	2	11	6
Similarity factor f_2 (profiles are similar when $f_2 \geq 50$)	71	51	65

4. Discussion

The BCS-based biowaiver guidelines take into account the rate of APIs release from the solid oral dosage forms, their solubility, and the in vitro transepithelial transport, thus describing the first stages of a drug LADME (liberation and absorption) [24,25]. To the best of the authors' knowledge, there is no data concerning the classification of NF to the BCS. NF is known to dissolve well in aqueous media and ethanol [5,27]. Based on this information, NF might be suggested to belong to BCS class I (high solubility, high permeability) or BCS class III (high solubility, low permeability). Thus, the present study aimed to determine the aqueous solubility of NF and its permeability through Caco-2 monolayers.

The determination of NF solubility was performed using the equilibrium solubility method. Based on EMA guideline, a substance is considered well soluble when the highest therapeutic dose dissolves in 250 mL or less of aqueous media within the pH range of 1.2–6.8 at 37 ± 1 °C [24]. According to FDA guideline, the solubility test should be evaluated based on the ionization characteristics of the tested substance in pH = pKa, pH = pKa + 1, and pH = pKa−1 [25]. The pKa value of NF has been reported as 8.2 [6,19], which is above the human gastrointestinal tract (GIT) physiological range. Therefore, we did not extend the pH condition above the physiological range. In the solubility studies, we used three media in ranges of gastrointestinal pH (1.2, 4.5, and 6.8) and the highest 200 mg NF dose strength. We showed that the minimum solubility of the NF highest single dose was 169.0 mg/mL at pH 4.5. The calculated D/S ratio was 1.2 mL, thus far below the critical value of 250 mL. Our results indicate that NF is a highly soluble substance in the entire examined pH range. The highest solubility value at pH 6.8 suggests that NF might be well soluble in intestinal pH conditions positively affecting drug absorption from the GIT.

According to BCS-based protocols, the permeability of a drug substance throughout the GIT can be assessed by in vitro methods using a monolayer of cultured epithelial cells [24,25]. Hence, to determine the absorption of NF, the permeability test using the Caco-2 cell line was performed, and permeability coefficients (P_{app}) were determined in both directions. In the present study, the permeability test of CAF was performed to confirm the suitability of the Caco-2 cell line system applied to determine transepithelial transport. CAF is recognized as a BCS reference substance [24,25] for which high permeability (P_{app} = ~50 × 10^{-6} cm/s; concentration 0.06 mg/mL) has been well documented [31,32]. Since we observed high transepithelial transport of CAF in both directions, the usefulness of the Caco-2 cell model was confirmed. The permeability study of CAF was performed only at the highest concentration (0.5 mg/mL) without cytotoxic effects against Caco-2 cells. According to BCS requirements for permeability analysis, the concentration of drug substance should be used in the amount of 0.01, 0.1, and 1 times its highest strength dissolved in 250 mL [24,25]. Assuming the NF 200 mg as the highest dose dissolute in 250 mL, we obtained a concentration range as follows: 0.8 mg/mL, 0.08 and 0.008 mg/mL. We examined the cytotoxicity of NF starting on the highest 1.0 mg/mL concentration. The 0.250 mg/mL of NF concentration was observed to cause down-regulation of cell viability to ~67%. Therefore, the bidirectional transport of NF was investigated at the two highest non-cytotoxic concentrations (0.125 mg/mL and 0.200 mg/mL), in the order of magnitude close to 0.08 mg/mL. We did not perform the permeability study of NF in the lowest concentration (0.008 mg/mL) since the analytical range of the NF assay method was validated for 0.01–0.3 mg/mL concentrations. According to literature data, when P_{aap} is lower than 1 × 10^{-6}, the substance is considered as poorly permeable (0–20%). Concomitantly, the highly permeable drug is characterized by P_{aap} > 10 × 10^{-6} [29,33]. Our results showed that the permeability of NF across the cells barrier is quite high since the estimated values of P_{app} for A-B transport direction in both doses were larger than 100 × 10^{-6} cm/s. Furthermore, we observed that the P_{app} values of NF within its non-cytotoxic concentrations were almost as good as highly permeable CAF results. Hence, a rapid and total in vivo epithelial transport of NF might be suggested.

In general, we suggest that NF might be assigned to BCS I class due to its high solubility and high permeability. However, to fully comply with BCS requirements, the permeability tests should be validated using several additional reference substances that represent different levels of permeability (high, moderate, low, zero, and efflux substrates).

A drug product is eligible for biowaiver procedure when the substance belongs to BCS I or III class and is an immediate-release oral dosage form [24,25]. Thus, we also examined the in vitro dissolution rate of in-house prepared NF capsules in accordance with the Praxilene® 100 mg formulation as a reference drug. The Praxilene product has a relatively simple composition with only two excipients (talc and magnesium stearate) that allowed us to closely define the quantity of each excipient in the dosage form. In our study, we showed that both products fulfil the IR requirements (>85% in not less than 15 min). Additionally, the similarity of the curves was confirmed statistically ($f_1 \leq 15$; $f_2 \geq 50$) in all media used in the range of pH 1.2–6.8. Thus, we conclude that multisourced excipients used for NF capsules preparation had no or minimal effect on its release rate. Our observations are in agreement with Flangan et al. since the excipients used for BCS I class drugs have been generally shown not to affect the intestinal absorption rate [34]. Moreover, the IR status of analyzed products indicates high pharmaceutical availability of NF throughout the GIT. Thus, we suggest that NF oral dosage form in comparison with Praxilene as a reference product meets the pharmacological equivalence criteria.

5. Conclusions

NF is a highly soluble substance within a wide pH range of physiological GIT conditions and highly permeable across Caco-2 cell monolayer. Thus, in the present study, we suggest that NF might be classified into BCS class I. Furthermore, we showed high dissolution rate of encapsulated

NF based on Praxilene® 100 mg composition and, therefore, it might be considered as an IR. To the best of the authors' knowledge, this is the first attempt to classify NF based on BCS requirements. The experimental design of this study was based mainly on the BSC guidelines for the pharmaceutical industry. Hence, our paper could be useful for further developmental studies on NF containing drugs.

Author Contributions: Conceptualization, H.P.-K., A.O., and I.I.; formal analysis, M.K.-S. and M.W.; data curation, M.W. and I.I.; writing—original draft preparation, M.K.-S.; writing—review and editing, H.P.-K., I.I., and A.O.; supervision, H.P.-K., A.O., and I.I.; project administration, P.I.C.; funding acquisition, H.P.-K. and P.I.C. All authors have read and agreed to the published version of the manuscript.

Funding: This research was funded by the Ministry of Science and Higher Education of Poland, grant number DWD/3/10/2019.

Conflicts of Interest: The authors declare no conflict of interest.

References

1. Amidon, G.L.; Lennernäs, H.; Shah, V.P.; Crison, J.R. A Theoretical Basis for a Biopharmaceutic Drug Classification: The Correlation of in Vitro Drug Product Dissolution and in Vivo Bioavailability. *Pharm. Res.* **1995**, *12*, 413–420. [CrossRef] [PubMed]
2. Manallack, D.T.; Prankerd, R.J.; Yuriev, E.; Oprea, T.I.; Chalmers, D.K. The significance of acid/base properties in drug discovery. *Chem. Soc. Rev.* **2013**, *42*, 485–496. [CrossRef] [PubMed]
3. Panakanti, R.; Narang, A.S. Impact of Excipient Interactions on Drug Bioavailability from Solid Dosage Forms. *Pharm. Res.* **2012**, *29*, 2639–2659. [CrossRef] [PubMed]
4. Hao, J.; Chen, B.; Yao, Y.; Hossain, M.; Nagatomo, T.; Yao, H.; Kong, L.; Sun, H. Practical access to four stereoisomers of naftidrofuryl and their binding affinity towards 5-hydroxytryptamine 2A receptor. *Bioorganic Med. Chem. Lett.* **2012**, *22*, 3441–3444. [CrossRef]
5. European Directorate for the Quality of Medicines. *European Pharmacopoeia*, 10th ed.; European Directorate for the Quality of Medicines: Strasbourg, France, 2019; pp. 3322–3323.
6. Waaler, P.; Graffner, C.; Müller, B. Biopharmaceutical studies of naftidrofuryl in hydrocolloid matrix tablets. *Int. J. Pharm.* **1992**, *87*, 229–237. [CrossRef]
7. Wiernsperger, N.F. Serotonin, 5-HT2 receptors, and their blockade by naftidrofuryl: A targeted therapy of vascular diseases. *J. Cardiovasc. Pharmacol.* **1994**, *23*, S37–S43. [CrossRef]
8. Verheggen, R.; Schrör, K. Effect of naftidrofuryl on platelet-induced vasospasm in vitro. Role of antiserotonergic actions. *Arzneimittelforschung* **1993**, *43*, 330–334.
9. Goldsmith, D.R.; Wellington, K. Naftidrofuryl. *Drugs Aging* **2005**, *22*, 967–977. [CrossRef]
10. Capon, A.; Lehert, P.; Opsomer, L. Naftidrofuryl in the treatment of subacute stroke. *J. Cardiovasc. Pharmacol.* **1990**, *16*, 62–66.
11. Lu, D.; Song, H.; Hao, Z.; Wu, T.; Mccleery, J. Naftidrofuryl for dementia. *Cochrane Database Syst. Rev.* **2011**, *12*, CD002955. [CrossRef]
12. Merck Serono Ltd. Praxilene 100 mg Capsules; Summary of Product Characteristics. Available online: https://www.medicines.org.uk/emc/product/990/smpc#companyDetails (accessed on 12 November 2020).
13. Brodie, R.; Chasseaud, L.; Taylor, T.; Hunter, J.; Ciclitira, P. Determination of naftidrofuryl in the plasma of humans by high-performance liquid chromatography. *J. Chromatogr.* **1979**, *164*, 534–540. [CrossRef]
14. Nishigaki, R.; Umemura, K.; Okui, K.; Hayashi, T.; Yamamoto, T.; Sakurai, Y. The pharmacokinetical analysis of the fate of naphtidrofuryl oxalate (LS121) in human subjects. II. Estimation of the first-pass effect after oral administration. *Yakugaku Zasshi.* **1986**, *106*, 916–923. [CrossRef] [PubMed]
15. Garrett, E.R. Bioanalyses and Pharmacokinetics of Nafronyl in the Dog. *J. Pharm. Sci.* **1984**, *73*, 635–649. [CrossRef] [PubMed]
16. Platt, D.; Mühlberg, W.; Rieck, W.; Horn, H.J.; Schmitt-Rüth, R. Pharmacokinetics of naftidrofuryl in multimorbidity in geriatric patients. *Z. Gerontol.* **1984**, *17*, 246–250.
17. Roth, K.; Hildebrand, M.; Beyer, K.-H. Metabolism of nafronyl in man. *Eur. J. Drug Metab. Pharmacokinet.* **1989**, *14*, 133–138. [CrossRef]
18. Sabry, S.M.; Belal, T.S.; Barary, M.H.; Ibrahim, M.E.A. A validated HPLC method for the simultaneous determination of naftidrofuryl oxalate and its degradation product (metabolite), naftidrofuryl acid: Applications to pharmaceutical tablets and biological samples. *Drug Test. Anal.* **2012**, *5*, 500–508. [CrossRef]

19. Moffat, A.C.; Osselton, M.D.; Widdop, B.; Watts, J. *Clarke's Analysis of Drugs and Poisons*, 4th ed.; Pharmaceutical Press: London, UK; Gurnee, IL, USA, 2011; pp. 1746–1747.
20. Riederer, P.; Laux, G.; Pöldinger, W. *Neuro-Psychopharmaka Ein Therapie-Handbuch*; Springer: Wien, Austria, 1999; p. 660.
21. Walmsley, L.M.; Taylor, T.; Wilkinson, P.A.; Brodie, R.R.; Chasseaud, L.F.; Alun-Jones, V.; Hunter, J.O. Plasma concentrations and relative bioavailability of naftidrofuryl from different salt forms. *Biopharm. Drug Dispos.* **1986**, *7*, 327–334. [CrossRef]
22. Hulot, T.; Gamand, S.; Dupain, T.; Ahtoy, P.; Bromet, M. Influence of age on the pharmacokinetics of naftidrofuryl after single oral administration in elderly versus young healthy volunteers. *Arzneimittelforschung* **1998**, *48*, 900–904. [PubMed]
23. Legallicier, B.; Barbier, S.; Bolloni, L.; Fillastre, J.-P.; Godin, M.; Kuhn, T.; Porte, F.; Chretien, P.; Dupainc, T.; Bromet-Petitd, M. Pharmacokinetics of Naftidrofuryl in Patients with Renal Impairment. *Arzneimittelforschung* **2011**, *55*, 370–375. [CrossRef] [PubMed]
24. European Medicines Agency (EMA). ICH M9 Guideline on Biopharmaceutics Classification System-Based Biowaivers. Available online: https://www.ema.europa.eu/en/documents/scientific-guideline/ich-m9-biopharmaceutics-classification-system-based-biowaivers-step-5_en.pdf (accessed on 10 February 2020).
25. U.S. Food and Drug Administration (FDA). Waiver of In Vivo Bioavailability and Bioequivalence Studies for Immediate-Release Solid Oral Dosage Forms Based on a Biopharmaceutics Classification System Guidance for Industry. Available online: https://www.fda.gov/media/70963/download (accessed on 26 December 2017).
26. Dahan, A.; Miller, J.M.; Amidon, G.L. Prediction of Solubility and Permeability Class Membership: Provisional BCS Classification of the World's Top Oral Drugs. *AAPS J.* **2009**, *11*, 740–746. [CrossRef]
27. The British Pharmacopoeia Commission. *British Pharmacopoeia*; The British Pharmacopoeia Commission: London, England, 2020.
28. Tavelin, S.; Gråsjö, J.; Taipalensuu, J.; Ocklind, G.; Artursson, P.; Wise, C. Applications of Epithelial Cell Culture in Studies of Drug Transport. *Methods Mol Biol.* **2002**, *188*, 233–272. [CrossRef] [PubMed]
29. Hubatsch, I.; E Ragnarsson, E.G.; Artursson, P. Determination of drug permeability and prediction of drug absorption in Caco-2 monolayers. *Nat. Protoc.* **2007**, *2*, 2111–2119. [CrossRef] [PubMed]
30. U.S. Food and Drug Administration (FDA). Dissolution Testing of Immediate Release Solid Oral Dosage Forms. Guidance for Industry. Available online: https://www.fda.gov/media/70936/download (accessed on 25 August 1997).
31. Volpe, D.A.; Faustino, P.J.; Ciavarella, A.B.; Asafu-Adjaye, E.B.; Ellison, C.D.; Yu, L.X.; Hussain, A.S. Classification of Drug Permeability with a Caco-2 Cell Monolayer Assay. *Clin. Res. Regul. Aff.* **2007**, *24*, 39–47. [CrossRef]
32. Smetanová, L.; Stetinova, V.; Kholova, D.; Kvetina, J.; Smetana, J.; Svoboda, Z. Caco-2 cells and Biopharmaceutics Classification System (BCS) for prediction of transepithelial transport of xenobiotics (model drug: Caffeine). *Neuro Endocrinol. Lett.* **2009**, *30*, 101–105. [PubMed]
33. Yee, S. In Vitro Permeability across Caco-2 Cells (Colonic) Can Predict In Vivo (Small Intestinal) Absorption in Man—Fact or Myth. *Pharm. Res.* **1997**, *14*, 763–766. [CrossRef]
34. Flanagan, T.R. Potential for pharmaceutical excipients to impact absorption: A mechanistic review for BCS Class 1 and 3 drugs. *Eur. J. Pharm. Biopharm.* **2019**, *141*, 130–138. [CrossRef]

pharmaceutics MDPI

Article

Dose-Dependent Solubility–Permeability Interplay for Poorly Soluble Drugs under Non-Sink Conditions

Kazuya Sugita [1,2], Noriyuki Takata [2] and Etsuo Yonemochi [1,*]

[1] Department of Physical Chemistry, Hoshi University, 2-4-41, Ebara, Shinagawa, Tokyo 142-8501, Japan; sugita.kazuya55@chugai-pharm.co.jp
[2] Quality Development Department, Chugai Pharma Manufacturing Co., Ltd., 5-5-1, Ukima, Kita, Tokyo 115-8543, Japan; takatanry@chugai-pharm.co.jp
* Correspondence: e-yonemochi@hoshi.ac.jp; Tel./Fax: +81-3-5498-5048

Abstract: We investigated the solubility–permeability interplay using a solubilizer additive under non-sink conditions. Sodium lauryl sulfate (SLS) was used as a solubilizer additive. The solubility and permeability of two poorly soluble drugs at various doses, with or without SLS, were evaluated by flux measurements. The total permeated amount of griseofulvin, which has high permeability, increased by the addition of SLS. On the other hand, triamcinolone, which has low permeability, showed an almost constant rate of permeation regardless of the SLS addition. The total permeated amount of griseofulvin increased by about 20–30% when the dose amount exceeded its solubility, whereas its concentration in the donor chamber remained almost constant. However, the total permeated amount of triamcinolone was almost constant regardless of dose amount. These results suggest that the permeability of the unstirred water layer (UWL) may be affected by SLS and solid drugs for high-permeable drugs. The effect of solid drugs could be explained by a reduction in the apparent UWL thickness. For the appropriate evaluation of absorption, it would be essential to consider these effects.

Keywords: non-sink condition; solubility–permeability interplay; unstirred water layer; poorly soluble drugs; solubilizer additive

check for updates

Citation: Sugita, K.; Takata, N.; Yonemochi, E. Dose-Dependent Solubility–Permeability Interplay for Poorly Soluble Drugs under Non-Sink Conditions. *Pharmaceutics* **2021**, *13*, 323. https://doi.org/10.3390/pharmaceutics13030323

Academic Editor: Im-Sook Song

Received: 1 February 2021
Accepted: 26 February 2021
Published: 2 March 2021

1. Introduction

In vitro tools that can assess the absorption performance of solid oral formulations, such as a dissolution test, play an important role in pharmaceutical development [1–8]. These in vitro tools have multiple purposes: selecting the formulation in the pre-clinical stage [2–5], optimizing both the formulation and the manufacturing process in the clinical stage [5], and conducting quality control and bioequivalence studies in the commercial stage [9–14]. Recent studies show that more than 70% of drug candidates have low solubility, classified in the Biopharmaceutical Classification System (BCS) as BCS class II or IV [3,4,15]. Their low solubility can dramatically limit their absorption. To increase the solubility of these drugs, various solubilizer additives, like surfactants and cyclodextrins (CDs), are often added to the formulations [16,17].

The most commonly used in vitro tool, dissolution testing, measures the dissolution rate and solubility of drugs to assess their absorption performance. However, some studies report that the results from the in vitro dissolution testing of formulations that include solubilizers often fail to predict the in vivo absorption [6,18–22]. A major reason for these inconsistent results may be found in the solubility–permeability interplay, wherein solubilizer additives increase drug solubility but decrease permeability. Some papers have reported that even though solubilizer additives successfully increase drug solubility, this interplay hinders in vivo absorption [23–26].

Intestinal membrane transport of drugs in the gastrointestinal tract (GIT) involves two processes: transcellular diffusion and paracellular diffusion [27,28] (pp. 297–307).

Transcellular diffusion is generally considered to determine drug permeability. Transcellular diffusion can be further divided into two processes: passive diffusion and active transport by carriers/transporters. Both processes affect the permeability of drugs, but the solubility–permeability interplay only occurs during passive diffusion; therefore, this study will focus only on passive diffusion.

Drug molecules dissolved in the GIT after oral administration can take on a variety of new forms; they can be ionized, captured in micelles, or drawn into complexes with other molecules. Among these, the un-ionized free molecules—those not tethered to complexes—are the ones that mainly affect permeability, and they are called un-ionized free drugs (UFDs) [29,30]. Solubilizer additives like surfactants and CDs increase the apparent solubility of drugs by forming micelles and trapping molecules within them or by directly binding to the molecules. However, solubilizers do not change the amount of UFDs, and therefore, the fraction of UFDs in the dissolved molecules decreases, which means the apparent permeability of drugs also decreases because of the solubilizers. The effect of the solubility–permeability interplay on drug absorption is a big issue that has been investigated in both in vitro and in vivo studies. Beig et al. examined the solubility–permeability interplay of CDs using in vitro studies [31–33]. Miller et al. confirmed a similar interplay effect by sodium lauryl sulfate (SLS) also using in vitro studies [34]. Hens et al. studied the effect of bile micelles on the solubility–permeability interplay by measuring the in vivo absorption of fenofibrate in healthy volunteers [35].

A lot of BCS class II and IV drugs cannot be dissolved completely in the gastrointestinal tract (GIT). When a drug is not completely dissolved, the condition is referred to a non-sink condition. Therefore, to appropriately evaluate drug absorption, we must understand the solubility–permeability relationship under realistic non-sink conditions. Unfortunately, most studies on the solubility–permeability interplay involve sink conditions in which drugs are dissolved completely. Under sink conditions, the effect of the solubility–permeability interplay on drug absorption can be explained by a mechanism involving two continuous processes in passive diffusion; the first is the diffusion of drug molecules in the unstirred water layer (UWL) on the membrane surface, and the second is diffusion in the membrane itself. As the membrane is composed of phospholipids, drug molecules should be in lipophilic form to be partitioned to the membrane. Because a UFD is far more lipophilic in the GIT than in any other form, it is thought that a UFD alone can permeate during passive diffusion. This theory has been confirmed by numerous studies over the years [30]. Therefore, it is assumed that the UFD amount alone determines permeability in the membrane. However, in the UWL, drug molecule diffusion could be affected by other forms, in addition to the UFD [36]. UWL diffusion may depend on the unique properties of drug molecules and solubilizer additives. Some studies have successfully confirmed the solubility–permeability interplay by solubilizer additives under sink conditions using the absorption mechanism described above [31–34]. However, it has also been reported that undissolved solid drugs could affect the diffusion of drug molecules in the UWL under non-sink conditions [37–39]. These studies suggest that the permeation of some drugs under non-sink conditions might be faster than that under sink conditions. Unfortunately, there have been too few studies on the solubility–permeability interplay under non-sink conditions.

The purpose of this study is to investigate the relationship between drug solubility, the amount of UFDs, and permeability under non-sink conditions. We used SLS, which is often used as a solubilizer additive in the formulations, and we used griseofulvin and triamcinolone, which have very different solubilities and lipophilicities, as model compounds (Figure 1 and Table 1). We measured the solubility and permeability of these compounds with or without SLS. To investigate the difference between sink and non-sink conditions, the sample dose was changed for each measurement.

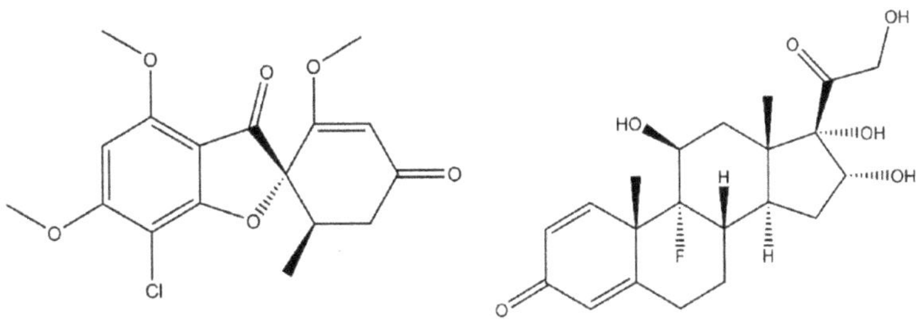

(a) griseofulvin (b) triamcinolone

Figure 1. The molecular structure of griseofulvin (**a**) and triamcinolone (**b**).

Table 1. Physicochemical properties of griseofulvin and triamcinolone.

Physicochemical Properties	Griseofulvin	Triamcinolone
Molecular weight (MW)	352.77	394.43
Ionization properties	Neutral	Neutral
Log P [1]	2.18 [40,41]	1.03 [40,42]
Aqueous solubility (μg/mL) [2]	29.9 [40,41]	158 [40,42]

[1] The partition coefficient is for partitioning between octanol and water. [2] Aqueous solubility was measured at 37 °C.

This study can clarify the effect of solubilizer additives and sample dosage on drug permeability and absorption under non-sink conditions.

2. Theoretical Basis

In discussing how the solubility–permeability interplay is mediated by solubilizer additives, such as surfactants, we assume that the drug permeability is determined by passive diffusion and that drug molecules are not ionized in the solvent. When solubilizer additives increase apparent solubility, the theoretical relationship between solubility and permeability is described as follows.

Based on Fick's first law, flux in the drug permeation can be expressed as shown in Equation (1): [36,43]

$$J(t) = P_{app}C_{app}(t) \quad (1)$$

where P_{app} is the effective or apparent permeability and $C_{app}(t)$ is the apparent drug concentration.

As described in the introduction, overall permeation can be divided into membrane permeation and UWL permeation. Thus, the apparent permeability (P_{app}) is calculated using both apparent membrane permeability ($P_{m\,(app)}$) and apparent UWL permeability ($P_{UWL\,(app)}$), as shown in Equation (2) [43,44]:

$$\frac{1}{P_{app}} = \frac{1}{P_{m\,(app)}} + \frac{1}{P_{UWL\,(app)}} \quad (2)$$

$P_{m\,(app)}$ is calculated using the fraction of UFDs (F_U) as shown in Equation (3) [45]:

$$P_{m\,(app)} = F_U P_{m\,(U)} \quad (3)$$

where $P_{m\,(U)}$ is the intrinsic permeability of UFDs. F_U is calculated by the solubility of drugs as shown in Equation (4):

$$F_U = \frac{S_U}{S} \quad (4)$$

where S_U is the intrinsic solubility of drugs in the absence of solubilizer additives and S is the apparent solubility of drugs.

$P_{UWL\,(app)}$ can be expressed using the apparent aqueous diffusivity ($D_{aq\,(app)}$) from Fick's first law as shown in Equation (5):

$$P_{UWL\,(app)} = \frac{D_{aq\,(app)}}{h_{UWL\,(app)}} \tag{5}$$

where $h_{UWL\,(app)}$ is the apparent thickness of the UWL. When there are no solubilizer additives in the drug formulation or test media in the permeability measurements, Equation (5) can be described as shown in Equation (6):

$$P_{UWL\,(U)} = \frac{D_{aq\,(U)}}{h_{UWL\,(U)}} \tag{6}$$

where $h_{UWL\,(U)}$ is the intrinsic thickness of the UWL and $D_{aq\,(U)}$ is the intrinsic aqueous diffusivity of UFDs. The thickness of the UWL can be determined based on rotation speed in the flux experiment [46,47]. If the rotation speed is constant, we can assume that the thickness of the UWL is constant, independent of the addition of solubilizer additives, as shown in Equation (7):

$$h_{UWL\,(app)} = h_{UWL\,(U)} \tag{7}$$

Substituting $h_{UWL\,(app)}$ of Equation (5) and $h_{UWL\,(U)}$ of Equation (6) for Equation (7), $P_{UWL\,(app)}$ is described as shown in Equation (8):

$$P_{UWL\,(app)} = P_{UWL\,(U)} \times \frac{D_{aq\,(app)}}{D_{aq\,(U)}} \tag{8}$$

The apparent aqueous diffusivity ($D_{aq\,(app)}$) is a combined total of each fraction of aqueous diffusivity as shown in Equation (9) [36]:

$$D_{aq\,(app)} = F_U D_{aq\,(U)} + (1 - F_U) D_{aq\,(B)} \tag{9}$$

where F_U is the same fraction of UFDs as in Equation (4) and $D_{aq\,(B)}$ is the aqueous diffusivity of drug molecules bound to solubilizer additives. $P_{UWL\,(app)}$ can be calculated by Equations (6), (8), and (9) as shown in Equation (10):

$$P_{UWL\,(app)} = \frac{1}{h_{UWL\,(app)}} \left\{ F_U D_{aq(U)} + (1 - F_U) D_{aq\,(B)} \right\} \tag{10}$$

If we know the aqueous diffusivity of each component and the thickness of the UWL, the apparent permeability P_{app} can be calculated based on the drug solubility using Equations (2), (3), and (10).

3. Materials and Methods

3.1. Materials

Griseofulvin and triamcinolone were purchased from Tokyo Chemical Industry Co., Ltd. (Tokyo, Japan). Buffer components (sodium dihydrogen phosphate (NaH_2PO_4), sodium hydroxide (NaOH), sodium chloride (NaCl)), acetonitrile (MeCN), trifluoroacetic acid (TFA), ethylene glycol, N,N-dimethylacetamide (DMA), and dimethyl sulfoxide (DMSO) were purchased from FUJI FILM Wako Pure Chemical Co. (Osaka, Japan). MeCN and TFA were HPLC grade. Ethylene glycol and DMA were Wako special grade. DMSO was a guaranteed reagent. The gastrointestinal tract (GIT) lipid and the acceptor sink buffer (ASB) were purchased from Pion Inc. (Billerica, MA, USA).

3.2. Methods

3.2.1. Flux Measurements

The flux was measured by MicroFlux^{TM} (Pion Inc., Billerica, MA, USA). Two chambers in this device were separated by a polyvinylidene fluoride (PVDF) membrane filter of 0.45 μm pore size with 25 μL of GIT lipid solution (Pion Inc., Billerica, MA, USA). Next, 20 mL of ASB (Pion Inc., Billerica, MA, USA) was added into each acceptor chamber, and 20 mL of the test sample solution was added to each donor chamber. Details of the test sample solution in the donor chambers are summarized in Table 2. The sample dose amount was set based on the preliminary solubility study. Then, 5 μg/mL of griseofulvin and 100 μg/mL of triamcinolone were evaluated under sink conditions, and other samples were evaluated under non-sink conditions. The SLS concentration was set based on the reported SLS amount used in the drug formulation and the reported solvent volume in human GIT. Japan's Ministry of Health, Labor and Welfare reported that the maximum SLS amount administered was 300 mg [48]. The solvent volume of the small intestine in a fasted condition, where most of orally administered drug is absorbed, was reported to be around 50–300 mL [49,50]. Therefore, the maximum SLS concentration in the human small intestine could be around 0.10–0.60% (*w/w*). If enough SLS was used in the drug formulation as solubilizer additive, more than 0.05% (*w/w*) SLS could be included in the solvent of the small intestine. To prepare 5 μg/mL of griseofulvin and 100 μg/mL of triamcinolone, 19.9 mL of test media and 0.1 mL of the concentrated sample solution prepared by DMSO were mixed. To prepare other test sample solutions, the determined test sample amount was added to a test tube containing test media. These samples were placed on the rotation stirrers in a water bath at 37 °C and stirred well. After stirring, these samples were suspended visually. The measurements were started by adding 20 mL of these test sample solutions to the donor chambers. Cross-bar magnetic stirrers were located in each chamber, rotating at 150 rpm. The media in the donor and the acceptor chambers were maintained at 37 °C during measurement. All flux measurements were performed in triplicate.

Table 2. List of test sample solution conditions in the donor chambers.

Compound	Test Media	Sample Dose Amount (μg/mL)
Griseofulvin	pH 6.5 phosphate buffer (pH 6.5 buffer)	5, 50, 200, and 1000
	pH 6.5 phosphate buffer with 0.05% (*w/w*) sodium lauryl sulfate (SLS) (pH 6.5 buffer + 0.05% SLS)	5, 50, 200, and 1000
Triamcinolone	pH 6.5 buffer	100, 500, 2000, and 10,000
	pH 6.5 buffer + 0.05% SLS	100, 500, 2000, and 10,000

The concentration–time profiles were determined via manual sampling from the donor chambers and acceptor chambers during flux measurements. At 0, 30, 60, 120, 240, and 360 min, 100 μL of the acceptor chamber solution was withdrawn and diluted to 100 μL (2× dilution) of 3:2 DMA:ethylene glycol (*v/v*). At the same time point, 400 μL of the donor chamber solution was withdrawn and filtered through a polytetrafluoroethylene (PTFE) membrane filter of 0.22 μm pose size. Then, 100 μL of the filtered solution was diluted to 100 μL (2× dilution) of 3:2 DMA:ethylene glycol (*v/v*). The sample concentration was determined by ultra-high-performance liquid chromatography (UHPLC).

The solubility of each model compound at 37 °C for each test medium was determined by using the donor chamber sample concentration at 0 min of 1000 μg/mL dose for griseofulvin and 10,000 μg/mL dose for triamcinolone.

From the obtained concentration–time profiles in the acceptor chambers, the flux (J) was calculated. The flux refers to the mass transfer through the membrane, and it is defined as the total amount of material crossing one unit area of the membrane per unit time, as described by Equation (11):

$$J\,(t) = \frac{1}{A}\cdot\frac{dm}{dt} = \frac{V}{A}\cdot\frac{dC(t)}{dt} \tag{11}$$

where dm/dt (μg/mL) is the total amount of material crossing the membrane per unit time, A is the area of the membrane (1.54 cm^2), V is the volume of the acceptor chamber (20 mL), and dC(t)/dt (μg/(mL·min)) is the slope of the concentration–time profiles in the acceptor chambers. Time intervals were selected in each test to exclude the lag time of the concentration–time profile and calculate the initial flux. The selected time intervals are described in the Results section. Based on Fick's first law, assuming the sink condition in the acceptor chambers, the flux can be described by Equation (12):

$$J\,(t) = P_{app}C_D(t) \tag{12}$$

where P_{app} is the apparent permeability of drugs and C_D (t) is the drug concentration in the donor chambers. As the initial flux was calculated in this study, C_D (t) at 0 min (=C_D (0)) was used to calculate P_{app} by Equation (12).

3.2.2. Sample Concentration Measurements by UHPLC

The sample concentrations were measured on a Waters (Milford, MA) Acquity UPLC H-Class system. An Acquity UPLC® BEH Shield RP18 1.7 μm, 2.1 × 50 mm, was used for chromatographic separation. A gradient mobile phase, spanning 95:5 to 0:100 (*v/v*) water:MeCN (both containing 0.05%TFA) over 2.0 min, was pumped at a flow rate of 1.0 mL/min. The injection volume and ultraviolet (UV) wavelength for griseofulvin were 5 μL and 240 nm, respectively. The injection volume and ultraviolet (UV) wavelength for triamcinolone were 1 μL and 292 nm, respectively.

4. Results

4.1. Effect of SLS on Griseofulvin Solubility and Triamcinolone Solubility

The solubility of griseofulvin and triamcinolone in each test medium at 37 °C is shown in Table 3. The solubility of griseofulvin increased by about 2.5-fold by the addition of 0.05% SLS. In contrast, the solubility of triamcinolone was mostly constant, independent of the addition of SLS. Compared with triamcinolone, griseofulvin is a lipophilic compound and is easy to solubilize using SLS.

Table 3. Solubility and un-ionized free drug (UFD) amount of griseofulvin and triamcinolone at 37 °C in each test medium.

Compound	Test Media	Solubility (μg/mL) [1]	UFD Amount (μg/mL)	Fraction of UFD (F_U)
Griseofulvin	pH 6.5 buffer	10.75 ± 0.38	10.75	1.00
	pH 6.5 buffer + 0.05% SLS	27.40 ± 0.07	10.75	0.39
Triamcinolone	pH 6.5 buffer	205.04 ± 10.34	205.04	1.00
	pH 6.5 buffer + 0.05% SLS	210.07 ± 6.54	205.04	0.98

[1] Results represent average solubility ± Standard deviation (SD) (n = 3). UFD, un-ionized free drug.

As both griseofulvin and triamcinolone are neutral compounds, we can assume that these drug molecules are not ionized in the aqueous test media. We can assume that these compounds formed only UFDs in pH 6.5 buffer and that UFDs and the drug molecules bound to SLS in pH 6.5 buffer + 0.05% SLS. Under non-sink conditions, the amount of UFDs would be constant regardless of the SLS amount. Therefore, the amount and fraction of UFDs were estimated by Equation (4) using the average solubility (Table 3).

4.2. Effect of Dose Amount and SLS on Flux and Permeability

4.2.1. Griseofulvin

The concentration–time profiles of griseofulvin in the acceptor chamber as determined by the flux measurements are shown in Figure 2. Those in the donor chamber as determined by the flux measurements are shown in Figure A1. The flux calculated using Equation (11) is shown in Figure 3.

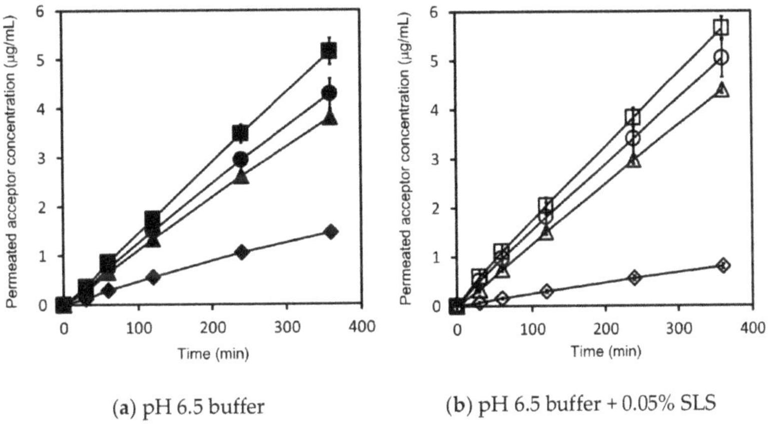

Figure 2. Griseofulvin concentration–time profile in the acceptor chamber as determined by flux measurements. Measurements in pH 6.5 buffer are represented by closed symbols for the 5 μg/mL sample dose (◆), 50 μg/mL sample dose (▲), 200 μg/mL sample dose (•), and 1000 μg/mL sample dose (■) (**a**). Measurements in pH 6.5 buffer + 0.05% Sodium lauryl sulfate (SLS) are represented by open symbols for the 5 μg/mL sample dose (◇), 50 μg/mL sample dose (△), 200 μg/mL sample dose (○), and 1000 μg/mL sample dose (□) (**b**). Results represent the average permeated griseofulvin concentration ± SD (n = 3).

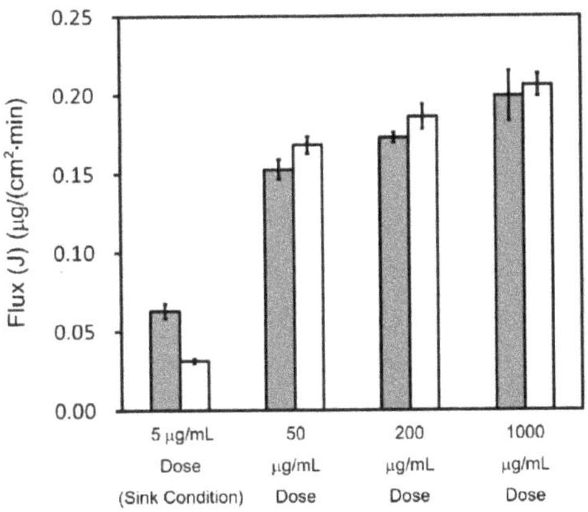

Figure 3. Calculated flux of griseofulvin. A time interval of 30–120 min was selected. The flux in pH 6.5 buffer is represented by gray bars. The flux in pH 6.5 buffer + 0.05% SLS is represented by white bars. Results represent the average griseofulvin flux ± SD (n = 3).

Based on the solubility in Table 3, as for both pH 6.5 buffer and pH 6.5 buffer + 0.05% SLS, the 5 μg/mL dose samples in the donor chamber were under sink conditions and the 50, 200, and 1000 μg/mL dose samples were under non-sink conditions. The sample concentration in the donor chambers for the 5 μg/mL dose correlated well with the prepared sample concentration, and the test samples were visually confirmed to be a transparent solution. On the other hand, the sample concentrations in the donor chamber for the 50, 200, and 1000 μg/mL doses was about 10 μg/mL in pH 6.5 buffer and about 25 μg/mL in pH 6.5 buffer + 0.05% SLS, which were lower than the prepared sample concentrations. These samples were visually confirmed to be suspensions.

The fluxes under sink conditions were smaller than those under non-sink conditions in both pH 6.5 buffer and pH 6.5 buffer + 0.05% SLS; this is because the sample concentrations in the donor chambers under sink conditions were lower than those under non-sink conditions. Under sink conditions, at the 5 μg/mL dose, the flux in pH 6.5 buffer + 0.05% SLS was almost half that in pH 6.5 buffer, even though the sample concentration at 0 min in the donor chamber showed almost the same value. Under non-sink conditions, at the 50, 200, and 1000 μg/mL doses, the flux in pH 6.5 buffer + 0.05% SLS was slightly higher than that in pH 6.5 buffer. Based on Equation (12), these results suggest that the apparent permeability in pH 6.5 buffer + 0.05% SLS was almost half that in pH 6.5 buffer.

In addition, in both pH 6.5 buffer and pH 6.5 buffer + 0.05% SLS, the flux increased by about 10–30%, depending on the dose amount under non-sink conditions, even though the sample concentration at 0 min in the donor chamber showed almost the same value.

4.2.2. Triamcinolone

The concentration–time profiles of triamcinolone in the acceptor chamber, as determined by the flux measurements, are shown in Figure 4, while those in the donor chamber, as determined by the flux measurements, are shown in Figure A2. The flux calculated using Equation (11) is shown in Figure 5.

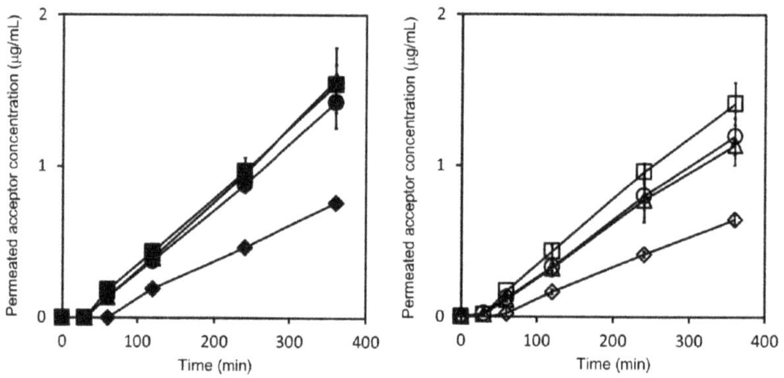

(**a**) pH 6.5 buffer (**b**) pH 6.5 buffer + 0.05% SLS

Figure 4. Triamcinolone concentration–time profile in the acceptor chamber, as determined by flux measurements. Measurements in pH 6.5 buffer are represented by closed symbols for the 100 μg/mL sample dose (◆), 500 μg/mL sample dose (▲), 2000 μg/mL sample dose (•), and 10,000 μg/mL sample dose (■) (**a**). Measurements in pH 6.5 buffer + 0.05% SLS are represented by open symbols for the 100 μg/mL sample dose (◇), 500 μg/mL sample dose (△), 2000 μg/mL sample dose (○), and 10,000 μg/mL sample dose (□) (**b**). Results represent the average permeated triamcinolone concentration ± SD (n = 3).

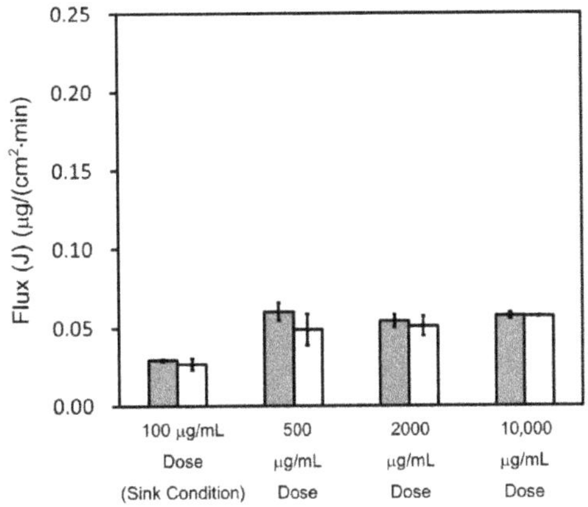

Figure 5. Calculated flux of triamcinolone. A time interval of 120–240 min was selected. The flux in pH 6.5 buffer is represented by gray bars. The flux in pH 6.5 buffer + 0.05% SLS is represented by white bars. Results represent the average triamcinolone flux ± SD (*n* = 3).

Based on the solubility in Table 3, for both pH 6.5 buffer and pH 6.5 buffer + 0.05% SLS, the 100 μg/mL dose test samples in the donor chamber were under sink conditions and the 500, 2000, and 10,000 μg/mL dose test samples in the donor chamber were under non-sink conditions. The sample concentration in the donor chamber for the 100 μg/mL dose correlated well with the prepared sample concentration, and the test samples were visually confirmed to be a transparent solution. On the other hand, the sample concentrations in the donor chamber for 500, 2000, and 10,000 μg/mL doses showed about 200 μg/mL in pH 6.5 buffer and pH 6.5 buffer + 0.05% SLS, which were lower than the prepared sample concentrations. These samples were visually confirmed to be suspensions.

The fluxes under sink conditions were smaller than those under non-sink conditions in both pH 6.5 buffer and pH 6.5 buffer + 0.05% SLS; this is because the sample concentrations in the donor chambers under sink conditions were lower than those under non-sink conditions. Under sink conditions, at the 100 μg/mL dose, the flux in pH 6.5 buffer + 0.05% SLS and pH 6.5 buffer showed almost similar values. Under non-sink conditions, in pH 6.5 buffer, the flux at all doses was also similar. In pH 6.5 buffer + 0.05% SLS, the flux at 500 and 2000 μg/mL doses was similar. At the 10,000 μg/mL dose, the flux and the donor concentration were about 10% higher than those at the 500 and 2000 μg/mL doses. Based on Equation (12), unlike griseofulvin, in both pH 6.5 buffer and pH 6.5 buffer + 0.05% SLS, the apparent permeability was mostly constant and not dependent on the sample dose amount under non-sink conditions.

4.3. Theoretical Calculation about Permeability

In this section, we calculated the permeabilities of compounds theoretically using the results and the physicochemical properties of compounds, also applying the equations in the Theoretical Basis section.

In pH 6.5 buffer under sink conditions, because both griseofulvin and triamcinolone are neutral compounds, all the drug molecules in the donor chamber would be UFDs. The intrinsic permeability of UFDs ($P_{app\,(U)}$) was calculated by Equation (12) using the drug concentration in the donor chamber and the measured flux (measured $P_{app\,(U)}$ in Table 4). It is reported that the intrinsic aqueous diffusivity of UFDs ($D_{aq\,(U)}$) depends on the molecular weight (MW) and can be empirically estimated by Equation (13) [51] (p. 381):

$$\text{Log } D_{aq\,(U)} = -4.131 - 0.4531 \text{Log MW} \tag{13}$$

Table 4. Measured and calculated permeability in pH 6.5 buffer.

Compound	Griseofulvin	Triamcinolone
MW	352.77	394.43
Measured $P_{app\,(U)}$ (cm/min) [1]	0.0148 ± 0.0007	0.000304 ± 0.000010
Calculated $D_{aq\,(U)}$ (cm^2/s)	5.18×10^{-6}	4.93×10^{-6}
Calculated $P_{UWL\,(U)}$ (cm/min)	0.0311	0.0296
Calculated $P_{m\,(U)}$ (cm/min)	0.0284	0.000307
Calculated $P_{app\,(U)}$ (cm/min)	0.0148	0.000304

[1] Results represent the average $P_{app\,(U)}$ ± SD (n = 3). MW, molecular weight. UWL, unstirred water layer.

Using the MW of the model compounds, each $D_{aq\,(U)}$ was calculated (calculated $D_{aq\,(U)}$ in Table 4). The UWL thickness ($h_{UWL\,(app)}$ or $h_{UWL\,(U)}$) for the MicroFlux^{TM} measurements in this study was estimated to be around 100 μm based on previous studies [43,44,51]. The intrinsic UWL permeability of UFDs ($P_{UWL\,(U)}$) was then calculated by Equation (6) (calculated $P_{UWL\,(U)}$ in Table 4). Substituting $P_{app\,(U)}$ and $P_{UWL\,(U)}$ in Equation (2), the intrinsic membrane permeability of UFD ($P_{m\,(U)}$) was calculated (calculated $P_{m\,(U)}$ in Table 4). The results suggested that the permeability of griseofulvin is affected by not only $P_{m\,(U)}$ but also $P_{UWL\,(U)}$, and that of triamcinolone can be determined by only $P_{m\,(U)}$. With triamcinolone, $P_{UWL\,(U)}$ is much smaller than $P_{m\,(U)}$.

For both model compounds, in pH 6.5 buffer + 0.05% SLS under sink conditions, the drug molecules in the donor chamber were UFDs and bound to SLS. The apparent permeability (P_{app}) was calculated by Equation (12) using the drug concentration in the donor chamber and the measured flux (measured P_{app} in Table 5). The apparent membrane permeability ($P_{m\,(app)}$) was calculated by Equation (3) using the fraction of UFDs (F_U) in Table 3 and $P_{m\,(U)}$ (calculated $P_{m\,(app)}$ in Table 5). Substituting P_{app} and $P_{m\,(app)}$ in Equation (2), the apparent UWL permeability ($P_{UWL\,(app)}$) was calculated (calculated $P_{UWL\,(app)}$ in Table 5). The apparent aqueous diffusivity ($D_{aq\,(app)}$) was calculated by Equation (5) using $P_{UWL\,(app)}$ and $h_{UWL\,(app)}$ = 100 μm (calculated $D_{aq\,(app)}$ in Table 5). Substituting F_U, $D_{aq\,(app)}$, and $D_{aq\,(U)}$ in Equation (9), the aqueous diffusivity of drug molecules bound to SLS ($D_{aq\,(B)}$) was calculated (calculated $D_{aq\,(B)}$ in Table 5). As for triamcinolone, $D_{aq\,(B)}$ was not calculated in this study. The reason for this is the fraction of the drug molecules bound to SLS in the donor chamber would be too small to calculate the impact of SLS-bound molecules on the apparent permeability using the method described above. As for griseofulvin, assuming that Equation (13) applies to SLS-bound drug molecules, their sizes were estimated to be around MW 20,000 Da. As the aggregated number of SLS in aqueous solutions was reported to be 62, their micellar weight appeared to be around 18,000 Da [52]. Therefore, the calculated $D_{aq\,(B)}$ agreed roughly with the reported micellar size formed by SLS. Assuming this micellar size is constant, permeability and flux could be calculated by Equation (10) and Equation (12) using the apparent solubility. The apparent solubility increased in proportion to the amount of SLS. When the sample concentration in the donor chamber remained at 5 μg/mL under sink conditions, flux and apparent permeability decreased as apparent solubility increased, as shown in Figure 6. For example, if the apparent solubility increased by 5 and 10 times, the apparent permeability and flux reduced to about 1/4 and 1/7, respectively.

Table 5. Measured and calculated permeability in pH 6.5 buffer + 0.05% SLS.

Compound	Griseofulvin	Triamcinolone
Measured P_{app} (cm/min) [1]	0.00648 ± 0.00026	0.000263 ± 0.000028
Calculated $P_{m\ (app)}$ (cm/min)	0.0112	0.000300
Calculated $P_{UWL\ (app)}$ (cm/min)	0.0153	0.0212
Calculated P_{app} (cm/min)	0.00648	0.000263
Calculated $D_{aq\ (app)}$ (cm^2/s)	2.56×10^{-6}	3.54×10^{-7}
Calculated $D_{aq\ (B)}$ (cm^2/s)	8.37×10^{-7}	-

[1] Results represent the average P_{app} ± SD (n = 3).

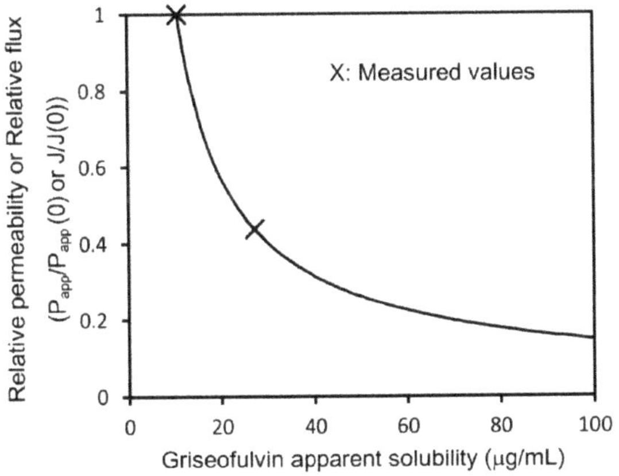

Figure 6. Calculated relationship between flux/apparent permeability and apparent solubility under sink conditions for griseofulvin. It was assumed that the sample concentration in the donor chamber remained at 5 μg/mL during the measurements. P_{app} (0) is the apparent permeability in the absence of solubilizer additives. J (0) is the flux in the absence of solubilizer additives.

5. Discussion

The results of this study suggest that the impact of SLS on permeability and flux under sink conditions is different from that under non-sink conditions. Additionally, we confirmed that permeability and flux could increase depending on the sample dose amount in the donor chamber. In this section, we discuss the solubility–permeability relationship and the absorption mechanism under non-sink conditions.

Under non-sink conditions, the apparent solubility of griseofulvin increased by the addition of SLS, and flux was calculated using Equations (10) and (12) (Figure 7). The equations express the increase in the drug amount diffusing in the UWL, which was due to the SLS-bound drug molecules. The enhancement of flux by the addition of SLS was consistent with the measured values at each sample dose.

In addition to UFDs and SLS-bound drugs, solid drugs in the donor chamber are also under non-sink conditions. Some studies indicate that solid drugs can exist in the UWL on the membrane [37,53–56]. A nearly saturated high-concentration layer is known to form on the surface of solid drugs [57] (pp. 263–264). If solid drugs are in the UWL under non-sink conditions, then the drug diffusion mechanism in the UWL may be different under sink and non-sink conditions (Figure 8). Under sink conditions, drug molecules in the UWL would be diffused from the UWL interface to the membrane. Under non-sink conditions, in addition to diffusion in the UWL, the drug molecules could also be diffused from the high-concentration layer on the solid drugs in the UWL to the membrane. This solid drug diffusion could decrease the apparent UWL thickness, as described in Figure 8. Because the drug molecules could be diffused from the surface of solid drug, the apparent UWL thickness reduction could depend on the total surface area of solid drugs in the UWL.

If the amount of solid drug increases or the particle size decreases, the apparent UWL thickness could also decrease, increasing permeability and flux as a result. Some studies have proposed a similar absorption mechanism, demonstrating this solid drug effect on in vivo and in vitro absorption [37–39].

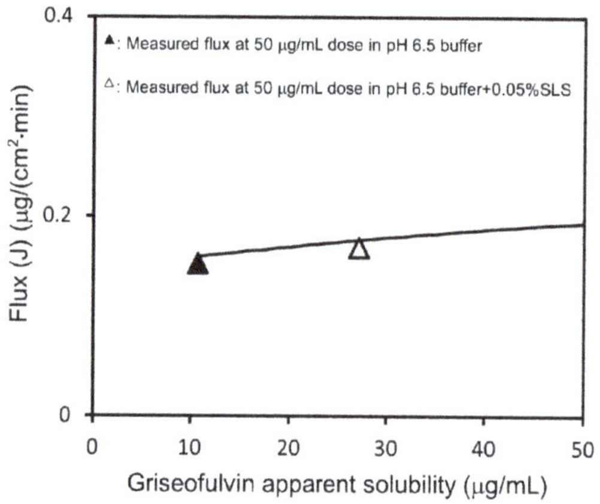

Figure 7. Calculated flux–apparent solubility relationship under sink conditions for griseofulvin. It is assumed that the UWL thickness remained constant. The results of flux measurement at a 50 μg/mL sample dose in pH 6.5 buffer and pH 6.5 buffer + 0.05% SLS were plotted.

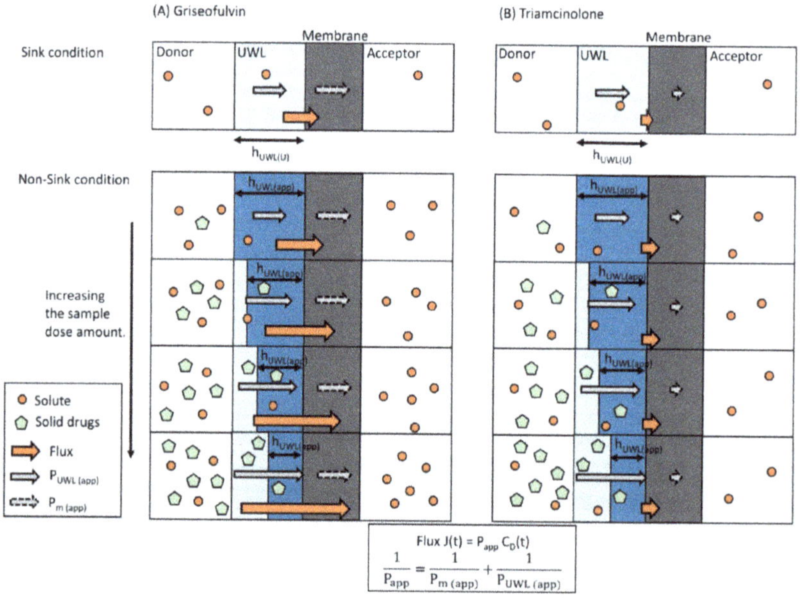

Figure 8. Proposed drug absorption mechanism under sink conditions and non-sink conditions for griseofulvin (**A**) and triamcinolone (**B**). Longer arrows represent higher flux, $P_{UWL\,(app)}$, or $P_{m\,(app)}$.

Based on this absorption mechanism, the apparent UWL thickness in this study decreased as the sample dose increased in the donor chamber. As shown in Figures 2 and 3, griseofulvin permeability and flux in both pH 6.5 buffer and pH 6.5 buffer + 0.05% SLS increased with the sample dose under non-sink conditions. When pH 6.5 buffer is in the donor chamber, the apparent UWL thickness is expressed using Equations (2) and (6) as shown in Equation (14):

$$h_{UWL\ (app)} = D_{aq\ (U)} \left(\frac{1}{P_{app}} - \frac{1}{P_{m\ (U)}} \right) \quad (14)$$

When pH 6.5 buffer + 0.05% SLS is in the donor chamber, the apparent UWL thickness is expressed using Equations (2) and (5) as shown in Equation (15):

$$h_{UWL\ (app)} = D_{aq\ (app)} \left(\frac{1}{P_{app}} - \frac{1}{P_{m\ (app)}} \right) \quad (15)$$

As for griseofulvin, substituting measured P_{app}, $P_{m\ (U)}$, $P_{m\ (app)}$, $D_{aq\ (U)}$, and $D_{aq\ (U)}$ in Equations (14) and (15), the apparent UWL thickness for each test condition was calculated, as shown in Figure 9. When the sample dose increased from 50 μg/mL to 1000 μg/mL, the apparent UWL thickness reduced from 100 μm to around 60–70 μm. When the apparent solubility increased by SLS, the effect of UWL thinning on the P_{app} of griseofulvin was calculated using Equations (2), (3), and (9) as shown in Equation (16):

$$P_{app} = \frac{1}{F_U P_{m\ (U)}} - \frac{h_{UWL\ (app)}}{F_U D_{aq(U)} + (1 - F_U) D_{aq\ (B)}} \quad (16)$$

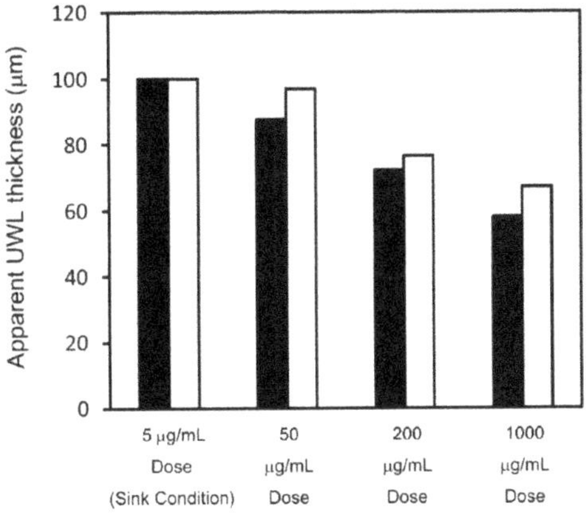

Figure 9. The calculated apparent UWL thickness ($h_{UWL\ (app)}$) of griseofulvin for each flux measurement. $h_{UWL\ (app)}$ in pH 6.5 buffer is represented by black bars. $h_{UWL\ (app)}$ in pH 6.5 buffer + 0.05% SLS is represented by white bars.

If the test sample in the donor chamber was under non-sink conditions, the sample concentration would be equal to the apparent solubility. Therefore, the effect of UWL thinning on the flux of griseofulvin could be estimated using Equation (1) and Equation (16), as shown in Figure 10. This explains how SLS addition and an increase in dose enhance flux.

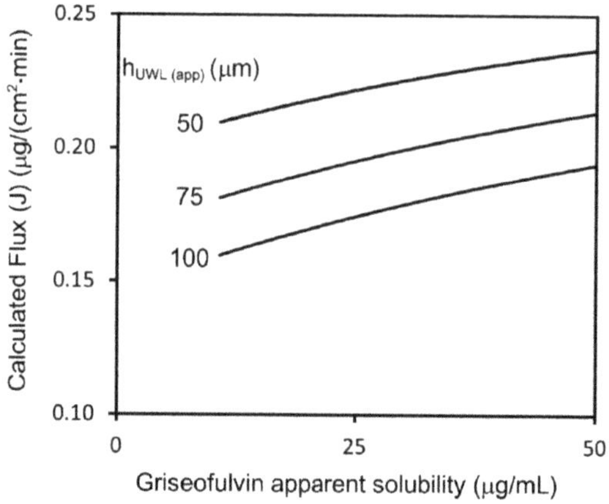

Figure 10. Calculated flux of griseofulvin for 50–100 μm apparent UWL thickness.

As the MW of oral pharmaceutical drugs is generally reported to be around 200–1000 Da, the variability of $D_{aq\ (U)}$ might be very small, based on Equation (13), compared with the variability of $P_{m\ (U)}$. $P_{m\ (U)}$ is generally known to show a large variation. To simply calculate the effect of UWL thinning on the permeability and flux of various drugs, we used a neutral model compound with an MW of 400 Da and pH 6.5 buffer as the donor chamber test media for the following calculations. When the $P_{m\ (U)}$ of this model compound was 0.001–1 cm/min, the relationship between UWL thickness and flux/permeability was calculated by Equation (17), as shown in Figure 11:

$$P_{app} = \frac{1}{P_{m\ (U)}} - \frac{h_{UWL\ (app)}}{D_{aq\ (U)}} \quad (17)$$

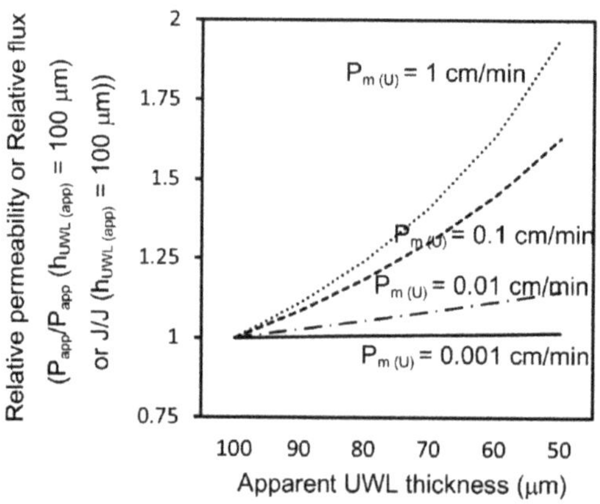

Figure 11. Calculated relationship between apparent permeability/flux and apparent UWL thickness for model compounds with $P_{m\ (U)}$ of 0.001–1 cm/min. It was assumed that the MW of the model compounds was 400 Da.

The $P_{m\ (U)}$ of triamcinolone was around 0.0003 cm/min. According to Figure 11, the permeability and flux for triamcinolone would be constant even if the apparent UWL thickness decreased. Therefore, the results for triamcinolone under non-sink conditions are concordant with the absorption model described above.

In addition, Figure 11 indicates that the permeability and flux of highly permeable drugs can be strongly affected by the presence of solid drugs in the UWL. If the UWL thickness reduces by 50% for a drug with a $P_{m\,(U)}$ of 1 cm/min, its permeability and flux would increase by about twofold. However, it is difficult to directly predict the in vivo absorption amount using the solubility–permeability relationship estimated by MicroFlux^{TM}. Factors like movement, surface area, and solvent volume in the human GIT differ from MicroFlux^{TM} conditions. Thus, the effect of solid drugs on UWL permeability may differ in vitro and in vivo. As for griseofulvin, Sugano suggested that solid drugs in the UWL could increase the in vivo permeability and in vivo drug absorption at a 500 mg dose by about twofold [37]. According to this study, the in vivo effect of solid drugs on permeability and drug absorption is larger than the in vitro effect seen in the flux measurements. The in vitro $P_{m\,(U)}$ of griseofulvin was 0.0284 cm/min in this study. Thus, it could be roughly predicted that the in vivo permeability and drug absorption of a drug with an in vitro $P_{m\,(U)}$ = 0.005 cm/min would increase by about 20–30% if the UWL thickness was reduced by half at the higher sample dose.

6. Conclusions

In this study, we examined the relationship between drug solubility, the amount of UFDs, and permeability under non-sink conditions. We found that drug molecules bound to solubilizer additives and solid drugs can enhance UWL permeability, resulting in increased flux or permeability under non-sink conditions. Conventional methods of measuring permeability, like Caco-2 or Parallel Artificial Membrane Permeability Assay (PAMPA), are performed under sink conditions. On the other hand, a lot of BCS class II and IV drugs cannot be adequately dissolved in the GIT, meaning that they are under non-sink conditions there. If we use conventional methods to predict the absorption of highly permeable drugs, the predicted amount could be much lower than the actual amount. Therefore, as the results of this study suggest, it is necessary to understand how the solubility–permeability relationship under non-sink conditions reflects the clinical context. MicroFlux^{TM} and the test conditions used in this study may be effective tools for assessing such effects on drug absorption. Not enough is known about the correlation between in vivo permeability and permeability, as estimated by MicroFlux^{TM}. However, by combining flux measurements with physiologically based pharmacokinetics (PBPK) modeling, we will be able to accurately predict the in vivo absorption for BCS class II and IV drugs in the future.

Author Contributions: Conceptualization, K.S. and N.T.; data curation, K.S.; formal analysis, K.S.; funding acquisition, K.S.; investigation, K.S.; methodology, K.S.; project administration, K.S.; resources, K.S.; software, K.S.; supervision, N.T. and E.Y.; validation, K.S.; visualization, K.S.; writing–original draft, K.S.; writing–review and editing, N.T. and E.Y. All authors have read and agreed to the published version of the manuscript.

Funding: This research was funded by Chugai Pharma Manufacturing Co., Ltd.

Institutional Review Board Statement: Not applicable.

Informed Consent Statement: Not applicable.

Data Availability Statement: The data presented in this study are available in this article.

Acknowledgments: We are deeply grateful to the members of our laboratories for giving us the chance to do this exciting work. We thank our colleagues in Chugai for their support and technical advice. We thank Kazutoshi Tabata for his assistance in setting flux measurements.

Conflicts of Interest: K.S. and N.T. are researchers currently employed by Chugai Pharma Manufacturing Co., Ltd. The funders/companies had no role in the design of the study; in the collection, analyses, or interpretation of data; in the writing of the manuscript, or in the decision to publish the results. The authors declare no conflict of interest.

Appendix A

See Figures A1 and A2.

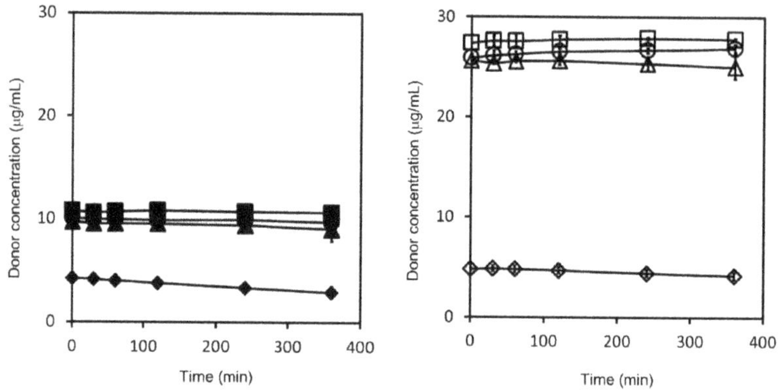

(**a**) pH 6.5 buffer (**b**) pH 6.5 buffer + 0.05% SLS

Figure A1. Griseofulvin concentration–time profile in the donor chamber, as determined by flux measurements. Measurements in pH 6.5 buffer are represented by closed symbols for the 5 µg/mL sample dose (◆), 50 µg/mL sample dose (▲), 200 µg/mL sample dose (•), and 1000 µg/mL sample dose (■) (**a**). Measurements in pH 6.5 buffer + 0.05% SLS are represented by open symbols for the 5 µg/mL sample dose (◇), 50 µg/mL sample dose (△), 200 µg/mL sample dose (○), and 1000 µg/mL sample dose (□) (**b**). Results represent the average griseofulvin concentration ± SD (*n* = 3).

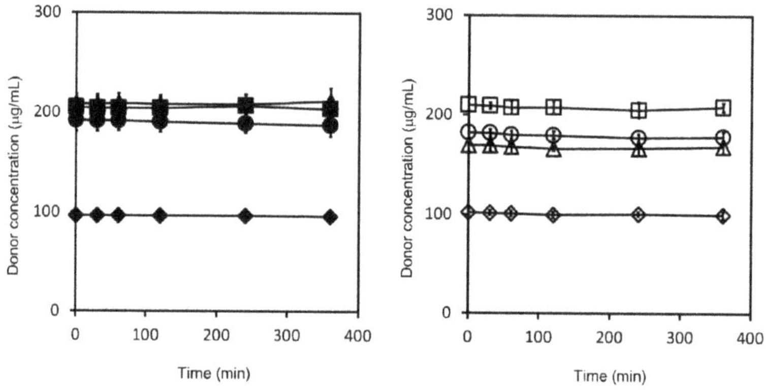

(**a**) pH 6.5 buffer (**b**) pH 6.5 buffer + 0.05% SLS

Figure A2. Triamcinolone concentration–time profile in the donor chamber, as determined by flux measurements. Measurements in pH 6.5 buffer are represented by closed symbols for the 100 µg/mL sample dose (◆), 500 µg/mL sample dose (▲), 2000 µg/mL sample dose (•), and 10,000 µg/mL sample dose (■) (**a**). Measurements in pH 6.5 buffer + 0.05% SLS are represented by open symbols for the 100 µg/mL sample dose (◇), 500 µg/mL sample dose (△), 2000 µg/mL sample dose (○), and 10,000 µg/mL sample dose (□) (**b**). Results represent the average triamcinolone concentration ± SD (*n* = 3).

References

1. Boyd, B.J.; Bergström, C.A.; Vinarov, Z.; Kuentz, M.; Brouwers, J.; Augustijns, P.; Brandl, M.; Bernkop-Schnürch, A.; Shrestha, N.; Préat, V.; et al. Successful oral delivery of poorly water-soluble drugs both depends on the intraluminal behavior of drugs and of appropriate advanced drug delivery systems. *Eur. J. Pharm. Sci.* **2019**, *137*, 104967. [CrossRef] [PubMed]
2. Butler, J.M.; Dressman, J.B. The Developability Classification System: Application of Biopharmaceutics Concepts to Formulation Development. *J. Pharm. Sci.* **2010**, *99*, 4940–4954. [CrossRef]
3. Rosenberger, J.; Butler, J.; Dressman, J. A Refined Developability Classification System. *J. Pharm. Sci.* **2018**, *107*, 2020–2032. [CrossRef]
4. Rosenberger, J.; Butler, J.; Muenster, U.; Dressman, J. Application of a Refined Developability Classification System. *J. Pharm. Sci.* **2019**, *108*, 1090–1100. [CrossRef]
5. Lennernäs, H.; Aarons, L.; Augustijns, P.; Beato, S.; Bolger, M.; Box, K.; Brewster, M.; Butler, J.; Dressman, J.; Holm, R.; et al. Oral biopharmaceutics tools—Time for a new initiative—An introduction to the IMI project OrBiTo. *Eur. J. Pharm. Sci.* **2014**, *57*, 292–299. [CrossRef]
6. Kostewicz, E.S.; Abrahamsson, B.; Brewster, M.; Brouwers, J.; Butler, J.; Carlert, S.; Dickinson, P.A.; Dressman, J.; Holm, R.; Klein, S.; et al. In vitro models for the prediction of in vivo performance of oral dosage forms. *Eur. J. Pharm. Sci.* **2014**, *57*, 342–366. [CrossRef]
7. Lennernäs, H.; Lindahl, A.; Van Peer, A.; Ollier, C.; Flanagan, T.; Lionberger, R.; Nordmark, A.; Yamashita, S.; Yu, L.; Amidon, G.L.; et al. In Vivo Predictive Dissolution (IPD) and Biopharmaceutical Modeling and Simulation: Future Use of Modern Approaches and Methodologies in a Regulatory Context. *Mol. Pharm.* **2017**, *14*, 1307–1314. [CrossRef]
8. Tsume, Y.; Mudie, D.M.; Langguth, P.; Amidon, G.E.; Amidon, G.L. The Biopharmaceutics Classification System: Subclasses for in vivo predictive dissolution (IPD) methodology and IVIVC. *Eur. J. Pharm. Sci.* **2014**, *57*, 152–163. [CrossRef]
9. Food and Drug Administration. *Guidance for Industry. Immediate Release Solid Oral Dosage Forms, Scale-Up and Post-Approval Changes: Chemistry, Manufacturing, and Controls, In Vitro Dissolution Testing, and In Vivo Bioequivalence Documentation*; FDA: Rockville, MD, USA, 1995.
10. Ministry of Health, Labour and Welfare (MHLW). *Guideline for Bioequivalence Studies of Generic Products (Revision)*; MHLW: Tokyo, Japan, 2012.
11. MHLW. *Guideline for Bioequivalence Studies of Generic Products for Different Strengths of Oral Solid Dosage Forms (Revision)*; MHLW: Tokyo, Japan, 2012.
12. European Medicines Agency. *Guideline on the Investigation of Bioequivalence*; EMA: London, UK, 2010.
13. Kuribayashi, R.; Takishita, T.; Mikami, K. Regulatory Considerations of Bioequivalence Studies for Oral Solid Dosage Forms in Japan. *J. Pharm. Sci.* **2016**, *105*, 2270–2277. [CrossRef]
14. European Medicines Agency. *ICH Q6A Specifications: Test Procedures and Acceptance Criteria for New Drug Substances and New Drug Products: Chemical Substances*; European Medicines Agency: London, UK, 2000.
15. Amidon, G.L.; Lennernäs, H.; Shah, V.P.; Crison, J.R. A theoretical basis for a biopharmaceutic drug classification: The correlation of in vitro drug product dissolution and in vivo bioavailability. *Pharm. Res.* **1995**, *12*, 413–420. [CrossRef]
16. Van Der Merwe, J.; Steenekamp, J.; Steyn, D.; Hamman, J. The Role of Functional Excipients in Solid Oral Dosage Forms to Overcome Poor Drug Dissolution and Bioavailability. *Pharmaceutics* **2020**, *12*, 393. [CrossRef]
17. Williams, H.D.; Trevaskis, N.L.; Charman, S.A.; Shanker, R.M.; Charman, W.N.; Pouton, C.W.; Porter, C.J.H. Strategies to Address Low Drug Solubility in Discovery and Development. *Pharmacol. Rev.* **2013**, *65*, 315–499. [CrossRef]
18. Sun, D.D.; Wen, H.; Taylor, L.S. Non-Sink Dissolution Conditions for Predicting Product Quality and In Vivo Performance of Supersaturating Drug Delivery Systems. *J. Pharm. Sci.* **2016**, *105*, 2477–2488. [CrossRef]
19. Sun, D.D.; Lee, P.I. Haste Makes Waste: The Interplay Between Dissolution and Precipitation of Supersaturating Formulations. *AAPS J.* **2015**, *17*, 1317–1326. [CrossRef]
20. Phillips, D.J.; Pygall, S.R.; Cooper, V.B.; Mann, J.C. Overcoming sink limitations in dissolution testing: A review of traditional methods and the potential utility of biphasic systems. *J. Pharm. Pharmacol.* **2012**, *64*, 1549–1559. [CrossRef]
21. Miyaji, Y.; Fujii, Y.; Takeyama, S.; Kawai, Y.; Kataoka, M.; Takahashi, M.; Yamashita, S. Advantage of the Dissolution/Permeation System for Estimating Oral Absorption of Drug Candidates in the Drug Discovery Stage. *Mol. Pharm.* **2016**, *13*, 1564–1574. [CrossRef]
22. Sun, D.; Hu, M.; Browning, M.; Friedman, R.L.; Jiang, W.; Zhao, L.; Wen, H. Dissolution Failure of Solid Oral Drug Products in Field Alert Reports. *J. Pharm. Sci.* **2017**, *106*, 1302–1309. [CrossRef]
23. Dahan, A.; Miller, J.M. The Solubility–Permeability Interplay and Its Implications in Formulation Design and Development for Poorly Soluble Drugs. *AAPS J.* **2012**, *14*, 244–251. [CrossRef]
24. Dahan, A.; Beig, A.; Lindley, D.; Miller, J.M. The solubility–permeability interplay and oral drug formulation design: Two heads are better than one. *Adv. Drug Deliv. Rev.* **2016**, *101*, 99–107. [CrossRef] [PubMed]
25. Porat, D.; Dahan, A. Active intestinal drug absorption and the solubility-permeability interplay. *Int. J. Pharm.* **2018**, *537*, 84–93. [CrossRef]
26. Nainwal, N.; Singh, R.; Jawla, S.; Saharan, V.A. The Solubility-Permeability Interplay for Solubility-Enabling Oral Formulations. *Curr. Drug Targets* **2019**, *20*, 1434–1446. [CrossRef]

27. Dahlgren, D.; Lennernäs, H. Intestinal Permeability and Drug Absorption: Predictive Experimental, Computational and In Vivo Approaches. *Pharmaceutics* **2019**, *11*, 411. [CrossRef] [PubMed]
28. Zhu, L.; Lu, L.; Wang, S.; Wu, J.; Shi, J.; Yan, T.; Xie, C.; Li, Q.; Hu, M.; Liu, Z. Chapter 11. Oral Absorption Basics: Pathways and Physicochemical and Biological Factors Affecting Absorption. In *Developing Solid Oral Dosage Forms*, 2nd ed.; Qiu, Y., Ed.; Academic Press: Cambridge, MA, USA, 2017; pp. 297–329.
29. Raina, S.A.; Zhang, G.G.Z.; Alonzo, D.E.; Wu, J.; Zhu, D.; Catron, N.D.; Gao, Y.; Taylor, L.S. Impact of Solubilizing Additives on Supersaturation and Membrane Transport of Drugs. *Pharm. Res.* **2015**, *32*, 3350–3364. [CrossRef] [PubMed]
30. Shore, P.A.; Brodie, B.B.; Hogben, C.A. The gastric secretion of drugs: A phpartition hypothesis. *J. Pharmacol. Exp. Ther.* **1957**, *119*, 361–369. [PubMed]
31. Beig, A.; Agbaria, R.; Dahan, A. Oral Delivery of Lipophilic Drugs: The Tradeoff between Solubility Increase and Permeability Decrease When Using Cyclodextrin-Based Formulations. *PLoS ONE* **2013**, *8*, e68237. [CrossRef]
32. Beig, A.; Miller, J.M.; Dahan, A. The interaction of nifedipine with selected cyclodextrins and the subsequent solubility–permeability trade-off. *Eur. J. Pharm. Biopharm.* **2013**, *85*, 1293–1299. [CrossRef] [PubMed]
33. Beig, A.; Agbaria, R.; Dahan, A. The use of captisol (SBE7-β-CD) in oral solubility-enabling formulations: Comparison to HPβCD and the solubility–permeability interplay. *Eur. J. Pharm. Sci.* **2015**, *77*, 73–78. [CrossRef] [PubMed]
34. Miller, J.M.; Beig, A.; Krieg, B.J.; Carr, R.A.; Borchardt, T.B.; Amidon, G.E.; Amidon, G.L.; Dahan, A. The Solubility–Permeability Interplay: Mechanistic Modeling and Predictive Application of the Impact of Micellar Solubilization on Intestinal Permeation. *Mol. Pharm.* **2011**, *8*, 1848–1856. [CrossRef]
35. Hens, B.; Brouwers, J.; Corsetti, M.; Augustijns, P. Gastrointestinal behavior of nano- and microsized fenofibrate: In vivo evaluation in man and in vitro simulation by assessment of the permeation potential. *Eur. J. Pharm. Sci.* **2015**, *77*, 40–47. [CrossRef] [PubMed]
36. Amidon, G.E.; Higuchi, W.I.; Ho, N.F.H. Theoretical and Experimental Studies of Transport of Micelle-Solubilized Solutes. *J. Pharm. Sci.* **1982**, *71*, 77–84. [CrossRef]
37. Sugano, K. Possible reduction of effective thickness of intestinal unstirred water layer by particle drifting effect. *Int. J. Pharm.* **2010**, *387*, 103–109. [CrossRef]
38. Imono, M.; Uchiyama, H.; Yoshida, S.; Miyazaki, S.; Tamura, N.; Tsutsumimoto, H.; Kadota, K.; Tozuka, Y. The elucidation of key factors for oral absorption enhancement of nanocrystal formulations: In vitro–in vivo correlation of nanocrystals. *Eur. J. Pharm. Biopharm.* **2020**, *146*, 84–92. [CrossRef]
39. Arce, F.A.; Setiawan, N.; Campbell, H.R.; Lu, X.; Nethercott, M.J.; Bummer, P.; Su, Y.; Marsac, P.J. Toward Developing Discriminating Dissolution Methods for Formulations Containing Nanoparticulates in Solution: The Impact of Particle Drift and Drug Activity in Solution. *Mol. Pharm.* **2020**, *17*, 4125–4140. [CrossRef] [PubMed]
40. Guo, J.; Elzinga, P.A.; Hageman, M.; Herron, J.N. Rapid Throughput Solubility Screening Method for BCS Class II Drugs in Animal GI Fluids and Simulated Human GI Fluids Using a 96-well Format. *J. Pharm. Sci.* **2008**, *97*, 1427–1442. [CrossRef] [PubMed]
41. Mithani, S.D.; Bakatselou, V.; TenHoor, C.N.; Dressman, J.B. Estimation of the Increase in Solubility of Drugs as a Function of Bile Salt Concentration. *Pharm. Res.* **1996**, *13*, 163–167. [CrossRef]
42. Bakatselou, V.; Oppenheim, R.C.; Dressman, J.B. Solubilization and Wetting Effects of Bile Salts on the Dissolution of Steroids. *Pharm. Res.* **1991**, *8*, 1461–1469. [CrossRef]
43. Tsinman, K.; Tsinman, O.; Lingamaneni, R.; Zhu, S.; Riebesehl, B.; Grandeury, A.; Juhnke, M.; Van Eerdenbrugh, B. Ranking Itraconazole Formulations Based on the Flux through Artificial Lipophilic Membrane. *Pharm. Res.* **2018**, *35*, 161. [CrossRef]
44. Avdeef, A. Leakiness and Size Exclusion of Paracellular Channels in Cultured Epithelial Cell Monolayers–Interlaboratory Comparison. *Pharm. Res.* **2010**, *27*, 480–489. [CrossRef] [PubMed]
45. Dahan, A.; Miller, J.M.; Hoffman, A.; Amidon, G.E.; Amidon, G.L. The Solubility–Permeability Interplay in Using Cyclodextrins as Pharmaceutical Solubilizers: Mechanistic Modeling and Application to Progesterone. *J. Pharm. Sci.* **2010**, *99*, 2739–2749. [CrossRef]
46. Sugano, K. Aqueous Boundary Layers Related to Oral Absorption of a Drug: From Dissolution of a Drug to Carrier Mediated Transport and Intestinal Wall Metabolism. *Mol. Pharm.* **2010**, *7*, 1362–1373. [CrossRef] [PubMed]
47. Korjamo, T.; Heikkinen, A.T.; Waltari, P.; Mönkkönen, J. The Asymmetry of the Unstirred Water Layer in Permeability Experiments. *Pharm. Res.* **2008**, *25*, 1714–1722. [CrossRef] [PubMed]
48. Safety Data in IPEC Japan. Available online: http://www.jpec.gr.jp/detail=normal&date=safetydata/ra/dara3.html (accessed on 30 November 2020).
49. Schiller, C.; Frohlich, C.-P.; Giessmann, T.; Siegmund, W.; Monnikes, H.; Hosten, N.; Weitschies, W. Intestinal fluid volumes and transit of dosage forms as assessed by magnetic resonance imaging. *Aliment. Pharmacol. Ther.* **2005**, *22*, 971–979. [CrossRef]
50. Mudie, D.M.; Murray, K.; Hoad, C.L.; Pritchard, S.E.; Garnett, M.C.; Amidon, G.L.; Gowland, P.A.; Spiller, R.C.; Amidon, G.E.; Marciani, L. Quantification of Gastrointestinal Liquid Volumes and Distribution Following a 240 mL Dose of Water in the Fasted State. *Mol. Pharm.* **2014**, *11*, 3039–3047. [CrossRef] [PubMed]
51. Avdeef, A. Chapter 7. Permeability—PAMPA. In *Absorption and Drug Development: Solubility, Permeability, and Charge State*, 2nd ed.; John Wiley & Sons, Inc.: Hoboken, NJ, USA, 2012; pp. 319–498.

52. Turro, N.J.; Yekta, A. Luminescent probes for detergent solutions. A simple procedure for determination of the mean aggregation number of micelles. *J. Am. Chem. Soc.* **1978**, *100*, 5951–5952. [CrossRef]
53. Doyle-McCullough, M.; Smyth, S.; Moyes, S.; Carr, K. Factors influencing intestinal microparticle uptake in vivo. *Int. J. Pharm.* **2007**, *335*, 79–89. [CrossRef]
54. Limpanussorn, J.; Simon, L.; Dayan, A.D. Transepithelial Transport of Large Particles in Rat: A New Model for the Quantitative Study of Particle Uptake. *J. Pharm. Pharmacol.* **1998**, *50*, 753–760. [CrossRef]
55. Norris, D.A.; Puri, N.; Sinko, P.J. The effect of physical barriers and properties on the oral absorption of particulates. *Adv. Drug Deliv. Rev.* **1998**, *34*, 135–154. [CrossRef]
56. Smyth, S.; Feldhaus, S.; Schumacher, U.; Carr, K. Uptake of inert microparticles in normal and immune deficient mice. *Int. J. Pharm.* **2008**, *346*, 109–118. [CrossRef] [PubMed]
57. Chen, Y.; Wang, J.; Flanagan, D.R. Chapter 9. Fundamentals of Diffusion and Dissolution. In *Developing Solid Oral Dosage Forms*, 2nd ed.; Qiu, Y., Ed.; Academic Press: Cambridge, MA, USA, 2017; pp. 253–270.

pharmaceutics

Article

Study of the L-Phenylalanine Ammonia-Lyase Penetration Kinetics and the Efficacy of Phenylalanine Catabolism Correction Using In Vitro Model Systems

Lyubov Dyshlyuk [1,2], Stanislav Sukhikh [2,3], Svetlana Noskova [3], Svetlana Ivanova [1,4,*], Alexander Prosekov [5] and Olga Babich [3]

1 Natural Nutraceutical Biotesting Laboratory, Kemerovo State University, Krasnaya Street 6, 650043 Kemerovo, Russia; soldatovals1984@mail.ru
2 Department of Bionanotechnology, Kemerovo State University, Krasnaya Street 6, 650043 Kemerovo, Russia; stas-asp@mail.ru
3 Institute of Living Systems, Immanuel Kant Baltic Federal University, A. Nevskogo Street 14, 236016 Kaliningrad, Russia; svykrum@mail.ru (S.N.); olich.43@mail.ru (O.B.)
4 Department of General Mathematics and Informatics, Kemerovo State University, Krasnaya Street 6, 650043 Kemerovo, Russia
5 Laboratory of Biocatalysis, Kemerovo State University, Krasnaya Street 6, 650043 Kemerovo, Russia; a.prosekov@inbox.ru
* Correspondence: pavvm2000@mail.ru

Abstract: The kinetics of L-phenylalanine ammonia-lyase (PAL) penetration into the monolayer of liver cells after its release from capsules was studied. The studies showed the absence of the effect of the capsule shell based on plant hydrocolloids on the absorption of L-phenylalanine ammonia-lyase in systems simulating the liver surface. After 120 min of incubation, in all variants of the experiment, from 87.0 to 96.8% of the enzyme penetrates the monolayer of liver cells. The combined analysis of the results concludes that the developed encapsulated form of L-phenylalanine ammonia-lyase is characterized by high efficiency in correcting the disturbed catabolism of phenylalanine in phenylketonuria, which is confirmed by the results of experiments carried out on in vitro model systems. PAL is approved for the treatment of adult patients with phenylketonuria. The encapsulated L-phenylalanine ammonia-lyase form can find therapeutic application in the phenylketonuria treatment after additional in vitro and in vivo studies, in particular, the study of preparation safety indicators. Furthermore, it demonstrated high efficacy in tumor regression and the treatment of tyrosine-related metabolic disorders such as tyrosinemia. Several therapeutically valuable metabolites biosynthesized by PAL via its catalytic action are included in food supplements, antimicrobial peptides, drugs, amino acids, and their derivatives. PAL, with improved pharmacodynamic and pharmacokinetic properties, is a highly effective medical drug.

Keywords: phenylketonuria; L-phenylalanine ammonia-lyase; enzyme; kinetics; catabolism disorder; biomedical drug

Citation: Dyshlyuk, L.; Sukhikh, S.; Noskova, S.; Ivanova, S.; Prosekov, A.; Babich, O. Study of the L-Phenylalanine Ammonia-Lyase Penetration Kinetics and the Efficacy of Phenylalanine Catabolism Correction Using In Vitro Model Systems. *Pharmaceutics* **2021**, *13*, 383. https://doi.org/10.3390/pharmaceutics13030383

Academic Editor: Im-Sook Song

Received: 21 February 2021
Accepted: 11 March 2021
Published: 13 March 2021

1. Introduction

Among hereditary metabolic diseases, a separate group includes diseases associated with amino acid metabolism disorders. To date, about 90 inborn errors in amino acid metabolism (primary aminoacidopathies) are known, including phenylketonuria (PKU). Although phenylketonuria is considered a rare hereditary disease, it is an urgent public health problem for the Russian Federation and many other countries [1]. The incidence of phenylketonuria among children in the world averages one in 10,000 newborns and ranges from 1:200,000 (Thailand) to 1:4370 (Turkey). The higher the level of consanguinity in the population, the higher the incidence of genetic diseases, including phenylketonuria [2]. In Russia, according to neonatal screening data, the frequency of phenylketonuria averages

1:7000 and varies by region from 1:4735 in the Kursk region to 1:18,000 in the Tyva Republic. The most common form is the classic phenylketonuria, in which diet therapy is currently the only effective treatment method [3].

Research on the approaches to phenylketonuria treatment has been conducted quite actively for over 50 years [4]. Nevertheless, the main possibility for phenylketonuria patients to maintain health remains a rigid diet that limits the consumption of protein foods not only of animal but also of plant origin. According to William B. Hanley (2012), the cost of such food per person is 20–40 thousand dollars per year. Therefore, the major directions of research on this issue, carried out in many countries of the world (USA, Germany, Great Britain, Brazil, Bulgaria, India, China, Russia, and many others), are limited to the creation of special products and the reduction in the cost of technologies for their production [5].

There have been reports of alternative therapy methods for patients with phenylketonuria (pharmacological treatment, enzyme therapy, transplantation, and gene modification) in recent decades. However, they are not used in the Russian Federation due to the lack of developed and available technologies. The most promising treatment is the use of the enzyme L-phenylalanine ammonia-lyase (PAL), both in the form of injections and capsules/tablets, which breaks down phenylalanine to safe products. Biomarin Pharmaceutical Inc. obtained the most significant results as part of the US national program. Despite many years of research on this disease, Biomarin Pharmaceutical Inc. was the first to order a survey among PKU patients on their quality of life and their therapy development expectations [6]. The survey showed that most respondents are interested in the development of new drugs and treatments, giving preference to oral administration of pharmaceuticals with the option of not following a rigid diet. These results confirm that the problem has not yet been resolved and remains relevant [7].

There are patents in the open press describing methods of obtaining PAL by cultivating the yeast *Rhodotorula* and other microbial cells (US4757015, US4636466, EP0140714, EP0321488), PAL purification (JP60172282, JP58086082), stabilization (US5753487, EP0703788, WO/1995/000151), application (US7531341, US20070048855, US20020102712, US7537923), etc.

On the Russian market, the PAL enzyme preparation can be purchased only from foreign manufacturers: a commercial preparation (EC 4.3.1.5), Sigma-Aldrich (USA), cost about 800 euros/10 units (~290 g). BioMarin Pharmaceutical Inc., which began the third stage of PEG-PAL clinical trials (a pegylated preparation of recombinant L-phenylalanine ammonia-lyase), achieved significant results in the development of technologies for PAL production. If this drug enters the pharmaceutical market, the drug's cost will limit its availability, especially when imported into other countries [8].

The therapeutic use of PAL is limited due to its proteolytic instability and immunogenicity. There are no proven technologies for purification and stabilization, as well as a stable form that guarantees the preservation of the enzyme before direct reaction with phenylalanine, especially in the acidic environment of the stomach [9,10].

Earlier, we obtained an encapsulated L-phenylalanine ammonia-lyase form, for which the degradation dynamics in model biological fluids (gastric and intestinal juices) [11] and storage stability [12] were studied. The main goal of PAL encapsulation in shells based on plant hydrocolloids is to stabilize it and ensure the possibility of subsequent therapeutic use.

This work aims to study the encapsulated L-phenylalanine ammonia-lyase penetration kinetics and the efficacy of phenylalanine catabolism correction using in vitro model systems.

2. Materials and Methods

2.1. Objects of Research

The object of this research was L-phenylalanine-ammonia-lyase (powder, activity from 1.5 to 5.0 U mg^{-1}, density 1192 kg m^{-3}, thermal conductivity 3.36 W $(m\ K)^{-1}$), obtained from the pigment yeast cultivation [12]. Encapsulated PAL was obtained as described in [11], sample No. 6: the capsule shell contains 10.0 wt % carrageenan, 10.0 wt % agar–agar, 10.0 wt % carboxymethyl cellulose, 5.0 wt % glycerin, and 65.0 wt % water.

To study the kinetics of PAL (encapsulated and not encapsulated) penetration into the liver cell monolayer, human cell lines (hepatomas Huh-7 and monocytes THP-1) (All-Union (Russian) collection of cell cultures, Institute of Cytology of the Russian Academy of Sciences, St. Petersburg, Russia) were used.

Human monocyte suspension THP-1 was grown in RPMI-1640 medium (Dia-m, Moscow, Russia) containing 10% heat-inactivated bovine serum albumin (FBS), 1 mM sodium pyruvate, 0.05 mM 2-mercaptoethanol, penicillin (100 IU/mL) and streptomycin (100 μg/mL). Human hepatoma cells Huh-7 were grown in DMEM medium (Dia-m, Moscow, Russia) containing 10% FBS, penicillin (100 IU/mL), and streptomycin (100 μg/mL). In co-cultures, cells were grown in a mixed medium (1:1) in a trans-well, where the cells were separated by a porous membrane (pore size 3 μm, distance 1 mm). In co-cultures, Huh-7 cells were planted at an initial concentration of 75×10^4 cells per well, cultured overnight, after which THP-1 cells (30×10^4 cells per well) were added. All cells were cultured in Costar 12-well plates (Corning-Costar, Corning, CA, USA). After the monolayer formation, the cells were passaged using a Versene dissociating solution and 0.25% trypsin solution. Cells were passaged every 3–4 days. The differentiated cells were cultured for 20–30 passages.

To create an in vitro model of the liver plate, 6-well plates (Corning-Costar, Corning, CA, USA) were used, into which BD Falcon™ Cell culture inserts with a pore size of 0.4 μm and a surface area of 4.2 cm^2 were inserted (BD Falcon™, Toronto, ON, Canada). The THP-1 and Huh-7 cell lines were removed from the surface of the culture plastic with Versene solutions and 0.25% trypsin solution with Hanks' salts. After obtaining the THP-1 cell suspension, 1.5 mL of the cell suspension with a cytosis of 2×10^5 cells/cm^2 was passed into the apical compartment (AC) of the test system, which is membrane wells. The number of cells in the suspension was counted in a Goryaev chamber. Similarly, a suspension of Huh-7 cells in a volume of 1.5 mL with a cytosis of 5×10^5 cells/cm^2 was sub-cultured onto membrane inserts.

The 2.5 mL of culture medium was added to the basolateral compartment (BC) of the test systems, which was the wells of a 6-well plate. The culture medium in the apical compartment (AC) and BC was changed by gentle pipetting every 24–48 h.

Model media simulating blood serum was used to analyze the efficiency of correction of disturbed phenylalanine catabolism by the developed form [11,12] of encapsulated L-phenylalanine ammonia-lyase on in vitro model systems. The model solution contained 5.5 mg bovine serum albumin, BSA (molecular weight 68,000 g/mol, isoelectric point 4.9), and 1.6 mg γ-globulin (molecular weight 200,000 g/mol, isoelectric point 6.0). The stock solution contained 1000 μmol/L of phenylalanine. Three series of experiments were carried out. In the first series, phenylalanine hydroxylase (PAH, number in the numerical classification of enzymes based on the chemical oxidation reactions they catalyze: EC 1.14.16.1), as well as tetrahydrobiopterin and ferrous salt, were added to the stock model solution. In the second series, phenylalanine transaminase (PAH, number in the numerical classification of enzymes based on the chemical transfer reactions of functional groups they catalyze: EC 2.6.1.58) was added to the stock model solution, in the third series—L-phenylalanine ammonia-lyase in the encapsulated form [11,12]. The enzyme activity varied in the range from 1.5 to 5.0 U/mg. All solutions were incubated for 4 h at 37 °C, taking samples every 30 min and recording the content of such substances as phenylalanine, tyrosine, trans-cinnamic acid, phenylpyruvate, phenyl lactate, and phenylacetate.

2.2. Determination of the Kinetics of PAL Penetration into the Monolayer of Liver Cells

Test systems in the form of membrane wells with 1.5 mL of cell suspension with a cytosis of 2×10^5 cells/cm^2 were preliminarily prepared. For this purpose, the cells were sub-cultured onto membrane inserts BD Falcon™ Cell culture inserts (Thermo fisher, Moscow, Russia).

Working concentrations of encapsulated [11,12] and not encapsulated L-phenylalanine ammonia-lyase (25, 50, and 100 mg) were prepared in Hanks' salt solution immediately before the experiments. The working concentrations of the solutions were selected based on the experiments carried out to determine the PAL hepatotoxicity. After complete dissolution, the working solutions were sterilized in a cleanroom before being added to the cells using MS PES Syringe Filters (Membran solutions, Tokyo, Japan) with 0.22 μm pore diameter syringe filters.

To assess the interaction of capsules with the test preparation, the PAL solution was incubated with a solution prepared from crushed capsules after their complete dissolution. Further, the obtained values of the kinetics of penetration through the monolayer of cells were compared with the kinetics of penetration of the enzyme without added capsule solution.

The apical and basolateral compartments were washed twice with Hanks' salt solution. Then, 2.5 mL of salt solution was added to the basolateral compartment and 1.5 mL of working PAL solutions to the apical compartment to determine the kinetics of drug penetration in the absence of capsules, or 750 μL of twice the concentration of PAL solution and 750 μL of salt solution to determine the kinetics of drug penetration in the presence of capsules.

The kinetics of encapsulated [11,12] and not encapsulated PAL penetration through monolayers of cells was assessed after 60 and 90 min, for which Hanks' salt solution was aspirated from BC and AC with the further determination of the enzyme concentration in solutions. The L-phenylalanine ammonia-lyase concentration was determined spectrophotometrically at a wavelength of 280 nm.

2.3. *Quantification of Phenylalanine and Tyrosine in Model Solutions*

In model solutions simulating blood serum, the amount of phenylalanine and tyrosine was determined by HPLC using an LC-20 liquid chromatograph (Shimadzu, Kyoto, Japan). The method involves deproteinization of a small volume (300 μL) of a solution simulating blood serum, followed by HPLC on a PEEK cation exchange column (lithium form, 9 μm, 46 × 250 mm). We used the reaction of amino acids with ninhydrin with the formation of colored compounds, which were recorded on a UV detector at 570 nm. The flow rate was 25 mL/h in a gradient of six mobile phases (pH 2.80, pH 3.00, pH 3.15, pH 3.50, pH 3.55, LiOH); the duration of each analysis was 170 min.

2.4. *Quantification of Trans-Cinnamic Acid*

The quantitative content of trans-cinnamic acid was determined by capillary electrophoresis on a Kapel-105 device (Lumex, St. Petersburg, Russia). Conditions for the electrophoretic determination of cinnamic acid: working electrolyte—10 mM $Na_2B_4O_7$ solution containing 40 mM sodium dodecyl sulfate; sample injection 5 s, 30 mbar; voltage +20 kV; the detection wavelength is 205 nm [13].

2.5. *Quantification of Phenylpyruvate, Phenyllactate, and Phenylacetate*

The quantitative content of phenylpyruvate, phenyl lactate, and phenylacetate was determined spectrophotometrically based on the ability of these compounds to form complex colored compounds with ferric iron ions.

3. Results

The phenylalanine hydroxylation system is shown in Figure 1; the scheme of metabolic processes that determine the development mechanism of PKU and some hyperphenylalaninemias in the case of BH_4 deficiency is presented in Figure 2.

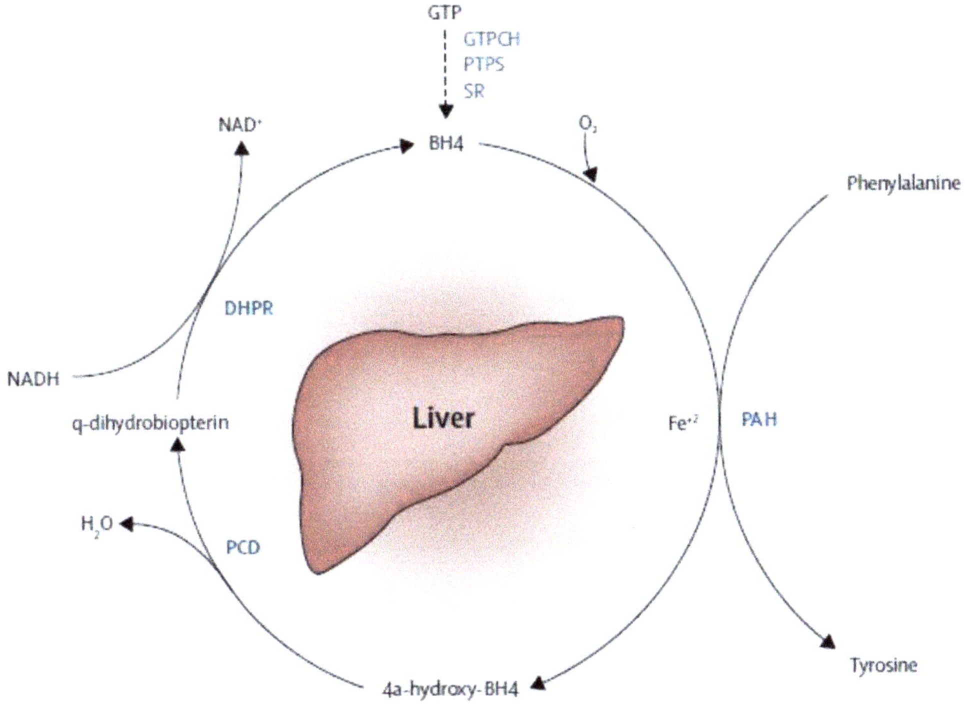

Figure 1. Phenylalanine hydroxylation system.

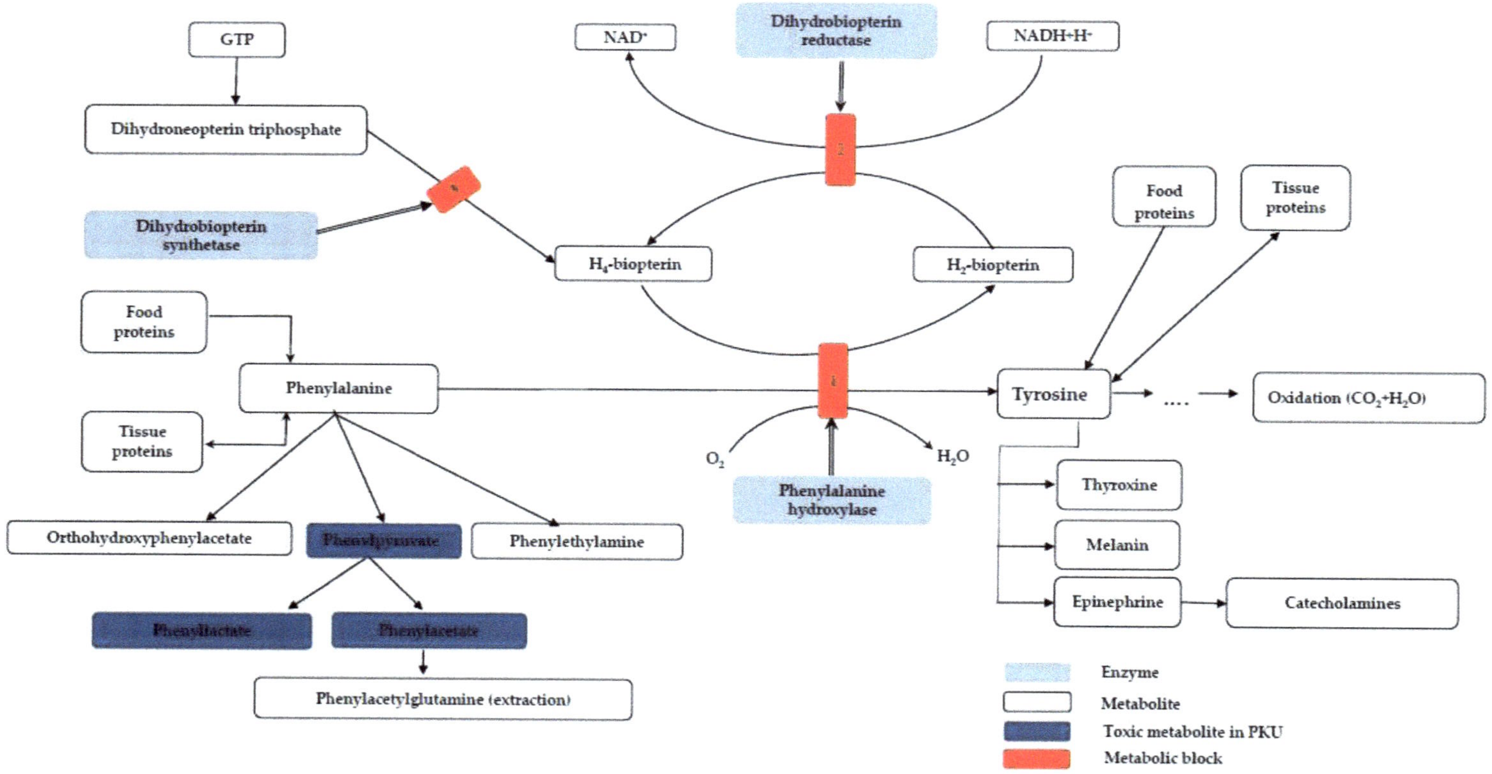

Figure 2. Scheme of metabolic processes that determine the mechanism of phenylketonuria development [14]: metabolic block 1—in case of phenylalanine hydroxylase deficiency (classical phenylketonuria); metabolic blocks 2–3—in case of various forms of BH_4 deficiency (phenylalanine hydroxylase-independent hyperphenylalaninemia).

In BH_4-dependent PKU forms, the metabolic block does not extend to the phenylalanine hydroxylation process itself but one of the stages of biosynthesis and regeneration of the active form of tetrahydrobiopterin [15].

PAH is a non-heme, homotetrameric, iron-containing enzyme that requires BH_4, molecular oxygen, and an active site-bound Fe^{2+} ion to convert phenylalanine to tyrosine (Scheme 1).

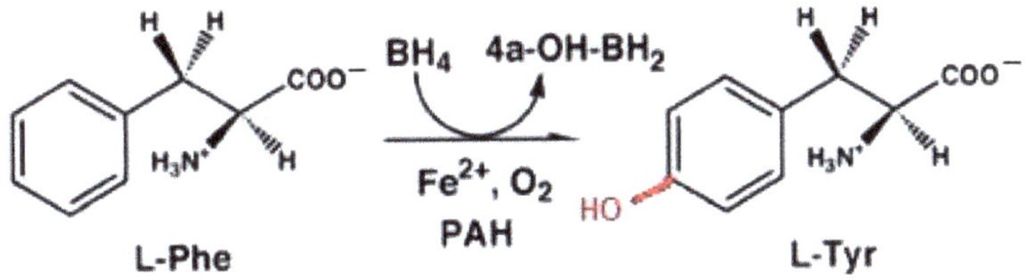

Scheme 1. PAH-catalyzed reaction.

This enzyme plays an essential role in most catabolism reactions of phenylalanine from food and is localized mainly in the liver [12].

One of the promising PKU treatments is enzyme replacement therapy using two enzyme systems: PAH and L-phenylalanine ammonia-lyase (PAL). Compared to PAH, PAL therapy has many advantages. PAL does not require cofactors for phenylalanine degradation, and the reaction product, trans-cinnamic acid (Scheme 2), has low toxicity.

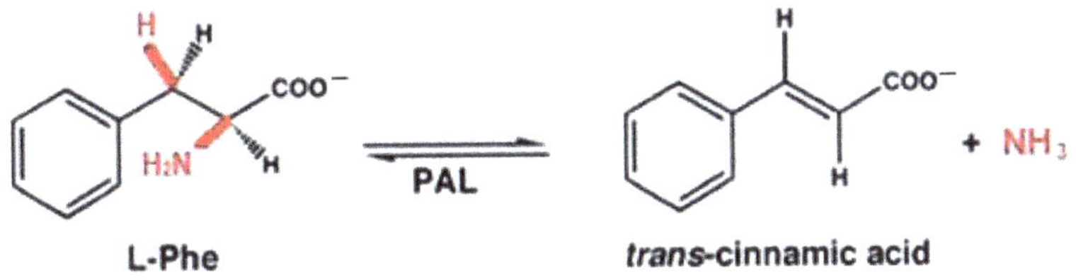

Scheme 2. PAL-catalyzed reaction.

The calculated data on the kinetics of the encapsulated [11,12] and not encapsulated L-phenylalanine ammonia-lyase penetration into the monolayer of liver cells (cell line Huh-7, cell line THP-1, and co-culture Huh-7 + THP-1) at incubation times of 60, 90, and 120 min are presented in Table 1.

Table 1. PAL content (%) in the basolateral compartment of test systems based on Huh-7 and THP-1 cell monolayers.

Cell Line	Incubation Conditions	Incubation Duration, min		
		60	90	120
The initial concentration of PAL 25 mg				
I	A	35.6 ± 1.8	68.9 ± 3.4	94.5 ± 4.7
	B	37.2 ± 1.9	67.3 ± 3.4	93.8 ± 4.7
II	A	41.4 ± 2.1	72.0 ± 3.6	95.2 ± 4.8
	B	39.8 ± 2.0	70.5 ± 3.5	95.0 ± 4.8
III	A	38.7 ± 1.9	69.5 ± 3.5	93.5 ± 4.7
	B	39.3 ± 2.0	68.4 ± 3.4	94.1 ± 4.7

Table 1. *Cont.*

Cell Line	Incubation Conditions	Incubation Duration, min		
		60	90	120
The initial concentration of PAL 50 mg				
I	A	33.2 ± 1.7	65.7 ± 3.3	87.0 ± 4.3
	B	31.8 ± 1.6	66.1 ± 3.3	88.3 ± 4.4
II	A	34.2 ± 1.7	66.3 ± 3.3	89.4 ± 4.5
	B	33.5 ± 1.7	67.8 ± 3.4	87.3 ± 4.4
III	A	36.7 ± 1.8	68.4 ± 3.4	90.2 ± 4.5
	B	35.5 ± 1.8	68.0 ± 3.4	88.6 ± 4.4
The initial concentration of PAL 100 mg				
I	A	45.6 ± 2.3	77.6 ± 3.9	96.8 ± 4.8
	B	47.2 ± 2.4	78.9 ± 3.9	95.7 ± 4.8
II	A	44.3 ± 2.2	79.0 ± 4.0	95.5 ± 4.8
	B	45.0 ± 2.3	78.3 ± 3.9	96.4 ± 4.8
III	A	46.6 ± 2.3	76.7 ± 3.8	96.4 ± 4.8
	B	48.1 ± 2.4	78.0 ± 3.9	96.7 ± 4.8

I—hepatoma Huh-7; II—monocytes -1; III—co-culture Huh-7 + -1; A—without capsules; B—with capsules. The experiments were carried out in triplicate.

The results of determining the phenylalanine concentration dynamics in model solutions of three series are shown in Figure 3.

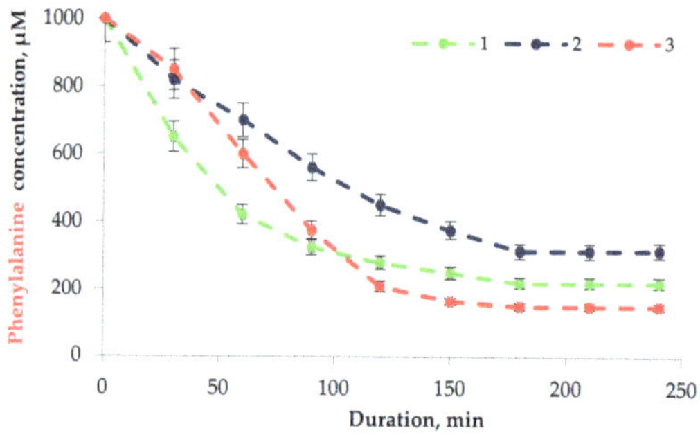

(a)

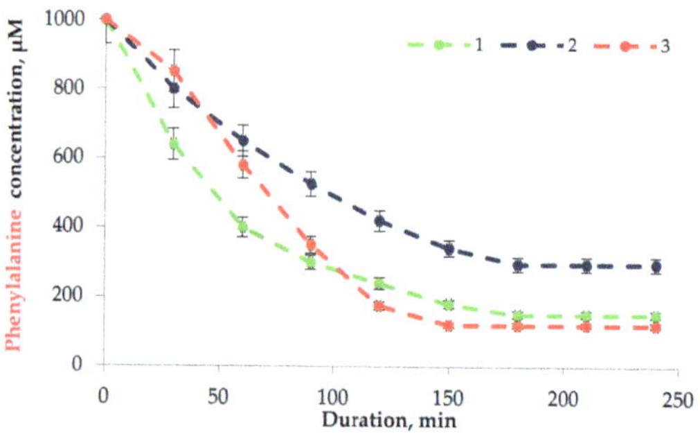

(b)

Figure 3. *Cont.*

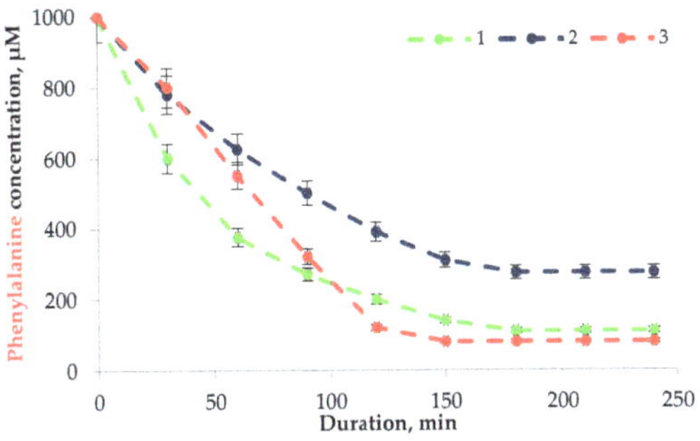

(c)

Figure 3. The phenylalanine concentration dynamics in a model medium (imitating blood serum) containing enzymes with activity (**a**) 1.5 U/mg; (**b**) 3.0 U/mg; (**c**) 5.0 U/mg depending on incubation duration: 1—PAH; 2—phenylalanine transaminase; 3—encapsulated L-phenylalanine ammonia-lyase. The experiments were carried out in triplicate.

The results of determining the content of phenylalanine metabolism products after incubation of model solutions with enzymes are presented in Table 2.

Table 2. Results of determination of the content of phenylalanine metabolism products after incubation of model solutions with enzymes.

Incubation Duration, min	The Concentration of Phenylalanine Metabolic Products, μM														
	1	2	3	4	5	1	2	3	4	5	1	2	3	4	5
	PAH					Phenylalanine Transaminase					Encapsulated PAL				
activity 1.5 U/mg															
0	0.0 ± 0.0	–*	–	–	–	–	–	0.0 ± 0.0	0.0 ± 0.0	0.0 ± 0.0	–	0.0 ± 0.0	–	–	–
30	12.5 ± 0.6	–	–	–	–	–	–	10.6 ± 0.5	6.3 ± 0.3	7.8 ± 0.4	–	8.6 ± 0.4	–	–	–
60	23.4 ± 1.2	–	–	–	–	–	–	15.4 ± 0.8	9.5 ± 0.5	11.2 ± 0.6	–	15.0 ± 0.8	–	–	–
90	28.7 ± 1.4	–	–	–	–	–	–	19.0 ± 1.0	12.7 ± 0.6	14.5 ± 0.7	–	24.2 ± 1.2	–	–	–
120	33.2 ± 1.7	–	–	–	–	–	–	27.6 ± 1.4	15.2 ± 0.8	17.6 ± 0.9	–	31.5 ± 1.6	–	–	–
150	36.7 ± 1.8	–	–	–	–	–	–	34.5 ± 1.7	18.8 ± 0.9	21.3 ± 1.1	–	38.3 ± 1.9	–	–	–
180	41.2 ± 2.1	–	–	–	–	–	–	38.9 ± 1.9	21.0 ± 1.1	24.5 ± 1.2	–	46.7 ± 2.3	–	–	–
210	48.5 ± 2.4	–	–	–	–	–	–	42.1 ± 2.1	23.4 ± 1.2	27.7 ± 1.4	–	59.0 ± 3.0	–	–	–
240	56.0 ± 2.8	–	–	–	–	–	–	45.7 ± 2.3	25.3 ± 1.3	30.2 ± 1.5	–	77.8 ± 3.9	–	–	–
activity 3.0 U/mg															
0	0.0 ± 0.0	–	–	–	–	–	–	0.0 ± 0.0	0.0 ± 0.0	0.0 ± 0.0	–	0.0 ± 0.0	–	–	–
30	14.6 ± 0.7	–	–	–	–	–	–	13.3 ± 0.7	7.8 ± 0.4	10.5 ± 0.5	–	14.1 ± 0.7	–	–	–
60	27.0 ± 1.4	–	–	–	–	–	–	17.0 ± 0.9	11.0 ± 0.6	15.6 ± 0.8	–	22.5 ± 1.1	–	–	–
90	31.2 ± 1.6	–	–	–	–	–	–	21.3 ± 1.1	14.7 ± 0.7	17.2 ± 0.9	–	46.9 ± 2.3	–	–	–
120	36.7 ± 1.8	–	–	–	–	–	–	30.8 ± 1.5	17.3 ± 0.9	19.0 ± 1.0	–	62.8 ± 3.1	–	–	–
150	41.0 ± 2.1	–	–	–	–	–	–	37.8 ± 1.9	22.0 ± 1.1	24.4 ± 1.2	–	87.2 ± 4.4	–	–	–
180	52.0 ± 2.6	–	–	–	–	–	–	44.5 ± 2.2	26.7 ± 1.3	29.8 ± 1.5	–	95.3 ± 4.8	–	–	–
210	64.3 ± 3.2	–	–	–	–	–	–	57.0 ± 2.9	29.8 ± 1.5	35.1 ± 1.8	–	107.4 ± 5.4	–	–	–
240	75.8 ± 3.8	–	–	–	–	–	–	65.0 ± 3.3	32.1 ± 1.6	44.5 ± 2.2	–	116.0 ± 5.8	–	–	–
activity 5.0 U/mg															
0	0.0 ± 0.0	–	–	–	–	–	–	0.0 ± 0.0	0.0 ± 0.0	0.0 ± 0.0	–	0.0 ± 0.0	–	–	–
30	25.6 ± 1.3	–	–	–	–	–	–	16.0 ± 0.8	12.4 ± 0.6	13.6 ± 0.7	–	19.5 ± 1.0	–	–	–
60	48.9 ± 2.4	–	–	–	–	–	–	22.4 ± 1.1	17.8 ± 0.9	19.5 ± 1.0	–	30.8 ± 1.5	–	–	–
90	55.3 ± 2.8	–	–	–	–	–	–	25.6 ± 1.3	23.0 ± 1.2	25.6 ± 1.3	–	54.6 ± 2.7	–	–	–
120	60.7 ± 3.0	–	–	–	–	–	–	34.8 ± 1.7	26.9 ± 1.3	34.1 ± 1.7	–	68.2 ± 3.4	–	–	–
150	74.2 ± 3.7	–	–	–	–	–	–	40.6 ± 2.0	31.4 ± 1.6	39.2 ± 2.0	–	77.3 ± 3.9	–	–	–
180	88.0 ± 4.4	–	–	–	–	–	–	55.9 ± 2.8	36.2 ± 1.8	44.8 ± 2.2	–	95.2 ± 4.8	–	–	–
210	102.4 ± 5.1	–	–	–	–	–	–	67.4 ± 3.4	42.1 ± 2.1	47.9 ± 2.4	–	115.6 ± 5.8	–	–	–
240	118.7 ± 5.9	–	–	–	–	–	–	88.0 ± 4.4	48.7 ± 2.4	51.2 ± 2.6	–	138.2 ± 6.9	–	–	–

1—tyrosine; 2—trans-cinnamic acid; 3—phenylpyruvate; 4—phenyllactate; phenylacetate; * "–"—not found. The experiments were carried out in triplicate.

4. Discussion

Phenylketonuria is a genetic autosomal recessive disease. Classic phenylketonuria occurs due to mutations in the q22–24 region of chromosome 12, which affects the structure and function of phenylalanine hydroxylase. This enzyme is responsible for converting phenylalanine (Phe) to tyrosine (Tyr) in the liver. The decreased activity of phenylalanine hydroxylase, as a rule, causes phenylalanine accumulation in the blood and body tissues, including the central nervous system. The exact mechanism of the increase in phenylalanine levels, which can damage the brain, is still unclear. The same can be said about direct damage and a decrease in tyrosine levels, as well as a lack of other large neutral amino acids that interfere with neurotransmitter formation and neuronal development [16–18].

From the perspective of the pathogenetic links underlying hyperphenylalaninemia development, several forms of this pathology are distinguished. A classic PKU caused by several mutations in the phenylalanine hydroxylase gene, the general result of which is a deficiency of the enzyme activity [17,19,20], and PKU forms, previously called atypical, which are associated with impaired metabolism of tetrahydrobiopterin (BH_4), a coenzyme involved in the hydroxylation of several amino acids, including phenylalanine [21,22].

In classic PKU, a defect in the phenylalanine 4-hydroxylase activity leads to a metabolic block in the conversion of phenylalanine to tyrosine, which results in abnormal metabolic product accumulation in the patient's body in large quantities—phenylpyruvate, phenyllactate, and phenylacetate, the content of which is insignificant under normal conditions. These metabolites can penetrate the blood–brain barrier and exert neurotoxic effects, especially on the developing central nervous system of a child. It is assumed that they contribute to the disruption of the myelination processes of nerve fibers [23].

Since the main reactions of phenylalanine metabolism are happening in the liver, the study of the kinetics of L-phenylalanine ammonia-lyase penetration into the monolayer of liver cells after its release from capsules [11,12] is of considerable interest in this study.

In recent years, various in vitro models have been developed for performing experiments on liver cells. In this regard, three main, fundamentally different approaches can be distinguished: precision-cut liver tissue slice, cell cultures, and isolated perfused liver model. The advantage of using precision-cut liver slices is the ability to compare the analysis of cell and tissue morphology. Liver perfusion allows a range of physiological and morphological parameters to be assessed (tissue histology). Cell culture models can be effectively used to assess cell metabolism, cytotoxicity, and genotoxicity. However, such studies are complicated by the difficulty of maintaining the culture of hepatocytes [11,24,25].

Edling et al. proposed to use a system based on connecting human cell lines: hepatoma (Xa-7) and monocytes (THP-1) [15]. With the introduction of various substances, an increase in the expression of genes for anti-inflammatory mediators and genes associated with stress was observed in both types of cell.

In this work, human cell lines (Huh-7 hepatomas and THP-1 monocytes) were used to study the kinetics of encapsulated [11,12] and not encapsulated PAL penetration into the monolayer of liver cells.

The results presented in Table 1 indicate that the kinetics of PAL penetration into the cell monolayer in the three test systems under study are practically the same. Moreover, it follows from Table 1 that the presence of a capsule shell based on plant hydrocolloids does not significantly affect the absorption of L-phenylalanine ammonia-lyase in systems simulating hepatic laminae.

Analysis of Figure 3 indicates that in all the studied model systems, there is a decrease in the concentration of phenylalanine with an increase in the duration of incubation, and the decrease in the concentration of this amino acid is directly proportional to the activity of enzymes: phenylalanine hydroxylase, phenylalanine transaminase, and encapsulated L-phenylalanine ammonium lyase. The minimum content of phenylalanine was recorded in a simulated blood serum containing encapsulated PAL: from 80 μmol/L to 150 μmol/L after 4-h incubation. The maximum content of phenylalanine was found in the model solution containing phenylalanine transaminase: from 275 µmol/L to 316 µmol/L after 4-h incubation with the enzyme.

A detailed analysis of Figure 3a allows us to conclude that the concentration of phenylalanine in a model medium (simulating blood serum) containing enzymes with an activity of 1.5 U/mg decreases with an increase in the incubation duration. The most significant decrease in phenylalanine concentration is observed for PAH, the smallest—for phenylalanine transaminase.

Analysis of Figure 3b allows us to conclude that the concentration of phenylalanine in a model medium (imitating blood serum) containing enzymes with an activity of 3.0 U/mg also decreases with an increase in the incubation duration. The most significant phenylalanine concentration decrease is observed for PAH, and to lower concentrations than in Figure 3b, the smallest—for phenylalanine transaminase.

Analysis of Figure 3c allows us to conclude that the concentration of phenylalanine in a model medium (imitating blood serum) containing enzymes with an activity of 5.0 U/mg also decreases with an increase in the incubation duration. The greatest decrease in phenylalanine concentration is observed for PAH, and to the lowest concentrations of the three presented enzymes. The smallest decrease in concentration is observed for phenylalanine transaminase.

Analyzing the results presented in Table 2, we concluded that the patterns of phenylalanine catabolism in biological fluids under the action of such enzymatic systems as phenylalanine hydroxylases, phenylalanine transaminases, and L-phenylalanine ammonia-lyase are consistent with theoretical data. Thus, upon incubation of a model medium simulating blood serum with PAH, an accumulation of tyrosine in the medium was observed: after incubation for 4 h at an enzyme activity of 5.0 U/mg, the concentration of this amino acid was 118.7 µmol/L. Thus, the phenylalanine metabolism proceeds according to the scheme shown in Scheme 1.

We found [12] that PAL stability during storage is longer in the encapsulated form than in the un-encapsulated one. By the 4th month of storage, the PAL activity in the capsule is 25.4% higher than in the absence of the capsule. Furthermore, by the 6th month, the activity of PAL in the encapsulated form is 46.4% higher than in the un-encapsulated one. Thus, it can be concluded that PAL is stable in encapsulated form for 6 months, which proves its superiority compared to un-encapsulated.

In the presence of the phenylalanine transaminase enzyme in the model environment, the accumulation of such products as phenylpyruvate, phenyllactate, and phenylacetate (toxic products of phenylalanine catabolism) is noted. These processes are shown in Figure 2.

Finally, in the model medium containing the enzyme L-phenylalanine ammonia-lyase (encapsulated form), the accumulation of trans-cinnamic acid is observed, the concentration of which after a 4-h exposure at a PAL activity of 5.0 U/mg is 138.2 µmol/L. The obtained data indicate that phenylalanine undergoes degradation according to the scheme shown in Scheme 2.

The work [26] presents the results of studies of the accumulation of tyrosine, phenols, and cinnamic acid in the medium at enzyme activity 1.0, 2.0, 3.0, 4.0, 5.0, 6.0, and 8.0 U/mg during incubation for 1, 2, 4, and 8 h. It was found that the concentrations of tyrosine, phenols, and cinnamic acid were the highest at the activity of L-phenylalanine ammonia-lyase 5.0 U/mg after incubation for 4 h. In [27], the PAL activity in relation to the accumulation of trans-cinnamic acid, tyrosine, flavonoids, benzoids, and phenolic glycosides was studied. The results obtained in [27] are in good agreement with the data obtained in our studies.

5. Conclusions

L-phenylalanine ammonia-lyase has recently become an important therapeutic enzyme with several biomedical properties [25]. The enzyme catabolizes L-phenylalanine to transcinnamate and ammonia. PAL is widespread in higher plants, some algae, ferns, and microorganisms, but is absent in animals. Although microbial PAL has been widely used in the past to produce industrially important metabolites, its high substrate specificity and catalytic efficiency have recently stimulated interest in its biomedical applications. PAL is approved for the treatment of adult phenylketonuria patients. In addition, it showed high efficacy in tumor regression and the treatment of tyrosine-related metabolic disorders such as tyrosinemia. The encapsulated L-phenylalanine ammonia-lyase form can find therapeutic application in the phenylketonuria treatment after additional in vitro and in vivo studies, in particular, the study of preparation safety indicators. This is evidenced by the results of studying the kinetics of encapsulated PAL penetration into a monolayer of liver cells, as well as the results of evaluating the effectiveness of capsules with PAL in terms of correcting impaired phenylalanine catabolism in phenylketonuria. Another important advantage of using L-phenylalanine ammonia-lyase in the capsule form is its stability during storage compared to the un-encapsulated enzyme [12] and the stability of the encapsulated preparation in the acidic environment of the stomach [11], which allows PAL to be released mainly in the intestine. Several therapeutically valuable metabolites biosynthesized due to their catalytic action are included in food supplements, antimicrobial peptides, drugs, amino acids, and their derivatives. PAL with improved pharmacodynamic and pharmacokinetic properties is a highly effective biological agent.

Author Contributions: S.I., A.P. and O.B. conceived and designed the research; L.D., S.N. and S.S. analyzed and interpreted the data; L.D. and S.S. contributed reagents, materials, analysis tools or data; S.I., A.P. and O.B. wrote the paper. All authors have read and agreed to the published version of the manuscript.

Funding: This research was funded by RUSSIAN FOUNDATION FOR BASIC RESEARCH, grant number 18-08-00444.

Institutional Review Board Statement: Not applicable.

Informed Consent Statement: Not applicable.

Data Availability Statement: Not applicable.

Conflicts of Interest: The authors declare no conflict of interest.

References

1. Isabella, V.M.; Ha, B.N.; Castillo, M.J.; Lubkowicz, D.J.; Rowe, S.E.; Millet, Y.A.; Anderson, C.L.; Li, N.; Fisher, A.B.; West, K.A.; et al. Development of a synthetic live bacterial therapeutic for the human metabolic disease phenylketonuria. *Nat. Biotechnol.* **2018**, *36*, 857–864. [CrossRef]
2. Parmeggiani, F.; Weise, N.J.; Ahmed, S.T.; Turner, N.J. Synthetic and therapeutic applications of ammonia-lyases and aminomutases. *Chem. Rev.* **2018**, *118*, 73–118. [CrossRef]
3. Levy, H.L.; Sarkissian, C.N.; Scriver, C.R. Phenylalanine ammonia lyase (PAL): From discovery to enzyme substitution therapy for phenylketonuria. *Mol. Genet. Metab.* **2018**, *124*, 223–229. [CrossRef]
4. Tork, S.D.; Nagy, E.Z.A.; Cserepes, L.; Bordea, D.M.; Nagy, B.; Toşa, M.I.; Paizs, C.; Bencze, L.C. The production of L- and D-phenylalanines using engineered phenylalanine ammonia lyases from Petroselinum crispum. *Sci. Rep.* **2019**, *9*, 20123. [CrossRef]
5. Tomoiaga, R.B.; Tork, S.D.; Horváth, I.; Filip, A.; Nagy, L.C.; Bencze, L.C. Saturation mutagenesis for phenylalanine ammonia lyases of enhanced catalytic properties. *Biomolecules* **2020**, *10*, 838. [CrossRef]
6. Hendrikse, N.M.; Larsson, A.H.; Gelius, S.S.; Kuprin, S.; Nordling, E.; Syrén, P.-O. Exploring the therapeutic potential of modern and ancestral phenylalanine/tyrosine ammonia-lyases as supplementary treatment of hereditary tyrosinemia. *Sci. Rep.* **2020**, *10*, 1315. [CrossRef]
7. Wu, Y.; Wang, W.; Li, Y.; Dai, X.; Ma, G.; Xing, D.; Zhu, M.; Gao, L.; Xia, T. Six phenylalanine ammonia-lyases from *Camellia sinensis*: Evolution, expression, and kinetics. *Plant Physiol. Biochem.* **2017**, *118*, 413–421. [CrossRef]
8. De Sousa, I.P.; Gourmel, C.; Berkovska, O.; Burger, M.; Leroux, J.C. A microparticulate based formulation to protect therapeutic enzymes from proteolytic digestion: Phenylalanine ammonia lyase as case study. *Sci. Rep.* **2020**, *10*, 3651. [CrossRef]
9. De Jong, F.; Hanley, S.J.; Beale, M.H.; Karp, A. Characterisation of the willow phenylalanine ammonia-lyase (PAL) gene family reveals expression differences compared with poplar. *Phytochemistry* **2015**, *117*, 90–97. [CrossRef]
10. Acosta, P.B.; Yannicelli, S. *The Ross Metabolic Formula System. Nutrition Support Protocols*, 4th ed.; Ross Products Division, Division of Abbott Laboratories: Columbus, OH, USA, 2001.
11. Babich, O.; Dyshlyuk, L.; Prosekov, A.; Noskova, S.; Ivina, O.; Pavsky, V.; Ivanova, S.; Bulgakova, O. Study of the potential of the capsule shell based on natural polysaccharides in targeted delivery of the l-phenylalanine ammonia-lyase enzyme preparation. *Pharmaceuticals* **2020**, *13*, 63. [CrossRef]

12. Babich, O.; Dyshlyuk, L.; Noskova, S.; Prosekov, A.; Ivanova, S.; Pavsky, V. The effectiveness of plant hydrocolloids at maintaining the quality characteristics of the encapsulated form of L-phenylalanine-ammonia-lyase. *Heliyon* **2019**, *6*, e03096. [CrossRef]
13. Prosekov, A.Y.; Mudrikova, O.V.; Babich, O.O. Determination of cinnamic acid by capillary zone electrophoresis using ion-pair reagents. *J. Anal. Chem.* **2012**, *67*, 474–477. [CrossRef]
14. Dhondt, J.L. Laboratory diagnosis of phenylketonuria. In *PKU and BH4. Advances in Phenylketonuria and Tetra-Hydrobiopterin*; Blau, N., Ed.; SPS Publications: Heilbronn, Germany, 2006; pp. 161–179.
15. Edling, Y.; Sivertsson, L.K.; Buturaa, A.; Ingelman-Sundberga, M.; Eka, M. Increased sensitivity for troglitazone-induced cytotoxicity using a human in vitro co-culture model. *Toxicol. In Vitro* **2009**, *23*, 1387–1395. [CrossRef]
16. Varga, A.; Csuka, P.; Sonesouphap, O.; Bánóczi, G.; Toşa, M.I.; Katona, G.; Molnár, Z.; Bencze, L.C.; Poppe, L.; Paizs, C. A novel phenylalanine ammonia-lyase from Pseudozyma antarctica for stereoselective biotransformations of unnatural amino acids. *Catal. Today* **2020**. [CrossRef]
17. Gentile, J.K.; Ten Hoedt, A.E.; Bosch, A.M. Psychosocial aspects of PKU: Hidden disabilities—A review. *Mol. GenetMetab.* **2010**, *99*, 64–67. [CrossRef] [PubMed]
18. Guldberg, P.; Henriksen, K.F.; Sipila, I.; Guttler, F.; de la Chapelle, A. Phenylketonuria in a low incidence population: Molecular characterisation of mutations in Finland. *J. Med. Genet.* **1995**, *32*, 976–978. [CrossRef] [PubMed]
19. Kim, W.; Erlandsen, H.; Surendran, S.; Stevens, R.C.; Gamez, A.; Michols-Matalon, K.; Tyring, S.K.; Matalon, R. Trends in Enzyme Therapy for Phenylketonuria. *Mol. Ther.* **2004**, *10*, 220–224. [CrossRef] [PubMed]
20. Pietz, J.; Kreis, R.; Rupp, A.; Mayatepek, E.; Rating, D.; Boesch, C.; Bremer, H.J. Large neutral amino acids block phenylalanine transport into brain tissue in patients with phenylketonuria. *J. Clin. Investig.* **1999**, *103*, 1169–1178. [CrossRef] [PubMed]
21. Rebuff, A.; Harding, C.O.; Ding, Z.; Thony, B. Comparison of AAV pseudotype 1, 2, and 8 vectors administered by intramuscular injection in the treatment of murine phenylketonuria. *Hum. Gene Ther.* **2010**, *21*, 463–477. [CrossRef]
22. Mays, Z.J.S.; Mohan, K.; Trivedi, V.D.; Chappell, T.C.; Nair, N.U. Directed evolution of Anabaena variabilis phenylalanine ammonia-lyase (PAL) identifies mutants with enhanced activities. *BioRxiv* **2020**, 1–14. [CrossRef]
23. Feduraev, P.; Skrypnik, L.; Riabova, A.; Pungin, A.; Tokupova, E.; Maslennikov, P.; Chupakhina, G. Phenylalanine and Tyrosine as Exogenous Precursors of Wheat (*Triticum aestivum L.*) Secondary Metabolism through PAL-Associated Pathways. *Plants* **2020**, *9*, 476. [CrossRef] [PubMed]
24. Thony, B.; Auerbach, G.; Blau, N. Tetrahydrobiopterin biosynthesis, regeneration and functions. *Biochem. J.* **2000**, *347*, 1–16. [CrossRef] [PubMed]
25. Van Rijn, M.; Jansma, J.; Brinksma, A.; Bakker, H.D.; Boers, G.H.J.; Carbasius-Weber, E.; Douwes, A.C.; van den Herberg, A.; Ter Horst, N.M.; de Klerk, J.B.C.; et al. A survey of natural protein intake in Dutch phenylketonuria patients: Insight into estimation or measurement of dietary intake. *J. Am. Diet Assoc.* **2008**, *108*, 1704–1707. [CrossRef] [PubMed]
26. Şirin, S.; Aydaş, S.B.; Aslım, B. Biochemical evaluation of phenylalanine ammonia lyase from endemic plant cyathobasis Fruticulosa (bunge) aellen. for the dietary treatment of phenylketonuria. *Food Technol. Biotechnol.* **2016**, *54*, 296–303. [CrossRef]
27. Lynch, J.H.; Orlova, I.; Zhao, C.; Guo, L.; Jaini, R.; Maeda, H.; Akhtar, T.; Cruz-Lebron, J.; Rhodes, D.; Morgan, J.; et al. Multifaceted plant reponses to circumvent phe hyperaccumulation by downregulation of flux through the shikimate pathway and by vacuolar phe sequestration. *Plant J.* **2017**, *92*, 939–950. [CrossRef] [PubMed]

pharmaceutics

Article

Estimating the Oral Absorption from Self-Nanoemulsifying Drug Delivery Systems Using an In Vitro Lipolysis-Permeation Method

Mette Klitgaard [1], Anette Müllertz [2] and Ragna Berthelsen [1,*]

[1] Department of Pharmacy, University of Copenhagen, 2100 Copenhagen, Denmark; mette.klitgaard@sund.ku.dk
[2] Bioneer: FARMA, Department of Pharmacy, University of Copenhagen, 2100 Copenhagen, Denmark; anette.mullertz@sund.ku.dk
* Correspondence: ragna.berthelsen@sund.ku.dk; Tel.: +45-35-33-65-13

Abstract: The aim of this study was to design an in vitro lipolysis-permeation method to estimate drug absorption following the oral administration of self-nanoemulsifying drug delivery systems (SNEDDSs). The method was evaluated by testing five oral formulations containing cinnarizine (four SNEDDSs and one aqueous suspension) from a previously published pharmacokinetic study in rats. In that study, the pharmacokinetic profiles of the five formulations did not correlate with the drug solubilization profiles obtained during in vitro intestinal lipolysis. Using the designed lipolysis-permeation method, in vitro lipolysis of the five formulations was followed by in vitro drug permeation in Franz diffusion cells equipped with PermeaPad® barriers. A linear in vivo–in vitro correlation was obtained when comparing the area under the in vitro drug permeation–time curve (AUC_{0-3h}), to the AUC_{0-3h} of the plasma concentration–time profile obtained from the in vivo study. Based on these results, the evaluated lipolysis-permeation method was found to be a promising tool for estimating the in vivo performance of SNEDDSs, but more studies are needed to evaluate the method further.

Keywords: in vivo–in vitro correlation; lipolysis-permeation; lipid-based drug delivery system; PermeaPad; cinnarizine; lipolysis

Citation: Klitgaard, M.; Müllertz, A.; Berthelsen, R. Estimating the Oral Absorption from Self-Nanoemulsifying Drug Delivery Systems Using an In Vitro Lipolysis-Permeation Method. *Pharmaceutics* **2021**, *13*, 489. https://doi.org/10.3390/pharmaceutics13040489

Academic Editor: Im-Sook Song

Received: 5 March 2021
Accepted: 30 March 2021
Published: 2 April 2021

1. Introduction

The majority of potential drug candidates in the pipelines of the industry today are challenged by their physicochemical properties, such as poor water-solubility, which directly affects the bioavailability of the drug candidates intended for oral administration [1–4]. Different enabling drug delivery systems have been developed and used to improve the bioavailability of such poorly water-soluble drugs (PWSDs) [2,3,5–8]. For lipophilic PWSDs, lipid-based drug delivery systems (LbDDSs) represent such enabling drug delivery systems, which have been shown to improve the bioavailability of a range of PWSDs [5,7–11]. LbDDSs, such as the self-nanoemulsifying drug delivery systems (SNEDDSs), consist of different mixtures of lipids, surfactants, and co-solvents. They bypass the dissolution rate-limiting step to oral drug absorption and exploit the endogenous routes of lipid digestion, i.e., lipolysis.

To aid the development of LbDDSs, multiple in vitro models have been designed to estimate the oral drug performance of LbDDSs. These in vitro models all simulate the human gastro-intestinal (GI) lipolysis process at different levels of complexity [8,12,13]. The most commonly used model is the intestinal in vitro lipolysis model, in which the porcine pancreatic lipase, pancreatin, is typically used as the source of digestive enzymes, because this has been shown to have similar digestive properties to human pancreatic lipase [8,12–16]. The enzyme-induced lipolysis breaks down the lipids and digestible surfactants present in LbDDSs and causes the formation of different colloidal structures that act as a drug solubilization reservoir in equilibrium with the free fraction of solubilized drug. When drugs are administrated in LbDDSs, the utilized excipients commonly need to be digested in order to release the incorporated drug [13,17]. When the intestinal in vitro lipolysis model is used to study the performance of LbDDSs, it is assumed that the amount of drug solubilized in the aqueous phase of the lipolysis medium is available for intestinal absorption, and therefore allows estimation of the drug performance in vivo [8,18,19]. Since its development in 2001 [20], several studies have tried to validate the predictive power of the in vitro lipolysis model. However, as recently described by Feeney et al., only few have succeeded in obtaining an in vivo–in vitro correlation (IVIVC) [8]. Several authors have stressed that the lack of an absorptive step might be an explanation for the general lack of IVIVCs when comparing in vitro lipolysis data with plasma concentration–time profiles, i.e., because the current intestinal in vitro lipolysis model is a closed system, it may not reflect the dynamic interaction between drug solubilization/dissolution, precipitation, and permeation with a continuous absorptive sink present in the human GI tract [3,8,13,21–29]. Based on these discussions, designing a method which combines the in vitro lipolysis model with in vitro permeation could possibly improve the estimation of the oral absorption of LbDDSs. There has in fact been an emerging interest in such combined methods, as covered in a review by Berthelsen et al. [12]. In recent studies by Keemink et al. [30,31] and Alskär et al. [32], in vitro lipolysis of LbDDSs was combined with permeation across a Caco-2 monolayer. In this setup, an immobilized microbial lipase was utilized, rather than the more commonly used pancreatin [15,16], because the Caco-2 monolayer was found to be incompatible with the porcine pancreatic extract [30–32]. Using their lipolysis-permeation setup, Keemink et al. and Alskär et al. obtained a rank order correlation between the amount of drug permeating the Caco-2 cell monolayer following in vitro lipolysis and the in vivo absorption of orally administered LbDDSs containing the lipophilic drugs fenofibrate and carvedilol [31,32].

The majority of drugs have been shown to be absorbed by passive transcellular diffusion [33–35]; therefore, an artificial permeation barrier is often considered a sufficiently appropriate alternative barrier for studying drug permeation. In the light of this, Bibi et al. studied the compatibility of an artificial biomimetic barrier, the PermeaPad®, which consists of a phospholipid layer sandwiched between two support sheets, in combination with in vitro lipolysis of an SNEDDS in side-by-side diffusion chambers [36]. The integrity of the PermeaPad®-barriers was evaluated by the permeation of the hydrophilic permeation marker, calcein, following a lipolysis-permeation study across the same barrier. In that study, it was concluded that the PermeaPad® was compatible with simulated intestinal lipolysis medium, the lipolysis products of the tested SNEDDS, and pancreatin [36].

Another important parameter in the development of lipolysis-permeation methods is the absorption surface area to donor volume (A/V) ratio. In most in vitro permeation models, this is far below that reported for the human intestine, i.e., <0.5 cm^{-1} in vitro vs. 1.9–2.3 cm^{-1} in vivo [35,37,38]. A small A/V ratio might cause an underestimation of drug permeation; therefore, an A/V ratio close to the in vivo A/V ratio might improve the level of in vivo mimicry, as well as the predictability of the in vitro model.

Based on the above, the purpose of the present study was to design and evaluate a simple in vitro lipolysis-permeation method using the PermeaPad® barrier to estimate the oral performance of PWSDs in SNEDDSs. The method was designed using existing equipment, namely, the in vitro lipolysis setup [20,39] and Franz diffusion cells equipped with PermeaPad® barriers. The application of the Franz cells enabled adjusting the donor volume to achieve a high A/V ratio, to simulate the in vivo conditions more closely. Furthermore, sink conditions were secured by applying an acceptor medium with a high drug solubility.

To evaluate the potential of the designed lipolysis-permeation method, a previously published study by Siqueira et al. was used as a frame of reference [39]. Siqueira et al. performed an in vitro lipolysis study and a pharmacokinetic (PK) study in rats of five oral cinnarizine formulations but were unable to correlate the in vitro and in vivo results [39]. The five studied cinnarizine formulations were four SNEDDSs and one aqueous suspension. In the SNEDDSs, cinnarizine was either dissolved at 80% (*w*/*w*) of its solubility in the preconcentrate ($SNEDDS_{80\%}$), suspended at 200% (*w*/*w*) of its solubility in the preconcentrate (superSNEDDS suspension), or dissolved in a supersaturated state corresponding to 200% (*w*/*w*) of its solubility in the preconcentrate (superSNEDDS solution). Additionally, cinnarizine was administrated as an aqueous suspension co-dosed with the blank SNEDDS in a ratio corresponding to administration of the $SNEDDS_{80\%}$ (the Chasing principle). While the *in vitro* lipolysis study predicted no difference in the performance of the four SNEDDSs, the PK study showed a different formulation rank-order when comparing the area under the plasma concentration–time curves (AUC), i.e., $SNEDDS_{80\%}$ = the Chasing principle > superSNEDDS suspension = superSNEDDS solution = aqueous suspension (Table S1 in the Supplementary Materials) [39]. In the present study, the five formulations from the reference study were tested using the lipolysis-permeation method to evaluate if (i) the in vitro lipolysis results could be reproduced; and if (ii) the method could be used to estimate the oral absorption of cinnarizine from SNEDDSs and thereby obtain an IVIVC for the tested formulations.

2. Materials and Methods

2.1. Materials

Bovine bile, bovine serum albumin (BSA), calcein, cinnarizine, 4-bromophenylboronic acid (4-BPBA), maleic acid, pancreatin from porcine pancreas (≥3 × USP specifications), propylene glycol, soybean oil, and tris(hydroxymethyl)aminomethane (Tris) were purchased from Sigma Aldrich (St. Louis, MO, USA) at analytical grade. Acetonitrile (ACN), ammonium phosphate monobasic, ethanol absolute, hydrochloric acid (37%), methanol, potassium dihydrogen phosphate, and sodium hydroxide were purchased from VWR Chemicals (Leuven, Belgium). Kolliphor RH 40 and Maisine 35-1 were kindly donated by BASF (Ludwigshafen, Germany) and by Gattefossé (Saint-Priest, France), respectively. Lipoid S PC was obtained from Lipoid (Ludwigshafen, Germany). The PermeaPad® barriers (25 mm) were generously donated by InnoME (Espelkamp, Germany). All water used in the experiments was of purified quality obtained from SG ultra-clear UV apparatus from Holm & Halby Service (Brøndby, Denmark).

2.2. Methods

2.2.1. Media Preparation

The blank simulated intestinal medium (SIM) was prepared by dissolving the components of Table 1 in purified water under stirring at 37 °C overnight. When all components were dissolved, the pH of the medium was adjusted to pH 6.5.

The hydrophilic marker calcein (logP -1.71, pK_a 1.8, 9.2 [40,41]) was dissolved in SIM to reach a concentration of 5 mM (SIM_{CAL}) and used to study the integrity of the PermeaPad® barrier in the lipolysis-permeation method. Calcein is an acidic compound; therefore, the pH of SIM_{CAL} was measured after the addition of calcein and re-adjusted to pH 6.5 by the addition of NaOH. SIM_{CAL} was used as the blank donor medium.

Table 1. Composition of simulated intestinal in vitro lipolysis medium (SIM) [39,42,43].

Component	Concentration (mM)
Bovine Bile	2.95
Phospholipids	0.26
NaCl	146.8
Tris	2
Maleic acid	2
$CaCl_2 \cdot 2H_2O$	1.4

The acceptor medium, PBS_{BSA}, was prepared as a 74 mM phosphate buffered saline solution (PBS) (29 mM KH_2PO_4 and 45 mM $Na_2HPO_4 \cdot 7H_2O$) with pH adjusted to 7.4 and supplemented with 4% (*w*/*v*) BSA. The donor and acceptor media were kept iso-osmotic at 290 ± 2 mOsmol/kg to avoid permeation caused by osmosis.

2.2.2. Preparation of Cinnarizine Formulations

To evaluate the designed lipolysis-permeation method, all five formulations from the reference study by Siqueira et al. [39] were tested: the $SNEDDS_{80\%}$, the superSNEDDS suspension, the superSNEDDS solution, the Chasing principle, and the aqueous suspension. The blank SNEDDS formulation was prepared from the components listed in Table 2. All formulations were loaded with the PWSD, cinnarizine (logP of 5.03 and pK_a of 1.9 and 7.47 [8,39,44,45]).

Table 2. Composition of the blank self-nanoemulsifying drug delivery system (SNEDDS) formulation.

Component	Ratio (% *w/w*)
Soybean oil: Maisine 35-1 (1:1, weight ratio)	55
Kolliphor RH 40	35
Ethanol	10

To prepare the blank SNEDDS, soybean oil, Maisine 35–1, and Kolliphor RH 40 were heated to 50 °C and mixed. After mixing, ethanol was added, and the blank formulation was set to stir at room temperature (25 ± 1 °C) overnight. The drug load was 20 mg/g for the $SNEDDS_{80\%}$, and 50 mg/g for the superSNEDDS suspension and superSNEDDS solution. The $SNEDDS_{80\%}$ and super-SNEDDS suspensions were prepared by weighing cinnarizine into a glass vial, adding the blank SNEDDS formulation, and stirring the mixture at room temperature overnight. The superSNEDDS solution was prepared by sonicating the cinnarizine with the blank SNEDDS at 60 °C for 2 h followed by storage at 60 °C for 24 h and stirring overnight at 37 °C. The superSNEDDS solution was used within 48 h after preparation to avoid precipitation. To prepare the aqueous suspension (10 mg/mL), cinnarizine was suspended in a 0.5% (*w/v*) methylcellulose solution with 5% (*v/v*) propylene glycol and set to stir at room temperature (25 ± 1 °C) overnight. For the Chasing principle, blank SNEDDS (with the same lipid load as the $SNEDDS_{80\%}$) was added to the lipolysis vessel prior to addition of the aqueous suspension.

2.2.3. The Lipolysis-Permeation Method

In the designed lipolysis-permeation method, the established in vitro intestinal lipolysis model was combined with a consecutive drug permeation step across PermeaPad® barriers in Franz diffusion cells (surface area 2 cm^2, acceptor compartment volume 7 mL) (Figure 1). The Franz diffusion cell acceptor compartment had continuous magnetic stirring and the temperature was kept at 37 °C.

Lipolysis Step

The intestinal in vitro lipolysis was carried out as described by Siqueira et al. with one minor modification [39], i.e., a bolus addition of calcium in the SIM (Table 1) was applied instead of the continuous addition of calcium described by Siqueira et al. [39]. In short, the experiments were carried out in a thermostated glass vessel (37 °C), which was set up with pH-stat apparatus (Titrando 804, Metrohm, Herisau, Switzerland) controlling pH input and titration in the Tiamo software v.2.4. Pancreatin from a porcine pancreas was weighed and suspended in SIM (Table 1), mixed, and centrifuged for 8 min at 5500 rpm (44,000× *g* at r_{max}) in a Heraeus Megafuge 16R centrifuge from Thermo Fisher Scientific (Osterode, Germany). The supernatant was collected and stored for up to 15 min prior to addition to the lipolysis vessel. The tested formulations were added to the lipolysis vessel to obtain a drug dose of 250 µg/mL cinnarizine and following 15 min of dispersion in 36 mL SIM_{CAL}, lipolysis was initiated by the addition of 4 mL of pancreatin, yielding a final lipase activity of 800 USPU/mL. Throughout the in vitro lipolysis, the pH was kept at 6.5 by automatic titration of 0.5 M NaOH. Samples of 2.6 mL were taken at times 0 min (following dispersion, but immediately prior to lipase addition), 15, 30 and 60 min. From each sample, 1 mL was taken out and inhibited with 5 µL lipase inhibitor (1 M 4-BPBA in methanol) to allow for quantification of the drug distribution at the specific time-point, and 1.5 mL of uninhibited sample was transferred to the Franz diffusion cell donor compartment for the permeation step. Each formulation was tested in triplicate (n = 3).

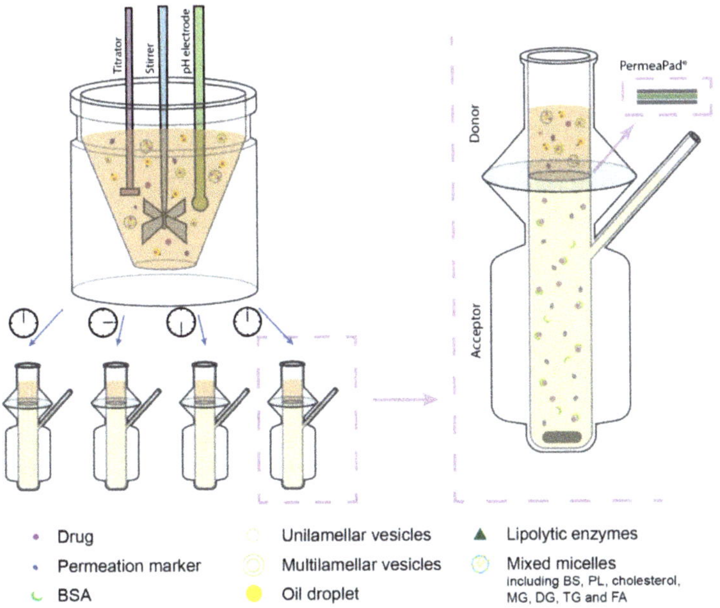

Figure 1. Schematic illustration of the designed lipolysis-permeation method: in vitro lipolysis of an SNEDDS was coupled with permeation across a PermeaPad® barrier in Franz diffusion cells with PBS_{BSA} in the acceptor compartment. Each lipolysis sample contained lipolysis products of the lipid-based drug delivery system (LbDDS) and the permeation marker (calcein) which was embedded in the simulated intestinal medium. Abbreviations: BS, bile salt; BSA, bovine serum albumin; DG, diglycerides; FA, fatty acids; MG, monoglycerides; PBS_{BSA}, phosphate-buffered saline (pH 7.4) with 4% (w/v) BSA; PL, phospholipids; TG, triglycerides.

Sample Treatment

A fraction (50 µL) of each inhibited lipolysis sample was directly diluted in ACN to determine the total amount of drug, i.e., the recovery of added drug. The remaining part of the samples underwent phase separation by centrifugation at 13,300 rpm (170,000× g at r_{max}) for 15 min in a Thermo Micro CL17 centrifuge from Thermo Fisher Scientific (Osterode, Germany). From each sample, 50 µL of the resulting supernatant (the aqueous phase) was appropriately diluted in ACN. The rest of the aqueous phase was removed, and the pellet was re-suspended in 1 mL ACN and sonicated for 15 min. The re-suspended pellet sample was centrifuged for 15 min at 13,300 rpm and 200 µL of the supernatant appropriately diluted in ACN. The amount of cinnarizine in each diluted sample was quantified by high-performance liquid chromatography (HPLC) (see Section 2.2.4).

Permeation Step

For the permeation step, the Franz diffusion cell acceptor compartment was filled with 7 mL of PBS_{BSA}. The PermeaPad® barriers (25 mm in diameter) were hydrated by adding 0.5 mL SIM (Table 1) to the donor compartment and allowing the system to equilibrate for 30 min. Following membrane hydration, the SIM was removed and 1.5 mL of uninhibited lipolysis samples (collected after 0, 15, 30, and 60 min of lipolysis, respectively) was added to initiate the permeation study. This way, the permeation from each formulation was tested across a total of twelve PermeaPad® barriers, i.e., drug permeation from each of the four samples collected from each lipolysis replicate was tested. Each permeation study ran for 3 h. Samples of 200 μL were collected from the acceptor compartment at 0, 5, 15, 30, 60, 90, 120, 150, and 180 min. The sample volume was replenished with fresh acceptor medium. Directly following collection, each sample was diluted with equal parts of ACN to precipitate the BSA and centrifuged for 15 min at 13,300 rpm (170,000× *g* at r_{max}) in a Thermo Micro CL17 centrifuge from Thermo Fisher Scientific (Osterode, Germany). The supernatants were immediately transferred to HPLC vials for the quantification of cinnarizine, and a 96-well plate for the quantification of calcein by fluorescence detection on a plate reader (see Section 2.2.4 for details).

Stability of the PermeaPad® Barrier

A control experiment was conducted to test the stability of the PermeaPad® barrier following prolonged contact with the blank donor medium (SIM_{CAL}), and acceptor medium (PBS_{BSA}), i.e., without drug formulations and digestive enzymes. The control experiment was conducted following the experimental procedure described in the previous section, using 1.5 mL of SIM_{CAL} as the donor medium. Following 3 h of permeation study, the calcein permeation was quantified as described in Section 2.2.4.

Cinnarizine Solubility

To evaluate if sink conditions were present for cinnarizine using the described lipolysis-permeation method, the apparent solubility of cinnarizine in PBS and PBS_{BSA} was determined by the shake-flask method with an incubation time of 48 h [46].

2.2.4. Quantification Methods

The amount of cinnarizine in the lipolysis-, and permeation samples was quantified by HPLC, using a Dionex Ultimate 3000 pump, an ASI 100 automated sample injector, a p680 pump, a Dionex PDA-100 Photodiode Array Detector and a Dionex Ultimate 3000 Detector from Thermo Scientific (Waltham, MA, USA). All samples were analyzed using a Phenomenex Kinetex C18 column (100 × 4.60 mm, 5 μm) (Torrance, CA, USA). The drug was eluted at 0.8 mL/min with 20 mM ammonium phosphate (pH 4.5):ACN (50:50 (*v*/*v*)). The amounts of cinnarizine in the lipolysis samples were quantified with UV detection at 253 nm. The amounts of cinnarizine in the permeation samples were quantified with fluorescence with excitation and emission wavelengths of 249 and 311 nm, respectively. The lipolysis samples were analyzed using an injection volume of 15 μL and a calibration curve in the range of 50–1000 ng/mL, while permeation samples were analyzed with an injection volume of 50 μL and a calibration curve with the range of 0.5–50 ng/mL.

The calcein content of the permeation samples was quantified on a Tecan Infinite M200 (Grödig, Austria) plate reader with Tecan Magellan software (ver. 6.5). The samples were analyzed with excitation and emission wavelengths of 485 and 520 nm, respectively, and a gain of 70. The samples were diluted appropriately with a 50:50 (*v*/*v*) mixture of PBS:ACN. The amount of calcein in 200 μL of each diluted sample was quantified with a calibration curve in the range 0.05–4.0 nmol/mL prepared in the same solvent mixture.

2.2.5. Data Processing

The steady-state flux (J) of calcein across the PermeaPad® barriers was determined from the slope of the linear section obtained by plotting the cumulative amount of permeated calcein per surface area of the membrane as a function of time [36,47]. The apparent permeability coefficient (P_{app}) was calculated from the obtained steady-state flux and the initial concentration of calcein (5 mM) in the donor compartment (C_0), according to Equation (1) [36,47].

$$P_{app} = \frac{J}{C_0} \quad (1)$$

In the case of cinnarizine administrated in the different SNEDDSs, the measured concentration in the aqueous phase of the lipolysis medium (i.e., the donor compartment concentration) represents both the free fraction of solubilized drug, and the amount of drug incorporated in the micelles and colloidal structures present in this phase. It is generally assumed that only the free fraction of the drug permeates the intestinal membrane [48]; therefore, the concentration of free drug should be used as C_0 in order to calculate the P_{app}. However, because it was not possible to quantify the free fraction of cinnarizine in the present setup, the P_{app} was not calculated for the cinnarizine permeation studies. Rather, the permeation profiles were used for the comparison of the different formulations.

The in vitro $AUC_{0\text{–}3h}$ (determined from Figure 4 displaying the mean cumulative permeated amount of cinnarizine as a function of time) was calculated by the linear trapezoidal method.

Statistical analysis of the obtained data was performed using GraphPad Prism ver. 7.04 (GraphPad Software, San Diego, CA, USA). Student's *t*-test and analysis of variance (ANOVA) were used to compare the means of two or more groups, respectively, with a significance level of $\alpha = 0.05$. All data are shown as the mean ± standard error of the mean (SEM) for easier comparison with the reference study. The PK parameters from the reference study were determined using WinNonLin ver. 5.2 (Pharsight Corporation, Mountain View, CA, USA). For the present study, the $AUC_{0\text{–}3h}$ of the in vivo plasma concentration-time profile was determined from the raw data granted by Siqueria, SD [39] (Table S1) in order to make a direct comparison to the in vitro $AUC_{0\text{–}3h}$.

3. Results and Discussions

In the present study, a lipolysis-permeation method was designed and evaluated based on: (i) the ability to reproduce the in vitro lipolysis results of the reference study; and (ii) the ability to apply the amount of permeated drug to obtain an IVIVC upon comparison to the in vivo data of the five cinnarizine formulations reported in the reference study by Siqueira et al. [39]. As a control of the permeation barrier integrity, the permeation of calcein was studied throughout the permeation step. Additionally, the A/V ratio and sink conditions were evaluated for the designed method.

3.1. Reproducing In Vitro Lipolysis Results

The amount of cinnarizine found in the aqueous phase of the lipolysis samples is depicted in Figure 2a with the accompanying lipolysis profiles of the amount of free fatty acids neutralized with NaOH in Figure 2b. The mean cinnarizine recovery from all lipolysis experiments was 85 ± 3% (mean ± SEM, $n = 15$).

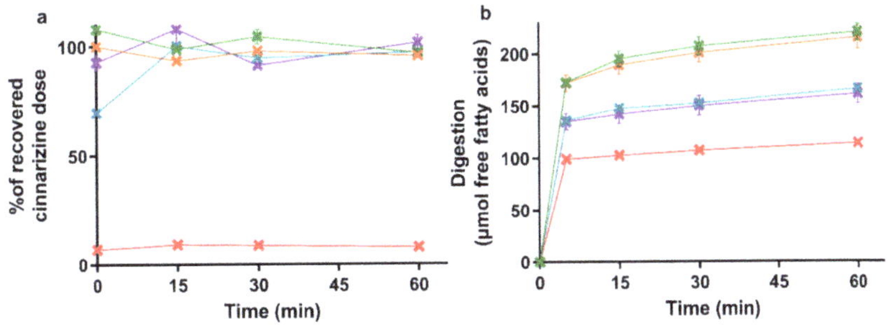

Figure 2. (**a**) Distribution of cinnarizine in the aqueous phase as percent of the total recovered dose after in vitro lipolysis of $SNEDDS_{80\%}$ (green), superSNEDDS suspension (blue), superSNEDDS solution (purple), the Chasing principle (orange), and aqueous suspension (red). (**b**) Lipolysis profiles of in vitro lipolysis at pH 6.5 of the same formulations. All data are represented as the mean ± SEM ($n = 3$).

The drug distribution profiles obtained during 60 min of in vitro lipolysis (Figure 2a) are similar to those obtained in the reference study [39]. In both studies, the entire recovered dose was found in the aqueous phase following lipolysis of the four SNEDDS formulations, while the majority of the cinnarizine dose was recovered in the pellet phase for the aqueous suspension. The lipolysis profiles of the titrated amount of free fatty acids released upon digestion of the five formulations (Figure 2b) was rank-ordered according to the amount of lipids added to the lipolysis vessel, i.e., $SNEDDS_{80\%}$ = the Chasing principle > superSNEDDS suspension = superSNEDDS solution > aqueous suspension. This is in accordance with the reference study [39], with the only difference being that the continuous calcium addition in the reference study resulted in a higher and more continuous rate of lipolysis.

3.2. Permeation Barrier Integrity

The integrity of the PermeaPad® barrier was tested following prolonged contact with the blank donor medium containing calcein (SIM_{CAL}) and acceptor medium (PBS_{BSA}), as well as during exposure to the lipolysis samples for each of the five formulations. Barrier integrity was evaluated based on the observed P_{app} of calcein depicted in Figure 3. The barrier integrity was tested for each formulation without (0 min lipolysis) and with enzymatic lipolysis (15–60 min lipolysis). The individual calcein permeation profiles can be found in the Supplementary Materials, Figure S1.

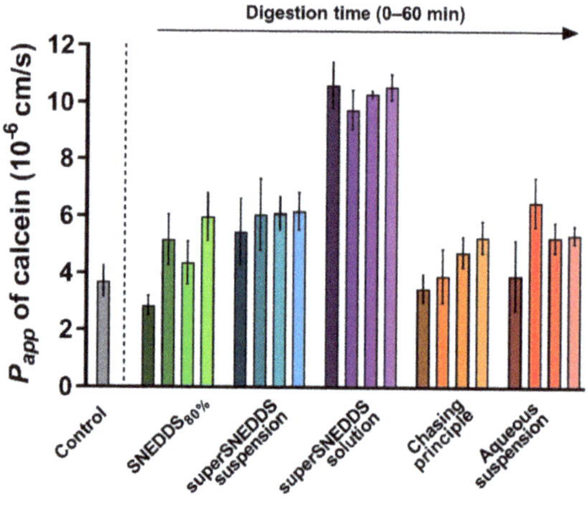

Figure 3. PermeaPad® stability depicted as calcein P_{app} values calculated from the 3 h of exposure to the different formulations before (0 min lipolysis time, darkest shade of every color) and after digestive enzyme addition (15, 30, and 60 min of lipolysis, the lightest shade of each color represents 60 min of lipolysis). The calcein P_{app} from the control experiments (grey bar) with no formulation or digestion is depicted for comparison. All data are depicted as the mean ± SEM ($n = 3$).

In the control experiment with SIM_{CAL} as the donor medium and PBS_{BSA} as the acceptor medium, the P_{app} of calcein across the PermeaPad® barrier was $3.7 \pm 0.6 \times 10^{-6}$ cm/s. This value is not significantly different from the values reported by Bibi et al. (P_{app} $3.4 \pm 0.5 \times 10^{-6}$ cm/s [36]), which indicates that PermeaPad® barrier was compatible with the selected donor and acceptor media.

When comparing the calcein P_{app} values obtained in the presence of each digesting formulation with the calcein P_{app} of the blank control (SIM_{CAL}), no difference was observed, except for a significantly higher P_{app} ($p \leq 0.05$) in the presence of the superSNEDDS solution (at all four time-points) (Figure 3). Generally, a slight tendency towards an increased P_{app} of calcein in the presence of the digestive enzymes (0 min lipolysis time compared to

15–60 min of lipolysis) was observed for all formulations, although this difference was not found to be significant (Figure 3, Figure S1).

The calcein P_{app} in the presence of the superSNEDDS solution was significantly higher when compared the calcein P_{app} from the present control study, which might indicate that the permeation barrier in these studies was disrupted to some degree. However, because all values were lower than the calcein P_{app} of $1.65 \pm 0.1 \times 10^{-5}$ cm/s previously reported for the PermeaPad® barrier with no lipid barrier layer [49], it was concluded that some barrier function was retained throughout the study. This was additionally based on the observation that the higher calcein P_{app} did not affect the permeation of cinnarizine (Section 3.3). Based on these results, it was concluded that permeation barrier function was sufficiently retained during all conducted studies.

3.3. Permeation Profiles

The permeation of cinnarizine across the PermeaPad® barrier was determined for lipolysis samples taken at each of the four time-points (0, 15, 30, and 60 min of lipolysis) for all five formulations. The individual cinnarizine permeation profiles for each formulation after each lipolysis time-point can be found in Figure S2. As can be seen in Figure S2, lipolysis had no significant effect on the permeation of cinnarizine and, therefore, the permeation profiles depicted in Figure 4 represent a pooled mean ± SEM for each formulation (n = 12).

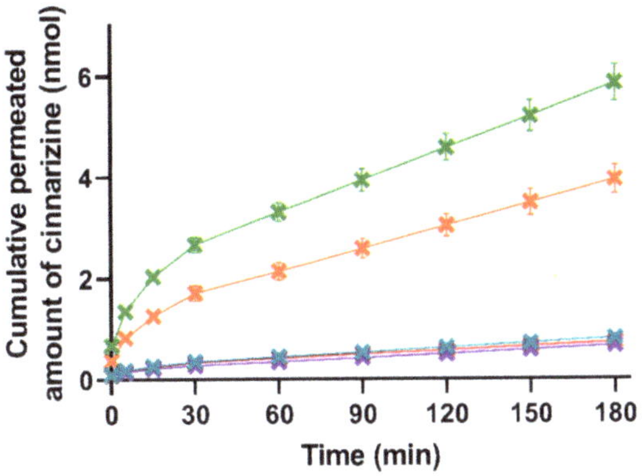

Figure 4. Mean cumulative permeated amount of cinnarizine as a function of time when studying the five formulations SNEDDS$_{80\%}$ (green), superSNEDDS suspension (blue), superSNEDDS solution (purple), the Chasing principle (orange), and aqueous suspension (red) in the lipolysis-permeation method. The data are presented as the mean ± SEM (n = 12).

The lipase-induced lipolysis seemingly did not affect the amount of cinnarizine permeation in the present study; therefore, the need for the lipolysis step could be challenged and perhaps rather substituted with a dispersion of the formulations in SIM, as has been used in other studies [22]. This is in accordance with studies by Michaelsen et al., who showed that addition of the lipase inhibitor Orlistat to SNEDDSs did not change the AUC of the plasma concentration–time profile of halofantrine and fenofibrate after oral dosing to rats [50,51]. However, other LbDDSs or drugs might be affected differently by lipid digestion.

As can be seen in Figure 4, there were no significant differences in the amount of permeated cinnarizine from the lipolysis samples of the superSNEDDS suspension, superSNEDDS solution, and the aqueous suspension at any given time point (t = 5–180 min). These results indicate that cinnarizine very likely precipitated in the donor compartment following administration of the superSNEDDS suspension and superSNEDDS solution. Following precipitation, the amount of cinnarizine in solution was expected to be close to that obtained following administration of the aqueous suspension, because the amount of permeated drug for these three formulations was comparable (i.e., the superSNEDDS suspension, superSNEDDS solution, and the aqueous suspension, Figure 4), and the concentration gradient across the permeation barrier, therefore, must be assumed to be similar. In the case of the $SNEDDS_{80\%}$ and the Chasing principle, a significantly higher amount of cinnarizine ($p \leq 0.05$) permeated from these formulations throughout the experiment (t = 5–180 min) when compared to the other three formulations (Figure 4). This observed difference is expected to be caused by the presence of a high amount of lipids and surfactants in these formulations, which inhibited the precipitation of cinnarizine following dispersion and digestion in SIM. The amount of permeated cinnarizine was higher from the $SNEDDS_{80\%}$ and the Chasing principle; thus, it is suggested that the distribution between the amount of drug solubilized in the SNEDDS and/or the colloidal structures formed during digestion of the SNEDDS and the amount of drug in aqueous solution (i.e., the free fraction) equilibrate much faster following drug absorption, as compared to the distribution between precipitated/undissolved cinnarizine and the amount of cinnarizine in aqueous solution (i.e., in the case if the superSNEDDS suspension, superSNEDDS solution, and the aqueous suspension).

Considering the PK parameters from the in vivo study (Table S1), only the $AUC_{0–3h}$ was significantly different between the formulations, making this parameter most relevant for the comparison with the in vitro lipolysis-permeation results. The rank-order of the formulations based on the $AUC_{0–3h}$ of the permeation profiles obtained from the in vitro lipolysis-permeation experiments is comparable to the rank order of the in vivo $AUC_{0–3h}$ (Figure 4, Table S1), i.e., $SNEDDS_{80\%}$ > the Chasing principle > superSNEDDS suspension = superSNEDDS solution = aqueous suspension. The $SNEDDS_{80\%}$ did, however, result in a significantly higher amount of in vitro permeation (higher in vitro $AUC_{0–3h}$) compared to the Chasing principle ($p \leq 0.05$), while there was no difference in the in vivo $AUC_{0–3h}$ values of these two formulations (Figure 4, Table S1). The observed lower drug permeation from the Chasing principle might be due to a lower dissolution/solubilization rate in vitro compared to in vivo. Specifically, this difference might be caused by the lack of a gastric step in the applied lipolysis-permeation method. A gastric step could increase the amount of drug available for permeation by increasing the amount of solubilized drug due to higher cinnarizine solubility at gastric pH, longer incubation time, and pre-lipolysis by gastric lipase. In a recent study by Klitgaard et al., the benefit of simulating the gastric lipolysis in combination with the intestinal lipolysis was shown [52]; however, the specific effect of this additional step in relation to the designed lipolysis-permeation method is for future studies to conclude.

3.4. *In Vivo–In Vitro Correlation*

Figure 5 depicts the in vivo $AUC_{0–3h}$ of the plasma concentration–time curve obtained following oral administration of the five tested formulations in rats, as a function of the in vitro $AUC_{0–3h}$ obtained from the permeated amount of drug from the same five formulations in the lipolysis-permeation method in this study.

As can be seen in Figure 5, a coefficient of determination (R^2) of 0.92 was obtained by linear correlation. The reason that the R^2 is not higher is the lower in vitro $AUC_{0–3h}$ observed for the Chasing principle compared to the $SNEDDS_{80\%}$, as described above. However, the amount of drug permeated using the lipolysis-permeation method (in vitro $AUC_{0\text{-}3h}$) displayed a good correlation with the in vivo $AUC_{0–3h}$. In the donor compartment, there will be an equilibrium between cinnarizine in the formed colloidal structures, e.g., vesicles and mixed micelles [53,54], and the free fraction available for absorption. The presence of the permeation barrier enables mass transfer of the free fraction, thereby enabling the dynamic interaction between the free fraction, solubilized fraction, and the permeated drug for which multiple studies have indicated a need [3,8,13,21–29,55,56].

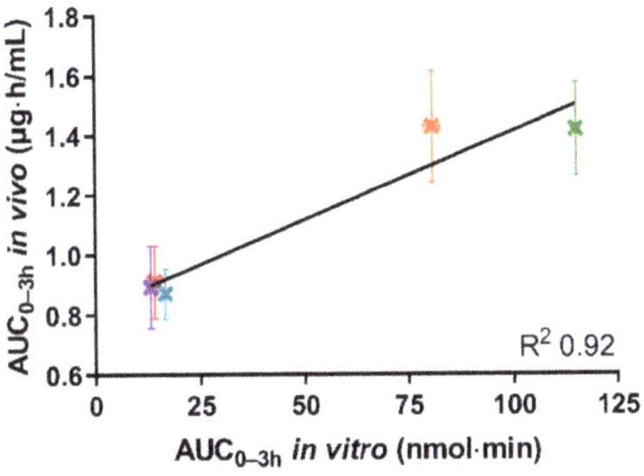

Figure 5. The correlation between in vitro $AUC_{0\text{-}3h}$ of permeated cinnarizine in the lipolysis-permeation method and in vivo $AUC_{0\text{-}3h}$ from the reference study of the $SNEDDS_{80\%}$ (green), superSNEDDS suspension (blue), superSNEDDS solution (purple), the Chasing principle (orange), and aqueous suspension (red). The in vitro data are presented as the mean ± SEM (n = 12), and the in vivo data as mean ± SEM (n = 6). Due to low variability of the in vitro data, these deviations are barely visible.

3.5. Absorption Surface Area to Donor Volume Ratio and Sink Conditions of the Lipolysis-Permeation Method

During the initial design of the lipolysis-permeation method, special focus was on (i) combining lipolysis and permeation in a way that ensured a high A/V ratio; and (ii) ensuring sink conditions in the acceptor compartment of the permeation module. Designing the lipolysis-permeation method using Franz diffusion cells with a vertical permeation setup prompted the possibility to use a low donor volume. It was thereby possible to obtain an A/V ratio of 1.34 cm^{-1}, which more closely simulated the in vivo A/V ratio (1.9–2.3 cm^{-1}) than previous permeation studies with A/V ratios of <0.5 cm^{-1} [35,37,38]. The addition of 4% (w/v) BSA to the acceptor medium (PBS) significantly improved the apparent solubility of cinnarizine ($p \leq 0.05$) with 1.30 ± 0.02 µg/mL in PBS_{BSA}, compared to 0.07 ± 0.02 µg/mL in PBS. With this increase in apparent drug solubility, sink conditions were ensured for the present experimental setup. This was confirmed because the highest amount of drug permeating resulted in a concentration of 13% (w/w) of the apparent saturation solubility in the acceptor medium PBS_{BSA}. In combination, the high A/V ratio and ensured sink conditions resulted in a permeation of 0.08–0.75% of the cinnarizine added to the donor compartment (Figure 4). This is a clear increase when compared to the similar setup used by Bibi et al., which resulted in a 0.00012% permeation from the dosed cinnarizine SNEDDS [36]. However, more studies are needed to evaluate the effect of a higher A/V ratio and improved sink conditions.

4. Conclusions

In the present study, an in vitro lipolysis-permeation method to estimate the oral drug absorption following administration of an SNEDDS was designed. The lipolysis-permeation method had an A/V ratio close to the in vivo conditions and enabled the use of physiologically relevant SIM and enzymes by applying the PermeaPad® barrier. Furthermore, sink conditions were ensured by the addition of 4% (w/v) BSA in the acceptor compartment. The predictability of the lipolysis-permeation method was evaluated using PK data from a reference study, in which five cinnarizine formulations were tested in rats [39]. No correlation was obtained between the $AUC_{0\text{–}60min}$ of the drug solubilization profiles during in vitro lipolysis and the in vivo PK data, which is in accordance with the reference study. However, the in vitro $AUC_{0\text{-}3h}$ of the permeation profiles from the five formulations showed a linear rank order correlation with the in vivo $AUC_{0\text{-}3h}$ of the plasma concentration time profiles. Based on this, the designed in vitro lipolysis-permeation method was found to be a promising tool for predicting the oral absorption of SNEDDSs, but further studies are needed to truly evaluate the method.

Supplementary Materials: The following are available online at https://www.mdpi.com/article/10.3390/pharmaceutics13040489/s1, Table S1: Pharmacokinetic parameters for cinnarizine after the administration of 25 mg/kg cinnarizine to rats, adapted from the reference study. Figure S1: The individual permeation graphs with the cumulative permeated amount of calcein after testing the five formulations in the lipolysis-permeation method. Figure S2: The individual permeation graphs with the cumulative permeated amount of cinnarizine after testing the five formulations in the lipolysis-permeation method. Reference [39] is cited in the Supplementary Materials.

Author Contributions: Conceptualization, M.K. and R.B.; Formal Analysis, M.K.; Investigation, M.K.; Methodology, M.K. and R.B.; Project Administration, R.B.; Resources, A.M. and R.B.; Supervision, A.M. and R.B.; Validation, M.K. and R.B.; Visualization, M.K.; Writing—Original Draft Preparation, M.K.; Writing—Review and Editing: A.M. and R.B. All authors have read and agreed to the published version of the manuscript.

Funding: This research received no external funding.

Institutional Review Board Statement: Not applicable.

Informed Consent Statement: Not applicable.

Data Availability Statement: Data is contained within the article or Supplementary Materials.

Acknowledgments: The authors thank InnoME (Espelkamp, Germany) for the kind donation of the PermeaPad® barriers.

Conflicts of Interest: The authors declare no conflict of interest.

References

1. Ruiz-Garcia, A.; Bermejo, M.; Moss, A.; Casabo, V.G. Pharmacokinetics in drug discovery. *J. Pharm. Sci.* **2008**, *97*, 654–690. [CrossRef] [PubMed]
2. Fagerberg, J.H.; Bergström, C.A.S. Intestinal solubility and absorption of poorly water soluble compounds: Predictions, challenges and solutions. *Ther. Deliv.* **2015**, *6*, 935–959. [CrossRef] [PubMed]
3. Kostewicz, E.S.; Abrahamsson, B.; Brewster, M.; Brouwers, J.; Butler, J.; Carlert, S.; Dickinson, P.A.; Dressman, J.; Holm, R.; Klein, S.; et al. In vitro models for the prediction of in vivo performance of oral dosage forms. *Eur. J. Pharm. Sci.* **2014**, *57*, 342–366. [CrossRef] [PubMed]
4. Zaki, N.M.; Artursson, P.; Bergstroöm, C.A.S. A Modified physiological BCS for prediction of intestinal absorption in drug discovery. *Mol. Pharm.* **2010**, *7*, 1478–1487. [CrossRef]
5. Porter, C.J.; Charman, W.N. In vitro assessment of oral lipid based formulations. *Adv. Drug Deliv. Rev.* **2001**, *50*, S127–S147. [CrossRef]
6. Carrière, F. Impact of gastrointestinal lipolysis on oral lipid-based formulations and bioavailability of lipophilic drugs. *Biochimie* **2016**, *125*, 297–305. [CrossRef]
7. Porter, C.J.; Pouton, C.W.; Cuine, J.F.; Charman, W.N. Enhancing intestinal drug solubilisation using lipid-based delivery systems. *Adv. Drug Deliv. Rev.* **2008**, *60*, 673–691. [CrossRef]
8. Feeney, O.M.; Crum, M.F.; McEvoy, C.L.; Trevaskis, N.L.; Williams, H.D.; Pouton, C.W.; Charman, W.N.; Bergström, C.A.; Porter, C.J. 50 years of oral lipid-based formulations: Provenance, progress and future perspectives. *Adv. Drug Deliv. Rev.* **2016**, *101*, 167–194. [CrossRef]
9. Christophersen, P.C.; Christiansen, M.L.; Holm, R.; Kristensen, J.; Jacobsen, J.; Abrahamsson, B.; Müllertz, A. Fed and fasted state gastro-intestinal in vitro lipolysis: In vitro in vivo relations of a conventional tablet, a SNEDDS and a solidified SNEDDS. *Eur. J. Pharm. Sci.* **2014**, *57*, 232–239. [CrossRef]
10. Dahan, A.; Hoffman, A. The effect of different lipid based formulations on the oral absorption of lipophilic drugs: The ability of in vitro lipolysis and consecutive ex vivo intestinal permeability data to predict in vivo bioavailability in rats. *Arbeitsgemeinschaft fur Pharmazeutische Verfahrenstechnik/Eur. J. Pharm. Biopharm.* **2007**, *67*, 96–105. [CrossRef]
11. Larsen, A.T.; Ohlsson, A.G.; Polentarutti, B.; Barker, R.A.; Phillips, A.R.; Abu-Rmaileh, R.; Dickinson, P.A.; Abrahamsson, B.; Østergaard, J.; Müllertz, A. Oral bioavailability of cinnarizine in dogs: Relation to SNEDDS droplet size, drug solubility and in vitro precipitation. *Eur. J. Pharm. Sci.* **2013**, *48*, 339–350. [CrossRef]
12. Berthelsen, R.; Klitgaard, M.; Rades, T.; Müllertz, A. In vitro digestion models to evaluate lipid based drug delivery systems; present status and current trends. *Adv. Drug Deliv. Rev.* **2019**, *142*, 35–49. [CrossRef]
13. Berthelsen, R.; Sassene, P.; Rades, T.; Müllertz, A. Evaluating oral drug delivery systems: Digestion models. In *Analytical Techniques in the Pharmaceutical Sciences*; Müllertz, A., Perrie, Y., Rades, T., Eds.; Springer: New York, NY, USA, 2016; pp. 773–790.

14. Williams, H.D.; Sassene, P.; Kleberg, K.; Bakala-N'Goma, J.-C.; Calderone, M.; Jannin, V.; Igonin, A.; Partheil, A.; Marchaud, D.; Jule, E.; et al. Toward the establishment of standardized in vitro tests for lipid-based formulations, part 1: Method parameterization and comparison of in vitro digestion profiles across a range of representative formulations. *J. Pharm. Sci.* **2012**, *101*, 3360–3380. [CrossRef]
15. Verger, R. Pancreatic lipases. In *Lipases*; Borgström, B., Brockman, H.L., Eds.; Elsevier: New York, NY, USA, 1984; pp. 84–150.
16. Capolino, P.; Guérin, C.; Paume, J.; Giallo, J.; Ballester, J.-M.; Cavalier, J.-F.; Carrière, F. In vitro gastrointestinal lipolysis: Replacement of human digestive lipases by a combination of rabbit gastric and porcine pancreatic extracts. *Food Dig.* **2011**, *2*, 43–51. [CrossRef]
17. Palin, K.J.; Wilson, C.G. The effect of different oils on the absorption of probucol in the rat. *J. Pharm. Pharmacol.* **1984**, *36*, 641–643. [CrossRef]
18. Larsen, A.; Holm, R.; Pedersen, M.L.; Müllertz, A. Lipid-based formulations for danazol containing a digestible surfactant, labrafil M2125CS: In vivo bioavailability and dynamic in vitro lipolysis. *Pharm. Res.* **2008**, *25*, 2769–2777. [CrossRef]
19. Dahan, A.; Hoffman, A. Use of a dynamic in vitro lipolysis model to rationalize oral formulation development for poor water soluble drugs: Correlation with in vivo data and the relationship to intra-enterocyte processes in rats. *Pharm. Res.* **2006**, *23*, 2165–2174. [CrossRef]
20. Zangenberg, N.H.; Mullertz, A.; Kristensen, H.G.; Hovgaard, L. A dynamic in vitro lipolysis model. I. Controlling the rate of lipolysis by continuous addition of calcium. *Eur. J. Pharm. Sci.* **2001**, *14*, 115–122. [CrossRef]
21. Lee, K.W.Y.; Porter, C.J.H.; Boyd, B.J. The effect of administered dose of lipid-based formulations on the in vitro and in vivo performance of cinnarizine as a model poorly water-soluble drug. *J. Pharm. Sci.* **2013**, *102*, 565–578. [CrossRef]
22. Griffin, B.T.; Kuentz, M.; Vertzoni, M.; Kostewicz, E.S.; Fei, Y.; Faisal, W.; Stillhart, C.; O'Driscoll, C.M.; Reppas, C.; Dressman, J.B. Comparison of in vitro tests at various levels of complexity for the prediction of in vivo performance of lipid-based formulations: Case studies with fenofibrate. *Arbeitsgemeinschaft fur Pharmazeutische Verfahrenstechnik/Eur. J. Pharm. Biopharm.* **2014**, *86*, 427–437. [CrossRef]
23. Stillhart, C.; Kuentz, M. Trends in the assessment of drug supersaturation and precipitation in vitro using lipid-based delivery systems. *J. Pharm. Sci.* **2016**, *105*, 2468–2476. [CrossRef]
24. Alskär, L.C.; Bergström, C.A.S. Models for predicting drug absorption from oral lipid-based formulations. *Curr. Mol. Biol. Rep.* **2015**, *1*, 141–147. [CrossRef]
25. Stillhart, C.; Imanidis, G.; Kuentz, M. Insights into drug precipitation kinetics during in vitro digestion of a lipid-based drug delivery system using in-line raman spectroscopy and mathematical modeling. *Pharm. Res.* **2013**, *30*, 3114–3130. [CrossRef]
26. Bevernage, J.; Brouwers, J.; Annaert, P.; Augustijns, P. Drug precipitation–permeation interplay: Supersaturation in an absorptive environment. *Arbeitsgemeinschaft fur Pharmazeutische Verfahrenstechnik/Eur. J. Pharm. Biopharm.* **2012**, *82*, 424–428. [CrossRef]
27. Thomas, N.; Holm, R.; Müllertz, A.; Rades, T. In vitro and in vivo performance of novel supersaturated self-nanoemulsifying drug delivery systems (super-SNEDDS). *J. Control. Release* **2012**, *160*, 25–32. [CrossRef]
28. Buckley, S.T.; Fischer, S.M.; Fricker, G.; Brandl, M. In vitro models to evaluate the permeability of poorly soluble drug entities: Challenges and perspectives. *Eur. J. Pharm. Sci.* **2012**, *45*, 235–250. [CrossRef]
29. Hens, B.; Brouwers, J.; Corsetti, M.; Augustijns, P. Gastrointestinal behavior of nano- and microsized fenofibrate: In vivo evaluation in man and in vitro simulation by assessment of the permeation potential. *Eur. J. Pharm. Sci.* **2015**, *77*, 40–47. [CrossRef]
30. Keemink, J.; Bergström, C.A.S. Caco-2 cell conditions enabling studies of drug absorption from digestible lipid-based formulations. *Pharm. Res.* **2018**, *35*, 1–11. [CrossRef]
31. Keemink, J.; Mårtensson, E.; Bergström, C.A.S. Lipolysis-permeation setup for simultaneous study of digestion and ab-sorption in vitro. *Mol. Pharm.* **2019**, *16*, 921–930. [CrossRef]
32. Alskär, L.C.; Parrow, A.; Keemink, J.; Johansson, P.; Abrahamsson, B.; Bergström, C.A. Effect of lipids on absorption of carvedilol in dogs: Is coadministration of lipids as efficient as a lipid-based formulation? *J. Control. Release* **2019**, *304*, 90–100. [CrossRef]
33. Mandagere, A.K.; Thompson, T.N.; Hwang, K.-K. Graphical model for estimating oral bioavailability of drugs in humans and other species from their caco-2 permeability and in vitro liver enzyme metabolic stability rates. *J. Med. Chem.* **2002**, *45*, 304–311. [CrossRef] [PubMed]
34. Florence, A.T. *Physicochemical Principles of Pharmacy*, 5th ed.; Pharmaceutical Press: London, UK, 2011.
35. Berben, P.; Bauer-Brandl, A.; Brandl, M.; Faller, B.; Flaten, G.E.; Jacobsen, A.-C.; Brouwers, J.; Augustijns, P. Drug permeability profiling using cell-free permeation tools: Overview and applications. *Eur. J. Pharm. Sci.* **2018**, *119*, 219–233. [CrossRef] [PubMed]
36. Bibi, H.A.; Holm, R.; Bauer-Brandl, A. Simultaneous lipolysis/permeation in vitro model, for the estimation of bioavailability of lipid based drug delivery systems. *Arbeitsgemeinschaft fur Pharmazeutische Verfahrenstechnik/Eur. J. Pharm. Biopharm.* **2017**, *117*, 300–307. [CrossRef] [PubMed]
37. Sironi, D.; Christensen, M.; Rosenberg, J.; Bauer-Brandl, A.; Brandl, M. Evaluation of a dynamic dissolution/permeation model: Mutual influence of dissolution and barrier-flux under non-steady state conditions. *Int. J. Pharm.* **2017**, *522*, 50–57. [CrossRef] [PubMed]
38. Mudie, D.M.; Shi, Y.; Ping, H.; Gao, P.; Amidon, G.L.; Amidon, G.E. Mechanistic analysis of solute transport in anin vitrophysiological two-phase dissolution apparatus. *Biopharm. Drug Dispos.* **2012**, *33*, 378–402. [CrossRef]

39. Siqueira, S.D.; Müllertz, A.; Gräeser, K.; Kasten, G.; Mu, H.; Rades, T. Influence of drug load and physical form of cinnarizine in new SNEDDS dosing regimens: In vivo and in vitro evaluations. *AAPS J.* **2017**, *19*, 587–594. [CrossRef]
40. Naderkhani, E.; Isaksson, J.; Ryzhakov, A.; Flaten, G.E. Development of a biomimetic phospholipid vesicle-based permeation assay for the estimation of intestinal drug permeability. *J. Pharm. Sci.* **2014**, *103*, 1882–1890. [CrossRef]
41. Flaten, G.E.; Dhanikula, A.B.; Luthman, K.; Brandl, M. Drug permeability across a phospholipid vesicle based barrier: A novel approach for studying passive diffusion. *Eur. J. Pharm. Sci.* **2006**, *27*, 80–90. [CrossRef]
42. Sassene, P.; Kleberg, K.; Williams, H.D.; Bakala-N'Goma, J.-C.; Carriere, F.; Calderone, M.; Jannin, V.; Igonin, A.; Partheil, A.; Marchaud, D.; et al. Toward the establishment of standardized in vitro tests for lipid-based formulations, part 6: Effects of varying pancreatin and calcium levels. *AAPS J.* **2014**, *16*, 1344–1357. [CrossRef]
43. Mosgaard, M.D.; Sassene, P.; Mu, H.; Rades, T.; Müllertz, A. Development of a high-throughput in vitro intestinal lipolysis model for rapid screening of lipid-based drug delivery systems. *Arbeitsgemeinschaft fur Pharmazeutische Verfahrenstechnik/Eur. J. Pharm. Biopharm.* **2015**, *94*, 493–500. [CrossRef]
44. Khan, J.; Rades, T.; Boyd, B.J. Lipid-based formulations can enable the model poorly water-soluble weakly basic drug cinnarizine to precipitate in an amorphous-salt form during in vitro digestion. *Mol. Pharm.* **2016**, *13*, 3783–3793. [CrossRef]
45. Gu, C.; Rao, D.; Gandhi, R.B.; Hilden, J.; Raghavan, K. Using a novel multicompartment dissolution system to predict the effect of gastric pH on the oral absorption of weak bases with poor intrinsic solubility. *J. Pharm. Sci.* **2005**, *94*, 199–208. [CrossRef]
46. Berthelsen, R.; Sjögren, E.; Jacobsen, J.; Kristensen, J.; Holm, R.; Abrahamsson, B.; Müllertz, A. Combining in vitro and in silico methods for better prediction of surfactant effects on the absorption of poorly water soluble drugs—A fenofibrate case example. *Int. J. Pharm.* **2014**, *473*, 356–365. [CrossRef]
47. Di Cagno, M.; Bibi, H.A.; Bauer-Brandl, A. New biomimetic barrier Permeapad™ for efficient investigation of passive permeability of drugs. *Eur. J. Pharm. Sci.* **2015**, *73*, 29–34. [CrossRef]
48. Dahan, A.; Miller, J.M. The solubility–Permeability interplay and its implications in formulation design and development for poorly soluble drugs. *AAPS J.* **2012**, *14*, 244–251. [CrossRef]
49. Bibi, H.A.; Di Cagno, M.; Holm, R.; Bauer-Brandl, A. Permeapad™ for investigation of passive drug permeability: The effect of surfactants, co-solvents and simulated intestinal fluids (FaSSIF and FeSSIF). *Int. J. Pharm.* **2015**, *493*, 192–197. [CrossRef]
50. Michaelsen, M.H.; Wasan, K.M.; Sivak, O.; Müllertz, A.; Rades, T. The effect of digestion and drug load on halofantrine absorption from self-nanoemulsifying drug delivery system (SNEDDS). *AAPS J.* **2015**, *18*, 180–186. [CrossRef]
51. Michaelsen, M.H.; Jørgensen, S.D.S.; Abdi, I.M.; Wasan, K.M.; Rades, T.; Müllertz, A. Fenofibrate oral absorption from SNEDDS and super-SNEDDS is not significantly affected by lipase inhibition in rats. *Eur. J. Pharm. Biopharm.* **2019**, *142*, 258–264. [CrossRef]
52. Klitgaard, M.; Beilles, S.; Sassene, P.J.; Berthelsen, R.; Müllertz, A. Adding a gastric step to the intestinal in vitro digestion model improves the prediction of pharmacokinetic data in beagle dogs of two lipid-based drug delivery systems. *Mol. Pharm.* **2020**, *17*, 3214–3222. [CrossRef]
53. Tran, T.; Siqueira, S.D.; Amenitsch, H.; Rades, T.; Müllertz, A. Monoacyl phosphatidylcholine inhibits the formation of lipid multilamellar structures during in vitro lipolysis of self-emulsifying drug delivery systems. *Eur. J. Pharm. Sci.* **2017**, *108*, 62–70. [CrossRef]
54. Tran, T.; Fatouros, D.G.; Vertzoni, M.; Reppas, C.; Müllertz, A. Mapping the intermediate digestion phases of human healthy intestinal contents from distal ileum and caecum at fasted and fed state conditions. *J. Pharm. Pharmacol.* **2017**, *69*, 265–273. [CrossRef]
55. Li, S.; He, H.; Parthiban, L.J.; Yin, H.; Serajuddin, A.T. IV-IVC considerations in the development of immediate-release oral dosage form. *J. Pharm. Sci.* **2005**, *94*, 1396–1417. [CrossRef]
56. Buch, P.; Langguth, P.; Kataoka, M.; Yamashita, S. IVIVC in oral absorption for fenofibrate immediate release tablets using a dissolution/permeation system. *J. Pharm. Sci.* **2009**, *98*, 2001–2009. [CrossRef] [PubMed]

pharmaceutics

MDPI

Article

Physico-Chemical and In Vitro Characterization of Chitosan-Based Microspheres Intended for Nasal Administration

Csilla Bartos *, Patrícia Varga, Piroska Szabó-Révész and Rita Ambrus

Faculty of Pharmacy, Institute of Pharmaceutical Technology and Regulatory Affairs, University of Szeged, 6726 Szeged, Hungary; varga.patricia@szte.hu (P.V.); revesz@pharm.u-szeged.hu (P.S.-R.); ambrus.rita@szte.hu (R.A.)

* Correspondence: bartos.csilla@szte.hu; Tel.: +36-6254-5575

Abstract: The absorption of non-steroidal anti-inflammatory drugs (NSAIDs) through the nasal epithelium offers an innovative opportunity in the field of pain therapy. Thanks to the bonding of chitosan to the nasal mucosa and its permeability-enhancing effect, it is an excellent choice to formulate microspheres for the increase of drug bioavailability. The aim of our work includes the preparation of spray-dried cross-linked and non-cross-linked chitosan-based drug delivery systems for intranasal application, the optimization of spray-drying process parameters (inlet air temperature, pump rate), and the composition of samples. Cross-linked products were prepared by using different amounts of sodium tripolyphosphate. On top of these, the micrometric properties, the structural characteristics, the in vitro drug release, and the in vitro permeability of the products were studied. Spray-drying resulted in micronized chitosan particles (2–4 μm) regardless of the process parameters. The meloxicam (MEL)-containing microspheres showed nearly spherical habit, while MEL was present in a molecularly dispersed state. The highest dissolved (>90%) and permeated (~45 $\mu g/cm^2$) MEL amount was detected from the non-cross-linked sample. Our results indicate that spray-dried MEL-containing chitosan microparticles may be recommended for the development of a novel drug delivery system to decrease acute pain or enhance analgesia by intranasal application.

Keywords: nasal administration; spray-drying; chitosan; microsphere; meloxicam

Citation: Bartos, C.; Varga, P.; Szabó-Révész, P.; Ambrus, R. Physico-Chemical and In Vitro Characterization of Chitosan-Based Microspheres Intended for Nasal Administration. *Pharmaceutics* **2021**, *13*, 608. https://doi.org/10.3390/pharmaceutics13050608

Academic Editor: Im-Sook Song

Received: 30 March 2021
Accepted: 19 April 2021
Published: 22 April 2021

1. Introduction

Nasal drug delivery provides an opportunity not merely to treat local pathological conditions (e.g., allergic rhinitis, nasal congestion) but also to deliver active pharmaceutical ingredients (APIs) to the systemic circulation or directly through the blood–brain barrier to the central nervous system [1]. The nose respiratory region is crucial from the aspect of systemic drug absorption. Drugs administered intranasally bypass the first-pass hepatic metabolism, thus side effects are avoided, and the large surface and the high vascularization of the mucosa cause the rapid onset of action [2,3]. Since it is an easily accessible, non-invasive, and painless option for systemic therapies, it is well accepted by patients [4]. However, there are some limitations that need to be taken into account. Firstly, mucosa sensitivity cannot be neglected, thus, drugs and excipients intended for intranasal delivery must not be irritants and definitely cannot be toxic [5]. The mucociliary clearance is a key determinant concerning the APIs residence time. The mucus layer renews in every 15–20 min interval, thus to prolong the APIs' contact time, the use of mucoadhesive polymers can be considered. The low permeability of the mucosa raises another problem that needs to be solved [6–8].

Nasal sprays, drops, gels, and ointments are extremely popular and widely used. Unfortunately, few nasal powders are accessible on the market, however, they have highly beneficial properties over the aforementioned formulations. Since nasal powders do not contain moisture and their physical stability is better concerning liquid and semi-solid formulations, they can be prepared without using preservatives [9,10]. Moreover, they are eliminated slowly from the nasal cavity, because the better adhesion allows a longer time period for the API absorption [11]. Particle size, morphology, or rheological features must be taken into consideration during the nasal powder formulation [12,13].

Chitosan is a semi-synthetic polymer that is obtained by chitin deacetylation, which is found mostly in crustaceans or mushroom cell walls [14]. It plays a key role in the biomedical field due to its advantageous properties. Chitosan and its derivatives as micro- or nanoparticles can be used for targeted or controlled delivery of antibiotics, antitumor drugs, proteins, or vaccines. They are highly suitable for tissue engineering and wound healing based on their stimulating effect on cell proliferation and tissue regeneration. In terms of nasal administration, chitosan's biocompatibility—which is due to the non-toxicity of its degradation products to the human body—and mucoadhesive characteristics are preferred [15–17]. Due to the cationic nature of chitosan, an ionic bond can be formed by the interaction between the negatively charged substructures of the mucus layer and chitosan, enabling mucoadhesion [18,19]. The positive charge interacts with tight junction-associated proteins as well, causing the distance growth between epithelial cells and enhancing the permeation property of chitosan [20]. Chitosan-based drug delivery systems are widely used for achieving controlled drug release. It has been reported that, by using cross-linking agents, an increased stability could be accomplished [21]. Glutaraldehyde and formaldehyde were used mainly as cross-linkers, but for their toxic quality, sodium tripolyphosphate (TPP) may be a more conspicuous alternative [22]. It possesses a negative charge, thus ionic bond is developed between TPP and chitosan [23,24].

Non-steroidal anti-inflammatory drugs (NSAIDs) are essential in relieving acute pain or enhancing analgesia as adjuvants to opioids [25,26]. The intranasal application of NSAIDs may offer an opportunity to attain a rapid analgesic effect by their absorption through the nasal mucosa to the systemic circulation [27]. During the formulation of NSAIDs, it is inevitable to solve their solubility problems, which can result in dose reduction that leads to decreased side effects together with their bioavailability improvement [28]. Several technological methods are available for modifying the physico-chemical properties and increasing the dissolution rate of NSAIDs [29–31]. Spray-drying is a one-step production method which can be applied to change the dissolution properties of a drug and provides an opportunity to prepare microspheres that match nasal requirements. This technique allows the control of particle properties such as their shape and size in a rapid and reproducible way [32,33]. It looks promising to create nasal formulations by spray-drying for pain relief with adequate dissolution properties, however, there is not any available literature on this topic thus far.

In our work, meloxicam (MEL) was chosen as an NSAID. It is used in joint disease therapy and serves as a favorable option because of its side effect profile. An MEL-containing nasal formulation may provide an opportunity to ease the pain alone or to potentiate the effects of opioids. In our previous research works, MEL- and meloxicam potassium monohydrate-containing spray and gel forms were prepared and investigated. The goal of this study was to design MEL-containing mucoadhesive intranasal microparticles to increase the residence time and the bioavailability of drugs by enhancing their dissolution and permeation. Chitosan microspheres were produced by spray-drying process, setting the parameters in order to acquire an energy-saving and quick preparation method. The effect of a lower inlet air temperature (90 °C)—lesser known in the literature—was compared with higher air temperatures. Furthermore, we optimized the composition of the formulation intended for nasal application by preparing MEL-incorporated chitosan-based microparticles and adding different amounts of TPP as a cross-linking agent. Particle size, morphological, and rheological properties of the products ensured nasal deposition. The physico-chemical properties as well as the in vitro dissolution and diffusion were determined and evaluated.

2. Materials and Methods

2.1. Materials

MEL was from EGIS Ltd. (Budapest, Hungary). Low molecular weight chitosan (Mw = 3800–20,000 Da) was obtained from Sigma Aldrich (Sigma Aldrich Co. LLC, St. Louis, MO, USA). TPP was purchased from Alfa Aeasar Co. (Alfa Aeasar GmbH & Co. KG, Karlsruhe, Germany). Dimethyl sulfoxide was from VWR Chemicals BDH Prolabo, and acetic acid was from Molar Chemicals Ltd. (Budapest, Hungary).

2.2. Methods

2.2.1. Preparation of Spray-Dried Products

Optimizing process parameters, 1% acetic acid chitosan solution was spray-dried using Büchi Mini Dryer B-191 (Büchi, Flawil, Switzerland) applying inlet air temperatures of 90, 120, and 150 °C and pump rates of 5, 10, and 15 mL/min. Aspirator capacity was 75% (Table 1). Afterwards, to optimize the composition of the formulation, the feeding emulsions were prepared of 50 mL 1% chitosan solution, 3.75 mL 4% MEL-dimethyl sulfoxide (DMSO) solution, and 0, 1, or 2 mL of 1% aqueous solution of TPP, applying the optimal parameters (Table 2). The physical mixtures (PMs) of chitosan, MEL, and TPP were produced as the control samples in the same mass ratio similarly to the spray-dried products. After spray-drying, the percentage yield was determined.

Table 1. Spray-drying process parameters.

Inlet Air Temperature (°C)	90	120	150
Pump Rate (mL/min)	5	10	15

Table 2. Composition of solutions for spray-drying.

1% Chitosan Solution (mL)	50	50	50	50	50	50
1% Aqueous TPP Solution (mL)	-	1	2	-	1	2
4% MEL-DMSO-Solution (mL)	-	-	-	3.75	3.75	3.75

2.2.2. Size Distribution by Laser Diffraction

The particle-size distribution of the spray-dried samples was measured by laser scattering (Malvern Mastersizer Sirocco 2000, Malvern Instruments Ltd., Worcestershire, UK). The measurements were carried out at 3 bar pressure and 75% frequency, and air was used as a dispersion medium. Approximately 1 g of product was tested in one measurement, and each measurement was performed 3 times. D0.1, D0.5, and D0.9 values were determined as the diameter of the particles below which 10, 50, and 90 volume percentages of the particles existed.

2.2.3. Scanning Electron Microscopy (SEM)

The shape and the surface morphology of the spray-dried particles were visualized by SEM (Hitachi S4700, Hitachi Scientific Ltd., Tokyo, Japan). Under an argon atmosphere, the samples were sputter-coated with gold-palladium in a high-vacuum evaporator with a sputter coater, and they were examined at 10 kV and 10 μA. The air pressure was 1.3–13 MPa.

2.2.4. Density Measurement

The bulked and the tapped densities of the formulations were measured using the Engelsmann Stampfvolumeter (Ludwigshafen, Germany) [34]. A 10 cm^3 cylinder was filled with 1.5–2.0 cm^3 powder to calculate bulk density. Then, it was tapped 1000 times. Compared to the volume before and after the taps, we calculated the tapped density of the samples. We calculated the flow characters of the samples from the bulk (ρ_b) and the tapped (ρ_t) density (Equation (1)):

$$\text{Carr index} = \frac{\rho_t - \rho_b}{\rho_t} \times 100 \tag{1}$$

2.2.5. Structural Analyses

The thermal analysis was executed with a Mettler Toledo DSC 821e (Schwerzenbach, Germany) system with the STARe program V9.1 (Mettler Inc., Schwerzenbach, Switzerland). Approximately 2–5 mg of samples were heated from 25 °C to 300 °C, applying 10 $°C \cdot min^{-1}$ heating rate under a constant argon flow of 10 $L \cdot h^{-1}$. Physical mixtures of chitosan, MEL, and TPP in the same mass ratio as the spray-dried samples contained were mixed in a Turbula mixer (Turbula WAB, Systems Schatz, Switzerland) at 50 rpm for 10 min and were applied as control samples.

XRPD was performed to investigate the physical state of MEL in the samples with a Bruker D8 Advance diffractometer (Bruker AXS GmbH, Karlsruhe, Germany) with Cu K λI radiation (λ = 1.5406 Å). The samples were scanned at 40 kV and 40 mA with an angular range of 3° to 40° 2θ. Si was used to calibrate the instrument. DIFFRACTPLUS EVA software was used to perform the manipulations: Kα2-stripping, background removal, and smoothing.

2.2.6. Fourier-Transformed Infrared Spectroscopy (FT-IR)

For the purpose of determining whether cross-linking and incorporation were successful, the FT-IR spectra of the samples was recorded on an AVATAR330 FT-IR spectrometer (Thermo Nicolet, Unicam Hungary Ltd., Budapest, Hungary) in the interval 400–4000 cm^{-1} at an optical resolution of 4 cm^{-1}. Samples were ground and compressed into pastilles at 10 t with 0.15 g of KBr.

2.2.7. Rheological Investigations

Rheological measurements were carried out at 32 °C with HAAKE RheoStress 1 Rheometer (HAAKE GmbH., Hamburg, Germany). Cone and plate geometry was used to study the rheological profile of the samples. The flow curve of the samples was determined by rotation tests controlled shear rate. The shear rate was increased from 0.1 to 100 1/s in controlled rate mode.

2.2.8. In Vitro Dissolution

The European Pharmacopoeia (6th Edition) paddle method (USP dissolution apparatus, type II Pharma Test, Heinburg, Germany) was applied to appoint the dissolution of MEL. A total of 50 mL of phosphate buffer solution (pH 5.6 ± 0.1) at 30 ± 0.5 °C was used as a dissolution medium. Taking into account the drug content of the microparticles, samples containing 6 mg of MEL were dispersed. The rotation speed of the paddles was 100 rpm. At predetermined intervals, the amount of dissolved MEL was determined by spectrophotometry (UNICAM UV/Vis Spectrometer, Cambridge, UK) at 364 nm. The in vitro drug release data of products were evaluated kinetically using various mathematical models such as zero order, first order, Higuchi, Hixon–Crowell, and Korsmeyer-Peppas model [35].

2.2.9. In Vitro Permeability

The in vitro permeability of MEL was studied on a modified horizontal diffusion model which simulated the nasal cavity circumstances (Figure 1). Samples containing 6 mg of MEL were added to the donor phase (9 mL), which was simulated with nasal electrolyte solution (SNES) of pH 6.0 ± 0.1 (represented the nasal cavity) [36]. Half the amount of the SNES was put into the donor chamber and, with its other half, the sample was washed in the donor phase. PB of pH 7.40, which corresponded with the pH of the blood, was used as the acceptor phase (9 mL). The two chambers were divided by a synthetic membrane

(Whatman® regenerated cellulose membrane filter with 0.45 µm pores) that was soaked in isopropyl myristate before the investigation. It modeled the lipophilic mucosa between the phases. The temperature of the phases was 30 °C (Thermo Haake C10-P5, Sigma, Aldrich Co. and the rotation rate of the stir-bars was set to 100 rpm. The amount of MEL diffused to the acceptor phase was determined spectrophotometrically at 364 nm in real time with an AvaLight DH-S-BAL spectrophotometer (AVANTES, Apeldoorn, The Netherlands). Each measurement was carried out in triplicate.

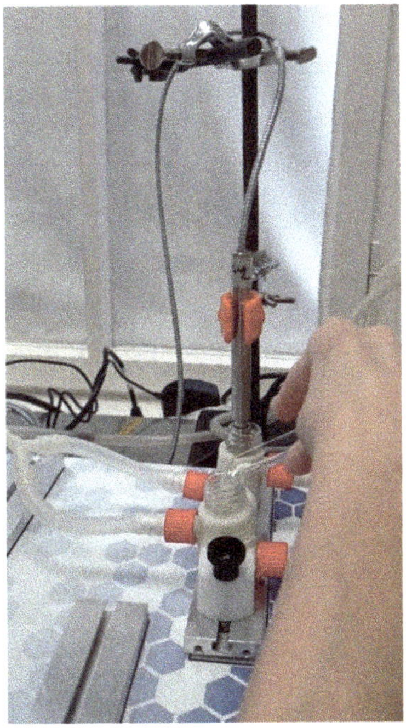

Figure 1. Illustration of in vitro permeability investigation.

3. Results and Discussion

3.1. Particle Size Distribution

The analysis of the results measured by laser diffraction revealed the fact that, by changing the process parameters, the average particle size of spray-dried products was approximately between 2–4 µm. Since the inlet air temperature and the pump rate did not have any effect on the size distribution of chitosan microspheres (Table 3), we chose the mild 90 °C inlet air temperature (requiring the lowest heat energy) and the relatively quick 10 mL/min pump rate to produce cross-linked and MEL-containing particles. At 15 mL/min pump rate, there was not sufficient time for the atomized drops to dry, thus they stuck to the column wall. The usage of TPP as a cross-linking material did not have any impact on the sizes of drug-free chitosan particles, however, there was a noticeable increase in the size of MEL-containing particles, especially when the volume of TPP solution was boosted (Table 4). Based on the literature data, the produced product size is considered to be an appropriate one for nasal administration [37]. The yields of the samples were between 38–64% concerning the MEL-free products, and they reached the 29–48% range regarding the MEL-containing microspheres.

Table 3. Optimization of the process parameters.

Sample	1	2	3	4	5	6	7	8	9
Inlet air temperature (°C)	90	120	150	90	120	150	90	120	150
Pump rate (mL/min)	5	5	5	10	10	10	15	15	15
Aspirator (%)	75	75	75	75	75	75	75	75	75
D0.1 (μm)	1.044	1.446	1.529	1.176	1.255	1.241	1.115	1.274	1.369
D0.5 (μm)	2.374	3.669	3.736	2.466	2.815	2.701	2.263	2.629	2.889
D0.9 (μm)	5.216	8.535	9.032	5.102	5.903	5.519	4.744	5.195	5.664

Table 4. Optimization of the composition.

Sample	4	10	11	12	13	14
Inlet air temperature (°C)	90	90	90	90	90	90
Pump rate (mL/min)	10	10	10	10	10	10
Aspirator (%)	75	75	75	75	75	75
1% aqueous TPP-solution (mL)	-	1	2	-	1	2
MEL-DMSO-solution (mL)	-	-	-	3.75	3.75	3.75
D0.1 (μm)	1.176	1.243	1.103	1.269	1.426	1.617
D0.5 (μm)	2.466	2.595	2.419	2.965	3.757	5.575
D0.9 (μm)	5.102	5.234	5.138	7.211	9.461	15.995

3.2. Morphology of the Samples

The SEM images provided an indication of the microspheres morphology. Products formulated by using different amounts of TPP solution (0, 1.0, 2.0 mL) were investigated. Drug-free particles (Samples 4, 10, 11) had a hollow structure. Nearly spherical microparticles were observed in case of MEL-containing samples (Samples 12, 13, 14). Drug-containing samples in the presence of 0 or 1.0 mL TPP solution revealed a depressed surface morphology with holes. Microspheres cross-linked with 2.0 mL TPP solution exhibited a smooth surface (Figure 2).

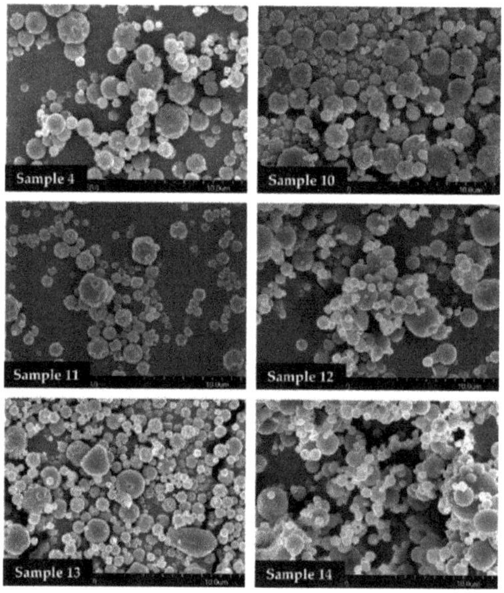

Figure 2. SEM images of spray-dried samples.

3.3. Powder Rheology Properties

The rheological properties of powders have a key role in their processability. Moreover, the deposition of particles in the nasal cavity is inversely proportional to the density. Hence, the density of microspheres has a key role in getting into the required nasal region. The lower density of particles could offer better flowability and an improved deposition. The bulked and the tapped densities and, furthermore, the Carr index values of formulations are shown in Table 5. In case of drug-containing products, the tapped density was around 0.15 g/cm^3, which was lower compared to the drug-free samples, predicting drug deposition in the required nasal regions. The Carr index results were in the range of 17 and 29, indicating the flowability, a parameter that is also responsible for the deposition.

Table 5. Powder rheology properties of the products.

Sample		4	10	11	12	13	14
Density	Bulk	0.2490	0.1384	0.3112	0.1256	0.1176	0.1193
(g/cm^3)	Tap	0.6225	0.2214	0.5187	0.1507	0.1470	0.1670
Carr index (%)		60	38	40	17	20	29

3.4. Structural Characterization by DSC and XRPD

DSC was applied to study the crystallinity and the melting of MEL in physical mixtures and in spray-dried products. Sharp endothermic peaks of MEL were observed in the physical mixtures (around 256 °C) that corresponded to the melting point of MEL, indicating that, in these cases, MEL was crystalline (Figure 3a). Chitosan is an amorphous additive. The endothermic peaks of crystalline MEL disappeared; only the characteristic curve of chitosan was recognized regarding the spray-dried products containing TPP, revealing the presence of MEL in a molecularly dispersed form. The non-cross-linked sample (Sample 12) presented a reduced MEL peak intensity referring to the presence of its crystalline fraction.

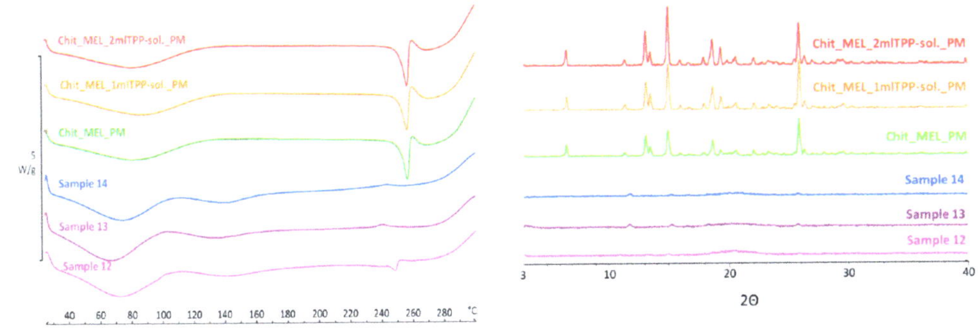

(**a**) (**b**)

Figure 3. (**a**) DSC curves of PMs (Chit_MEL_2mlTPP-sol., Chit_MEL_1mlTPP-sol., Chit_MEL) and MEL-containing spray-dried samples; (**b**) XRPD patterns of PMs and MEL-containing spray-dried samples.

XRPD was employed to investigate the physical state of drug-containing spray-dried samples and PMs as controls. The XRPD diffractograms of PMs demonstrated the crystalline structure of MEL, as established during DSC measurements. Its characteristic peaks were detected at 13.22, 15.06, and 25.7° (2Θ). The diffractograms of the spray-dried samples reconfirmed the presence of drugs, especially in the molecularly dispersed form. A few of the peaks of MEL appeared with a reduced but growing intensity with the decrease of TPP content, suggesting the presence of crystalline MEL (Figure 3b). The highest amount of crystalline MEL form was found where no cross-linking agent was applied.

3.5. FTIR Investigations

The intermolecular interactions of the microspheres were characterized by FT-IR (Figure 4a). Seven characterization peaks were observed in HMW chitosan–TPP microspheres at 3363.41, 2881.27, 1646.15 to 1653.24, 1376.47 to 1587.93, 1058.24 to 1064.48, 1026.87 to 1028.81, and 886.58 to 894.85 cm^{-1}. These peaks could be defined as O–H from H-bonded, C–H stretch form aldehyde, C=N and N–H from amine I and amide II, -CH_3 symmetrical deformation, C–N from amine, C–O stretching, and C–H from alkene or aromatic bonds, respectively [38,39]. Increasing the amount of TPP the peaks at 3363.41 cm^{-1} became broad, indicating an enhancement in hydrogen bonding. The peak at 1646.15 to 1650.20 cm^{-1} became larger in the presence of TPP compared to chitosan alone thanks to the electrostatic interaction between the amino groups in chitosan and the phosphoric groups in TPP [40]. The TPP peak at 1127.29 cm^{-1} disappeared after chitosan and TPP cross-linking due to the intermolecular interactions of chitosan and TPP. MEL-containing microparticles showed the characteristic absorption bands at specific wavenumbers (Figure 4b) The intensity of characteristic peaks of MEL at 3290.13, 1550.56, and 1265.14 cm^{-1} decreased because of drug incorporation to the microsphere.

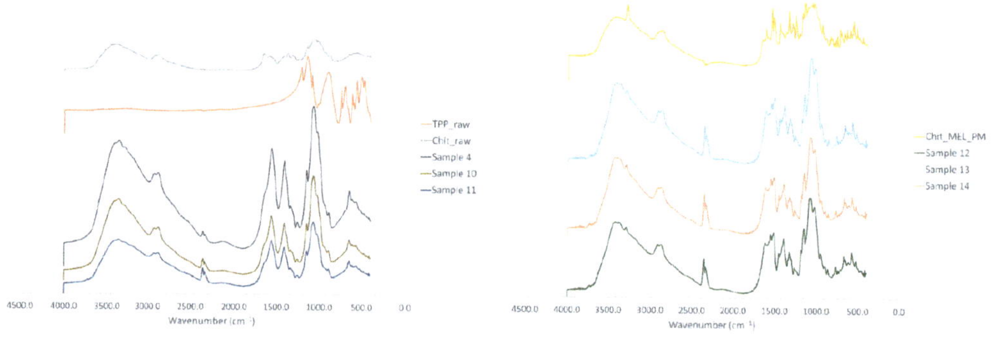

(a) (b)

Figure 4. (**a**) FT-IR curves of the raw materials and the spray-dried samples without MEL, (**b**) FT-IR curves of the PMs and the MEL-containing spray-dried samples.

3.6. In Vitro Dissolution Study

Before the dissolution studies, microspheres were dispersed in phosphate buffer (pH = 5.6), and the viscosity of samples was detected. Samples displayed shear-thinning behavior thanks to the orientation of the polimer chains in the flow direction. The viscosity of samples increased with increasing TPP amount.

The in vitro dissolution test was carried out at pH of 5.6 in phosphate buffer simulating the nasal conditions. The dissolution of raw MEL and of MEL from cross-linked and non-cross-linked samples was studied. Unprocessed MEL was used as a control; only 4.5% of it dissolved in 60 min (Table 6). The spray-dried samples revealed fast initial release in the first 15 min, which was followed by a slower stage. The presence of drugs in a molecularly dispersed form resulted in the rapid dissolution of API from the microspheres. The dissolved amount of MEL was decreased by the growth of TPP concentration. The lowest dissolved amount of drug was perceptible in the presence of 2 mL TPP. The highest amount of MEL—more than 90% during 1 h—was dissolved from the non-cross-linked Sample 12. This phenomena could be explained with the formation of cross-links only as the result of reaction between the phosphate and the amino groups of chitosan in the case of Sample 12 [41]. Adding TPP, the enhancement in hydrogen bonding and the electrostatic interaction between the amino and the phosphoric groups of chitosan and TPP kept MEL inside the microparticles.

Table 6. The percentage of dissolved drugs from raw MEL and MEL-containing spray-dried products.

Time (min)	Dissolved Drug (%)			
	Raw MEL	**Sample 12**	**Sample 13**	**Sample 14**
5	0.157 ± 0.01	50.15 ± 2.44	35.53 ± 2.51	48.85 ± 1.78
10	0.583 ± 0.03	60.24 ± 3.05	47.62 ± 3.01	60.96 ± 2.38
15	1.003 ± 0.05	68.18 ± 3.76	55.97 ± 3.41	75.20 ± 2.80
30	2.618 ± 0.13	78.37 ± 3.10	67.53 ± 3.92	79.93 ± 3.38
60	4.548 ± 0.23	82.38 ± 4.68	73.28 ± 4.1	93.65 ± 3.66

During the analyses of the kinetics of drug release, the data were evaluated by correlation coefficient (R^2). R^2 values were used as the criteria to choose the best model to describe drug release from the products (Table 7). Because of the low solubility, the dissolution of raw MEL was slow and fitted the zero order kinetics model. In the case of TPP-free spray-dried product (Sample 12), the strongest correlation was shown with the first order kinetics model (Equation (2)):

$$\frac{M_t}{M_\infty} = 1 - e^{-k*t} \quad (2)$$

where M_t is the cumulative amount of drug released at time "t"; M_∞ is the initial amount of drug in the dosage form; k is the release rate constant, revealing that the dissolution rate was concentration dependent. Approaching the saturation concentration, the dissolution slowed down. Concerning Samples 13 and 14, the drug release fit the Korsmeyer-Peppas model (Equation (3)):

$$\frac{M_t}{M_\infty} = k * t^n \quad (3)$$

where n is a constant, which characterizes the transport mechanism of diffusion, indicating that the drug release mechanism from these samples was diffusion controlled by gelling and the slow erosion of the chitosan [42].

Table 7. R^2 values of kinetic analysis of in vitro drug release using different models.

Model	**Raw MEL** R^2	**Sample 12** R^2	**Sample 13** R^2	**Sample 14** R^2
Zero order	0.9927	0.7658	0.7309	0.7787
First order	0.989	0.9685	0.8626	0.8732
Higuchi	0.8021	0.7799	0.6757	0.8234
Hixon–Crowell	0.9892	0.8304	0.6634	0.7354
Korsmeyer-Peppas	0.9756	0.945	0.9528	0.9496

3.7. *In Vitro Diffusion Study*

Modified diffusion horizontal cell model was used for diffusion investigations. Figure 5 demonstrates that the rapid dissolution of MEL from a molecularly dispersed state in the case of the spray-dried products resulted in a faster diffusion and a higher permeated drug concentration in the acceptor phase. The lowest drug amount permeated related to raw MEL. The highest diffused concentration was observed from the product which did not contain TPP in its composition (approximately 45 μg/cm^2). In the presence of TPP, chitosan formed a well-structured complex due to the intermolecular interactions, resulting in decreased swelling capacity of the polymer matrix and less drug dissolution and diffusion.

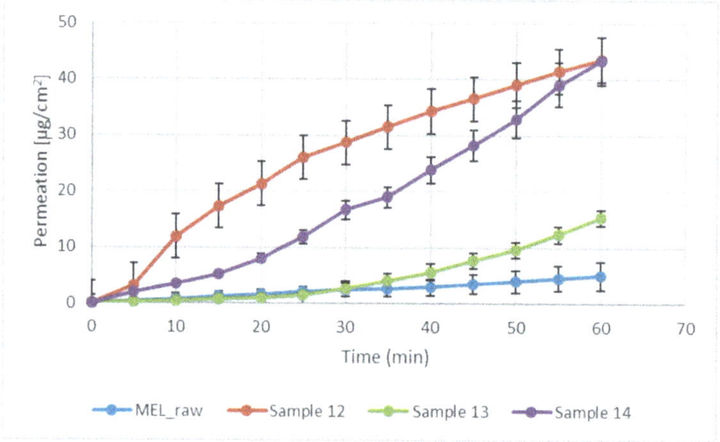

Figure 5. In vitro permeability of raw MEL and of MEL-containing spray-dried products.

4. Conclusions

The aim of our work was to prepare MEL-containing spray-dried chitosan microspheres for nasal administration. The effect of the process parameters (inlet air temperature and pump rate) on the particle size and the morphology of the microspheres was studied. As a novelty, a lower inlet air temperature (90 °C) was investigated than usual. With the chosen parameters, cross-linked and MEL-containing samples were formulated. The physicochemical (particles size, shape, crystalline- and chemical structure) and the rheological properties of the microspheres were characterized, and the dissolution rate and the diffusion through the artificial membrane of the drug-containing powders were investigated.

The inlet air temperature and the pump rate did not have an effect on particle size distribution and morphology, therefore, the parameters that required the least energy (90 °C) and resulted in fast drying (10 mL/min) were chosen. Hereinafter, applying these parameters, MEL-containing samples were prepared adding different amounts of TPP solutions (0, 1, or 2 mL). The size of spray-dried MEL containing microparticles increased compared to the drug-free particles, however, the average particle size was between 2.9–5.6 μm, and they had a spherical habit. The density of microspheres (around 0.15 g/cm^3) predicted drug deposition in the respiratory region of the nose. In the spray-dried samples, MEL was primarily in a molecularly dispersed state, however, concerning the non-cross-linked samples, a small crystalline fraction of MEL was observed. The MEL incorporation to the chitosan microparticles was successful. According to the in vitro dissolution and the permeability studies, the amounts of dissolved and diffused MEL were decreased by raising the concentration of TPP. In the case of microspheres that were formulated without TPP, more than 90% of drugs were dissolved during 1 h, and the same product showed the highest permeated drug amount (≈45 μg/cm^2). It can be explained by the formed cross-links, thus chitosan retained MEL from dissolution and diffusion. For all three samples, the initial rapid dissolution was followed by a decelerating drug release.

Because of mucoadhesive and permeability-enhancer features of chitosan and fast and continuous dissolution and diffusion of molecularly dispersed MEL, formulated microspheres prepared by spray-drying may be recommended for further optimization in order to develop nasal dosage forms. After the dose settings and the choice and the setting of the medical device suitable for nasal powder delivery are determined, the drug delivery system may be suggested for relieving acute pain or as an adjuvant of analgesia through the nasal mucosa.

Author Contributions: Conceptualization and Methodology, C.B., P.S.-R. and R.A.; Investigation, C.B., P.V.; Evaluation, C.B.; Writing—original draft, C.B. and P.V.; Writing—review and editing, P.S.-R. and R.A. All authors have read and agreed to the published version of the manuscript.

Funding: This research was funded by the University of Szeged Open Access Fund grant number 5223.

Institutional Review Board Statement: Not applicable.

Informed Consent Statement: Not applicable.

Data Availability Statement: Not applicable.

Acknowledgments: This work was supported by the Ministry of Human Capacities, Hungary grant TKP 2020 and 2.2.1-15-2016-00007 Project. Thanks to Tamás Kiss for his help in calculating the kinetic models.

Conflicts of Interest: The authors declare no conflict of interest. The founding sponsors had no role in the design of the study; in the collection, analyses, or interpretation of data; in the writing of the manuscript, and in the decision to publish the results.

References

1. Casettari, L.; Illum, L. Chitosan in Nasal Delivery Systems for Therapeutic Drugs. *J. Control. Release* **2014**, *190*, 189–200. [CrossRef] [PubMed]
2. Costantino, H.R.; Illum, L.; Brandt, G.; Johnson, P.H.; Quay, S.C. Intranasal Delivery: Physicochemical and Therapeutic Aspects. *Int. J. Pharm.* **2007**, *337*, 1–24. [CrossRef]
3. Mathias, N.R.; Hussain, M.A. Non-Invasive Systemic Drug Delivery: Developability Considerations for Alternate Routes of Administration. *J. Pharm. Sci.* **2010**, *99*, 1–20. [CrossRef] [PubMed]
4. Hao, J.; Zhao, J.; Zhang, S.; Tong, T.; Zhuang, Q.; Jin, K.; Chen, W.; Tang, H. Fabrication of an Ionic-Sensitive in Situ Gel Loaded with Resveratrol Nanosuspensions Intended for Direct Nose-to-Brain Delivery. *Colloids Surf. B Biointerfaces* **2016**, *147*, 376–386. [CrossRef] [PubMed]
5. Aulton, M.E.; Taylor, K. (Eds.) *Aulton's Pharmaceutics: The Design and Manufacture of Medicines*, 5th ed.; Elsevier: Edinburgh, UK; New York, NY, USA, 2018; ISBN 978-0-7020-7005-1.
6. Illum, L. Nasal Drug Delivery—Possibilities, Problems and Solutions. *J. Control. Release* **2003**, *87*, 187–198. [CrossRef]
7. Pires, A.; Fortuna, A.; Alves, G.; Falcão, A. Intranasal Drug Delivery: How, Why and What For? *J. Pharm. Pharm. Sci.* **2009**, *12*, 288. [CrossRef]
8. Jiang, L.; Gao, L.; Wang, X.; Tang, L.; Ma, J. The Application of Mucoadhesive Polymers in Nasal Drug Delivery. *Drug Dev. Ind. Pharm.* **2010**, *36*, 323–336. [CrossRef]
9. Marttin, E.; Romeijn, S.G.; Coos Verhoef, J.; Merkus, F.W.H.M. Nasal Absorption of Dihydroergotamine from Liquid and Powder Formulations in Rabbits. *J. Pharm. Sci.* **1997**, *86*, 802–807. [CrossRef]
10. Kublik, H.; Vidgren, M.T. Nasal Delivery Systems and Their Effect on Deposition and Absorption. *Adv. Drug Deliv. Rev.* **1998**, *29*, 157–177. [CrossRef]
11. Alhalaweh, A.; Andersson, S.; Velaga, S.P. Preparation of Zolmitriptan–Chitosan Microparticles by Spray Drying for Nasal Delivery. *Eur. J. Pharm. Sci.* **2009**, *38*, 206–214. [CrossRef]
12. Billotte, A.; Dunn, P.; Henry, B.; Marshall, P.; Woods, J. Intranasal Formulations for Treating Sexual Disorders. U.S. Patent Application No. 10/389,127, 21 August 2003.
13. Ahmadi, M.; Zubair, M.; Ahmad, K.A.; Riazuddin, V.N. Study on Nasal Deposition of Micro Particles and Its Relationship to Airflow Structure. *Int. J. Fluid Heat Transf.* **2016**, *1*, 1–11.
14. Sinha, V.R.; Singla, A.K.; Wadhawan, S.; Kaushik, R.; Kumria, R.; Bansal, K.; Dhawan, S. Chitosan Microspheres as a Potential Carrier for Drugs. *Int. J. Pharm.* **2004**, *274*, 1–33. [CrossRef] [PubMed]
15. Zhao, D.; Yu, S.; Sun, B.; Gao, S.; Guo, S.; Zhao, K. Biomedical Applications of Chitosan and Its Derivative Nanoparticles. *Polymers* **2018**, *10*, 462. [CrossRef]
16. Anitha, A.; Sowmya, S.; Kumar, P.T.S.; Deepthi, S.; Chennazhi, K.P.; Ehrlich, H.; Tsurkan, M.; Jayakumar, R. Chitin and Chitosan in Selected Biomedical Applications. *Prog. Polym. Sci.* **2014**, *39*, 1644–1667. [CrossRef]
17. Jătariu, A.N.; Holban, M.N.; Peptu, C.A.; Sava, A.; Costuleanu, M.; Popa, M. Double Crosslinked Interpenetrated Network in Nanoparticle Form for Drug Targeting—Preparation, Characterization and Biodistribution Studies. *Int. J. Pharm.* **2012**, *436*, 66–74. [CrossRef]
18. Bernkop-Schnürch, A.; Dünnhaupt, S. Chitosan-Based Drug Delivery Systems. *Eur. J. Pharm. Biopharm.* **2012**, *81*, 463–469. [CrossRef]
19. Kang, M.L.; Cho, C.S.; Yoo, H.S. Application of Chitosan Microspheres for Nasal Delivery of Vaccines. *Biotechnol. Adv.* **2009**, *27*, 857–865. [CrossRef] [PubMed]
20. Schipper, N.G.M.; Olsson, S.; Hoogstraate, J.A.; deBoer, A.G.; Vårum, K.M.; Artursson, P. Chitosans as Absorption Enhancers for Poorly Absorbable Drugs 2: Mechanism of Absorption Enhancement. *Pharm. Res.* **1997**, *14*, 923–929. [CrossRef] [PubMed]

21. Desai, K.G.H.; Park, H.J. Preparation of Cross-Linked Chitosan Microspheres by Spray Drying: Effect of Cross-Linking Agent on the Properties of Spray Dried Microspheres. *J. Microencapsul.* **2005**, *22*, 377–395. [CrossRef]
22. Bhumkar, D.R.; Pokharkar, V.B. Studies on Effect of PH on Cross-Linking of Chitosan with Sodium Tripolyphosphate: A Technical Note. *AAPS Pharmscitech* **2006**, *7*, E138–E143. [CrossRef]
23. Yang, W.; Fu, J.; Wang, T.; He, N. Chitosan/Sodium Tripolyphosphate Nanoparticles: Preparation, Characterization and Application as Drug Carrier. *J. Biomed. Nanotechnol.* **2009**, *5*, 591–595. [CrossRef]
24. Pan, C.; Qian, J.; Zhao, C.; Yang, H.; Zhao, X.; Guo, H. Study on the Relationship between Crosslinking Degree and Properties of TPP Crosslinked Chitosan Nanoparticles. *Carbohydr. Polym.* **2020**, *241*, 116349. [CrossRef]
25. Kumar, N. *WHO Normative Guidelines on Pain Management—Report of a Delphi Study to Determine the Need for Guidelines and to Identify the Number and Topics of Guidelines That Should Be Developed by WHO*; 2007. Available online: https://www.who.int/medicines/areas/quality_safety/delphi_study_pain_guidelines.pdf (accessed on 30 March 2021).
26. Horváth, T.; Ambrus, R.; Völgyi, G.; Budai-Szűcs, M.; Márki, Á.; Sipos, P.; Bartos, C.; Seres, A.B.; Sztojkov-Ivanov, A.; Takács-Novák, K.; et al. Effect of Solubility Enhancement on Nasal Absorption of Meloxicam. *Eur. J. Pharm. Sci.* **2016**, *95*, 96–102. [CrossRef]
27. Bartos, C.; Ambrus, R.; Kovács, A.; Gáspár, R.; Sztojkov-Ivanov, A.; Márki, Á.; Janáky, T.; Tömösi, F.; Kecskeméti, G.; Szabó-Révész, P. Investigation of Absorption Routes of Meloxicam and Its Salt Form from Intranasal Delivery Systems. *Molecules* **2018**, *23*, 784. [CrossRef]
28. Yong, C.S.; Jung, S.H.; Rhee, J.-D.; Choi, H.-G.; Lee, B.-J.; Kim, D.-C.; Choi, Y.W.; Kim, C.-K. Improved Solubility and In Vitro Dissolution of Ibuprofen from Poloxamer Gel Using Eutectic Mixture with Menthol. *Drug Deliv.* **2003**, *10*, 179–183. [CrossRef] [PubMed]
29. Bartos, C.; Ambrus, R.; Sipos, P.; Budai-Szűcs, M.; Csányi, E.; Gáspár, R.; Márki, Á.; Seres, A.B.; Sztojkov-Ivanov, A.; Horváth, T.; et al. Study of Sodium Hyaluronate-Based Intranasal Formulations Containing Micro- or Nanosized Meloxicam Particles. *Int. J. Pharm.* **2015**, *491*, 198–207. [CrossRef]
30. Ambrus, R.; Amirzadi, N.N.; Aigner, Z.; Szabó-Révész, P. Formulation of Poorly Water-Soluble Gemfibrozil Applying Power Ultrasound. *Ultrason. Sonochem.* **2012**, *19*, 286–291. [CrossRef] [PubMed]
31. Blagden, N.; de Matas, M.; Gavan, P.T.; York, P. Crystal Engineering of Active Pharmaceutical Ingredients to Improve Solubility and Dissolution Rates. *Adv. Drug Deliv. Rev.* **2007**, *59*, 617–630. [CrossRef] [PubMed]
32. Elversson, J.; Millqvist-Fureby, A.; Alderborn, G.; Elofsson, U. Droplet and Particle Size Relationship and Shell Thickness of Inhalable Lactose Particles During Spray Drying. *J. Pharm. Sci.* **2003**, *92*, 900–910. [CrossRef] [PubMed]
33. Kulkarni, A.D.; Bari, D.B.; Surana, S.J.; Pardeshi, C.V. In Vitro, Ex Vivo and in Vivo Performance of Chitosan-Based Spray-Dried Nasal Mucoadhesive Microspheres of Diltiazem Hydrochloride. *J. Drug Deliv. Sci. Technol.* **2016**, *31*, 108–117. [CrossRef]
34. 2.9. Bulk density and tapped density of powders. In *European Pharmacopoea 9.0*; Council of Europe: Strasbourg, France, 2016; p. 359.
35. Szabó, B.; Kállai, N.; Tóth, G.; Hetényi, G.; Zelkó, R. Drug Release Profiles and Microstructural Characterization of Cast and Freeze Dried Vitamin B12 Buccal Films by Positron Annihilation Lifetime Spectroscopy. *J. Pharm. Biomed. Anal.* **2014**, *89*, 83–87. [CrossRef]
36. Jug, M.; Hafner, A.; Lovrić, J.; Kregar, M.L.; Pepić, I.; Vanić, Ž.; Cetina-Čižmek, B.; Filipović-Grčić, J. An Overview of In Vitro Dissolution/Release Methods for Novel Mucosal Drug Delivery Systems. *J. Pharm. Biomed. Anal.* **2018**, *147*, 350–366. [CrossRef]
37. Pereswetoff-Morath, L. Microspheres as Nasal Drug Delivery Systems. *Adv. Drug Deliv. Rev.* **1998**, *29*, 185–194. [CrossRef]
38. Lawrie, G.; Keen, I.; Drew, B.; Chandler-Temple, A.; Rintoul, L.; Fredericks, P.; Grøndahl, L. Interactions between Alginate and Chitosan Biopolymers Characterized Using FTIR and XPS. *Biomacromolecules* **2007**, *8*, 2533–2541. [CrossRef]
39. Luo, Y.; Zhang, B.; Cheng, W.-H.; Wang, Q. Preparation, Characterization and Evaluation of Selenite-Loaded Chitosan/TPP Nanoparticles with or without Zein Coating. *Carbohydr. Polym.* **2010**, *82*, 942–951. [CrossRef]
40. Wu, Y.; Yang, W.; Wang, C.; Hu, J.; Fu, S. Chitosan Nanoparticles as a Novel Delivery System for Ammonium Glycyrrhizinate. *Int. J. Pharm.* **2005**, *295*, 235–245. [CrossRef] [PubMed]
41. Ma, Z.; Garrido-Maestu, A.; Jeong, K.C. Application, Mode of Action, and In Vivo Activity of Chitosan and Its Micro- and Nanoparticles as Antimicrobial Agents: A Review. *Carbohydr. Polym.* **2017**, *176*, 257–265. [CrossRef] [PubMed]
42. Wang, J.J.; Zeng, Z.W.; Xiao, R.Z.; Xie, T.; Zhou, G.L.; Zhan, X.R.; Wang, S.L. Recent Advances of Chitosan Nanoparticles as Drug Carriers. *Int. J. Nanomed.* **2011**, *6*, 765–774. [CrossRef]

pharmaceutics

MDPI

Article

Enhanced Bioavailability and Efficacy of Silymarin Solid Dispersion in Rats with Acetaminophen-Induced Hepatotoxicity

Im-Sook Song [1,*], So-Jeong Nam [1], Ji-Hyeon Jeon [1], Soo-Jin Park [2] and Min-Koo Choi [3,*]

1 BK21 FOUR Community-Based Intelligent Novel Drug Discovery Education Unit, Vessel-Organ Interaction Research Center (VOICE), Research Institute of Pharmaceutical Sciences, College of Pharmacy, Kyungpook National University, Daegu 41566, Korea; goddns159@nate.com (S.-J.N.); kei7016@naver.com (J.-H.J.)

2 College of Korean Medicine, Daegu Haany University, Daegu 38610, Korea; sjp124@dhu.ac.kr

3 College of Pharmacy, Dankook University, Cheon-an 31116, Korea

* Correspondence: isssong@knu.ac.kr (I.-S.S.); minkoochoi@dankook.ac.kr (M.-K.C.); Tel.: +82-53-950-8575 (I.-S.S.); +82-41-550-1438 (M.-K.C.); Fax: +82-53-950-8557 (I.-S.S.)

Abstract: We evaluated the bioavailability, liver distribution, and efficacy of silymarin-D-α-tocopherol polyethylene glycol 1000 succinate (TPGS) solid dispersion (silymarin-SD) in rats with acetaminophen-induced hepatotoxicity (APAP) compared with silymarin alone. The solubility of silybin, the major and active component of silymarin, in the silymarin-SD group increased 23-fold compared with the silymarin group. The absorptive permeability of silybin increased by 4.6-fold and its efflux ratio decreased from 5.5 to 0.6 in the presence of TPGS. The results suggested that TPGS functioned as a solubilizing agent and permeation enhancer by inhibiting efflux pump. Thus, silybin concentrations in plasma and liver were increased in the silymarin-SD group and liver distribution increased 3.4-fold after repeated oral administration of silymarin-SD (20 mg/kg as silybin) for five consecutive days compared with that of silymarin alone (20 mg/kg as silybin). Based on higher liver silybin concentrations in the silymarin-SD group, the therapeutic effects of silymarin-SD in hepatotoxic rats were evaluated and compared with silymarin administration only. Elevated alanine aminotransferase, aspartate aminotransferase, and alkaline phosphatase levels were significantly decreased by silymarin-SD, silymarin, and TPGS treatments, but these decreases were much higher in silymarin-SD animals than in those treated with silymarin or TPGS. In conclusion, silymarin-SD (20 mg/kg as silybin, three times per day for 5 days) exhibited hepatoprotective properties toward hepatotoxic rats and these properties were superior to silymarin alone, which may be attributed to increased solubility, enhanced intestinal permeability, and increased liver distribution of the silymarin-SD formulation.

Keywords: silymarin; D-α-Tocopherol polyethylene glycol 1000 succinate (TPGS); liver distribution; acetaminophen-induced hepatotoxicity

check for updates

Citation: Song, I.-S.; Nam, S.-J.; Jeon, J.-H.; Park, S.-J.; Choi, M.-K. Enhanced Bioavailability and Efficacy of Silymarin Solid Dispersion in Rats with Acetaminophen-Induced Hepatotoxicity. *Pharmaceutics* **2021**, 13, 628. https://doi.org/10.3390/pharmaceutics13050628

Academic Editor: José Martínez Lanao

Received: 17 March 2021
Accepted: 26 April 2021
Published: 28 April 2021

1. Introduction

Milk thistle has been used for over 2000 years as a general medicinal herb to treat liver, kidney, and gallbladder diseases [1,2]. Silymarin is an ethanol extract from milk thistle and is a complex mixture of flavonolignans, consisting of silibin, isosilibin, silydianin, silychristin and other compounds [3]. Silybin, a main component of silymarin, accounts for about 60–70%, followed by silychristin (20%), silydianin (10%), and isosilybin (5%) [4,5]. Silymarin is one of the most popular herbal supplementations that are known to be effective in liver disease [6]. It is also used to protect liver toxicity induced by acute ethanol exposure, carbon tetrachloride treatment, and high acetaminophen (APAP) doses [7]. Hepatoprotective effects of silymarin are mediated by reducing reactive oxygen species and increasing cellular glutathione and superoxide dismutase levels in the liver [8].

Despite the therapeutic benefits of silymarin, it is used at high doses (280–1000 mg) due to its low aqueous solubility (50–430 μg/mL), low bioavailability (23–47%), and limited absorption properties [9–11]. These poor biochemical characteristics may lead to unsatisfactory and nonreproducible clinical outcomes, in spite of the high doses, as there is an increased possibility of drug–drug interactions with other concomitantly administered drugs [6,12,13]. Therefore, formulation strategies to increase silymarin solubility and intestinal absorption have been investigated [14]. Widespread approaches include lipid-based formulations, including emulsions, liposomes, and solid lipid nanoparticles. Silymarin-loaded emulation-containing soybean lecithin and Tween 80 resulted in a 1.9-fold increase in the oral bioavailability of silymarin compared with silymarin suspended in polyethylene glycol (PEG) [15]. A self-emulsifying drug delivery system (SEDDS) has been applied to silymarin formulation. Silymarin-loaded SEDDS containing Tween 20, HCO-50, and Transcutol increased the silymarin bioavailability 3.6-fold [16]. A 2.7-fold increase in silymarin oral bioavailability has also been reported by using silymarin SEDDS composed of ethyl linoleate, Cremophor EL, and ethanol [17]. However, these emulations and SEDDS formulations had a high content of surfactant or other excipients. Silymarin nanoemulsions with reduced surfactant content have been reported to enhance silymarin oral bioavailability ranged from 1.3- to 4-fold [18–20]. Liposomes, proliposomes, and PEGylated liposomes of silymarin composed of phospholipid and cholesterol have been reported. These formulations showed a high encapsulation efficiency of more than 85% with increasing oral bioavailability of silymarin [14,21,22]. Moreover, surface-modified liposomes were reported to increase hepatoprotective efficacy. Hepatic-targeting ligand Sito-G-modified PEGylated silymarin liposomes were formulated and they enhanced hepatic uptake of silymarin in HeG2 cells [23]. Solid lipid nanoparticles of silymarin using Compritol 888 ATO, soybean lecithin, and poloxamer 188 showed a 2.8-fold higher oral bioavailability and enhanced liver distribution [24]. Besides the increased solubility and bioavailability of silymarin, in vivo liver-targeting and therapeutic efficiency await further investigation. Many other silymarin formulations, such as cyclodextrin inclusion complexes, solid dispersions (SDs), polymer-based nanocarriers, and so on [14], have focused on the linkage between the solubility enhancement and their oral bioavailability because the low silymarin solubility has been reported to limit its absorption [14,25].

In addition to low solubility, silymarin acts as a substrate for efflux pumps in the intestinal epithelium, and silymarin absorption is therefore restricted by these mechanisms, such as P-glycoprotein (P-gp), breast cancer resistance protein (BCRP), and multidrug resistance-related proteins (MRPs) [26]. Because of the nature of silymarin (e.g., low solubility and low permeability), it is classified under the Biopharmaceutics Classification System (BCS) as Category IV [14,27]. However, there have been controversies regarding the BCS category of silymarin. Many research papers consider it as BCS Category II [28,29]. Therefore, the objective of this study was to increase the oral bioavailability of silymarin by increasing its intestinal permeability through the inhibition of an efflux transporter, which is a strategy for the formulation of BCS Category III or IV drugs showing low intestinal permeability [30–32]. SD formulation was selected because it is a well-established technique for increasing the oral bioavailability by increasing the solubility of poorly-soluble drugs and by increasing permeability by modulating intestinal efflux pumps. Moreover, SD is easy to formulate with a reduced drug-to-excipient ratio and it is easy to change the kind of excipient [33].

Recently, various pharmaceutical excipients have emerged, not only as solubilizing agents, but also as potential alternatives to P-gp and metabolic inhibitors [32]. Polyethylene glycol 400 (PEG400), pluronic P85, pluronic F127, Tween 80, and vitamin E-D-α-tocopheryl polyethylene glycol 1000 succinate (TPGS) have been reported to inhibit in vitro P-gp-mediated efflux and intestinal metabolism when assessed using digoxin and verapamil as a substrate for P-gp and cytochrome P450 (CYP) 3A, resulting in enhanced oral bioavailability [30–32,34]. Among these excipients, TPGS is a nonionic water soluble vitamin E derivative, approved for pharmaceutical adjuvant use in drug formulations by the United States Food and Drug Administration [35]. TPGS has been used as an absorption enhancer, emulsifier, solubilizing agent, and permeation enhancer in pharmaceutics and cosmetics [36–38]. The molecule prolongs the half-life of drugs, and increases intestinal drug absorption by inhibiting ATPase activity of efflux pumps [30,39,40].

Therefore, we aimed to investigate the solubility and intestinal permeability of a silymarin-TPGS solid dispersion (silymarin-SD) formulation. We also aimed to investigate the pharmacokinetics and liver distribution, the target tissue of silymarin, as well as the efficacy of our silymarin-SD formulation in rats with acute hepatotoxicity. Concentrations of silymarin were monitored as silybin, the representative and major component of silymarin [3,41]. To induce acute hepatotoxicity, we used APAP overdosing, which is a widely used chemically-induced hepatoxic model [42]. At safe therapeutic doses, APAP is metabolized into glucuronide and sulfate via conjugation reactions at 60–90%. Approximately 5–10% of APAP is oxidized to N-acetyl-p-benzoquinone imine (NAPQI) by mixed-function oxidase enzymes. APAP is immediately conjugated with glutathione [16–21]. However, APAP overdoses produce the reactive intermediate, NAPQI [43], which binds to cellular proteins, induces oxidative stress, and promotes injury development during APAP-induced hepatotoxicity [30,44].

2. Materials and Methods

2.1. Reagents

Silymarin flabolignans (CAS No. 65666-07-1), Silybin (CAS No. 22888-70-6), TPGS (CAS No. 9002-96-4), Poloxamer 407 (CAS No. 9003-11-6), Tween 20 (CAS No. 9005-64-5), Tween 80 (CAS No. 9005-65-6), hydroxypropyl cellulose (HPC; CAS No. 9004-64-2), sodium dodecyl sulfate (SDS; CAS No. 151-21-3), pluronic F127 (CAS No. 9003-11-6), polyvinylpyrrolidone (PVP; CAS No. 9003-39-8), polyethylene glycol 400 (PEG 400) (CAS No. 25322-68-3), sodium carboxymethyl cellulose (CMC) (CAS No. 9004-32-4), naringenin (internal standard, IS) (CAS No. 67604-48-2), Hank's balanced salt solution (HBSS, pH 7.4), and acetaminophen (APAP; CAS No. 103-90-2) were purchased from Sigma-Aldrich (St. Louis, MO, USA). Distilled water, acetonitrile, and methanol were of high-performance liquid chromatography grade and purchased from J.T. Baker (Center Valley, PA, USA). All other chemicals and solvents were of reagent and analytical grade.

2.2. Selection of Excipients

The effect of various excipients on the silymarin solubility was measured. Silymarin (5 mg) and excipients such as TPGS, Poloxamer 407, Tween 20, Tween 80, HPC, SDS, pluronic F127, PVP (5 mg each) were sonicated for 5 min with 2 mL of distilled water and shaken at 25 °C for 12 h. Mixtures were centrifuged at 16,000× *g* for 10 min and supernatants filtered through a membrane filter (pore size; 0.22 μm). Filtrates were diluted in 85% acetonitrile and silybin concentrations analyzed using a liquid chromatography-tandem mass spectrometry (LC-MS/MS) system.

2.3. Preparation of Silymarin-SD

To determine the ratio of silymarin and TPGS, the solubility of silymarin (10 mg) was measured in the presence of various concentrations of TPGS (0.01–50 mg). After dissolving silymarin (10 mg) and varying concentrations of TPGS (0.01–50 mg) in 30 mL of 40% ethanol and freezing at −80 °C for 12 h, this mixture was then dried using a freeze dryer (FDCF-12012, operon, Seoul, Korea) at −120 °C for 72 h. The solubility of the silymarin formulation with varying ratios of TPGS was measured after dissolving these formulations in 2 mL of distilled water and shaken at 25 °C for 12 h. Mixtures were centrifuged at 16,000× *g* for 10 min and supernatants filtered through a membrane filter (pore size; 0.22 μm). Filtrates were diluted in 85% acetonitrile and silybin concentrations were analyzed using a liquid chromatography-tandem mass spectrometry (LC-MS/MS) system.

After deciding the ratio of silymarin and TPGS, SD formulation of silymarin-TPGS at a ratio of 1:1 (*w*/*w*) (silymarin-SD) was prepared for further characterization. Briefly, silymarin and TPGS were accurately weighed (0.5 g each), and dissolved in 300 mL of 40% ethanol and frozen at −80 °C for 12 h and this mixture was then dried using a freeze dryer (FDCF-12012, operon, Seoul, Korea) at −120 °C for 72 h. After freeze-drying, the resulting samples were passed through a KP sieve (mesh size = 0.84 μm) and stored in a thermo-hygrostat (25 °C, 20% relative humidity) until the use of silymarin-SD for the characterization and the pharmacokinetic and efficacy study.

2.4. Characterization of Silymarin-SD

Silymarin (5 mg) and silymarin-SD (10 mg) was dissolved with 2 mL of distilled water and shaken at 25 °C for 12 h. Mixtures were centrifuged at 16,000× *g* for 10 min and supernatants filtered through a membrane filter (pore size; 0.22 μm). Filtrates were diluted in 85% acetonitrile and silybin concentrations analyzed using an LC-MS/MS system.

Dissolution studies were conducted in 900 mL of distilled water for 120 min in a D-63150 dissolution test apparatus (Erweka, Heusenstamm, Germany) at 37 °C and 50 rpm using a paddle method. Briefly, silymarin powder (20 mg) and silymarin-SD formulation (equivalent to 20 mg silymarin) were packed into a gelatin capsule, and each capsule was placed inside the sinker. An aliquot (1 mL) of a medium was collected at 0, 10, 20, 30, 45, 60, 90, and 120 min and filtered through a membrane filter (pore size; 0.22 μm), and an equal volume of water replaced after each sampling. Silybin concentrations in filtrates were analyzed using an LC-MS/MS system.

X-ray diffraction (XRD) of silymarin, TPGS, and silymarin-SD was determined on an X-ray diffractometer (Ultima IV; Rigaku Co., Tokyo, Japan) using Cu Kα radiation, at 40 mA and 40 kV. Data were obtained from 5–60° (2θ) at a step size of 0.02° and a scanning speed of 5°/min.

Differential scanning calorimetry (DSC) of silymarin, TPGS, and silymarin-SD was determined using a DSC 131EVO (Setaram, Caluire, France). Sample weighing approximately 5 mg were placed in a closed aluminum pan and heated at a scanning rate of 5 °C/min from 10 °C to 200 °C, with nitrogen purging at 20 mL/min. Indium was used to calibrate the temperature scale.

Fourier-transform infrared spectroscopy (FTIR) spectra of silymarin, TPGS, physical mixture, and silymarin-SD were obtained in the spectral region of 4000–600 cm^{-1} using a resolution of 4 cm^{-1} and 64 scans using a Frontier FTIR spectrometer (PerkinElmer, Norwalk, CT, USA) in transmittance mode.

2.5. Intestinal Permeability Study

Male Wistar rats weighing 225–270 g (eight weeks old, n = 28) were purchased from Samtako Co. (Osan, Korea). Rats were housed in a 12-h light/dark cycle, and food and water were supplied ad libitum for one week prior to animal studies. Control rats (n = 4) received a vehicle (40% PEG 400) by oral administration for two days (4 p.m., 11 p.m., and 9 a.m.). APAP rats (n = 4) received an oral dose of APAP (3 g/kg dissolved in 40% PEG 400) for two days (4 p.m., 11 p.m., and 9 a.m.). Rats were fasted for 16 h, but had free access to water before study commencement. Rats were then anesthetized using isoflurane (isoflurane vaporizer to 2% with oxygen flow at 0.8 L/min) 24 h after the last APAP administration. Blood samples were collected from the abdominal aorta in heparinized blood tubes, and centrifuged at 16,000× *g* for 1 min to separate plasma. These were used to determine alanine aminotransferase (ALT) and aspartate aminotransferase (AST) levels using kits supplied by Young Dong Diagnostics (Yongin, Korea). A proximal jejunum section (approximately 10 cm) was excised and washed in prewarmed HBSS (pH 7.4). Segments were mounted on a tissue holder of a Navicyte Easy Mount Ussing Chamber (Warner Instruments, Holliston, MA, USA), with a surface area of 0.76 cm^2, and acclimated in HBSS for 15 min with continuous oxygenation (95% O_2/5% CO_2 gas). Intestinal permeability studies were commenced by changing HBSS on both sides of intestinal segments using 1 mL prewarmed HBSS containing silymarin or silymarin-SD (i.e., equivalent to 20 μM silybin) at the donor side and 1 mL prewarmed fresh HBSS at the receiver side. Sample aliquots (400 μL) were withdrawn every 30 min for 2 h from the receiver side, and an equal volume of prewarmed fresh HBSS was replaced at the receiver side.

To investigate whether efflux transporters were involved in this process, an apical to basal (A to B) and a basal to apical (B to A) transport of 20 μM silybin in the presence of representative inhibitors of P-gp, MRPs, and BCRPs such as 20 μM cyclosporine A (CsA), 100 μM MK-571, and 20 μM fumitremorgin C (FTC), respectively, were measured in a proximal jejunum section from control rats (n = 4) [45,46]. The effects of TPGS (0.01–1 mg/mL) on silybin permeability were also measured in a proximal jejunum section from control rats (n = 4) using the above method. For silybin analysis, sample aliquots (100 μL) were mixed for 5 min with 200 μL acetonitrile containing 20 ng/mL of naringenin (IS), and centrifuged at 16,000× g for 5 min. After this, a 5 μL supernatant was directly injected into an LC-MS/MS system.

To monitor intestinal integrity, Lucifer yellow (50 μM) permeability was measured in a proximal jejunum section from control rats (n = 12) as described previously [31,45]. Lucifer yellow fluorescence in 200 μL sample aliquots was measured using a fluorescence spectrophotometer (Infinite 200 PRO, Tecan, Switzerland) at an excitation wavelength of 425 nm and emission wavelength of 535 nm.

2.6. *Pharmacokinetics of Silymarin or Silymarin-SD in APAP-Induced Hepatotoxic Rats*

Pharmacokinetics of silymarin following single and repeated oral administration of silymarin and silymarin-SD for 5 days was measured in APAP-induced hepatotoxic rats. To induce hepatotoxicity, rats received an oral dose of APAP (3 g/kg) for 2 days, which was identical to the method described in Section 2.4. The dosing schedule for silymarin or silymarin-SD and APAP is shown in Figure 1.

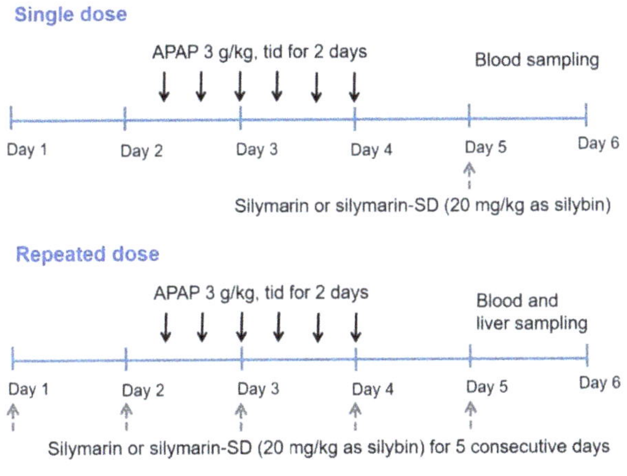

Figure 1. Dosing schedule for silymarin or silymarin-SD and APAP. Tid, three times per day.

For single administration of silymarin or silymarin-SD, rats with APAP-induced hepatotoxicity received silymarin (20 mg/kg as silybin, n = 4) or silymarin-SD (20 mg/kg as silybin, suspended in 0.5% CMC, n = 4) via oral gavage 24 h after the last APAP administration. Blood samples were taken from the cannulated femoral artery at 0.25, 0.5, 1, 2, 4, 8, and 24 h after silymarin and silymarin-SD administration (Figure 1). Bloods were centrifuged at 16,000× g for 1 min, and 50 μL plasma stored at −80 °C for silybin assay.

For the repeated administration of silymarin and silymarin-SD for five consecutive days, rats received silymarin (20 mg/kg as silybin, n = 4) or silymarin-SD (20 mg/kg as silybin, suspended in 0.5% CMC, n = 4) via oral gavage at 10 a.m. or five consecutive days. On the third and fourth day, rats received an oral APAP (3 g/kg dissolved in 40% PEG 400) dose at 4 p.m., 11 p.m., and 9 a.m.. Blood samples were taken from the cannulated femoral artery at 0.25, 0.5, 1, 2, 4, 8, and 24 h after the last administration of silymarin or silymarin-SD (Figure 1), centrifuged at 16,000× *g* for 1 min, and 50 μL plasma were stored at −80 °C for the silybin assay.

To investigate the liver distribution of silymarin and silymarin-SD, blood samples were collected from the abdominal artery at 0.5, 1, 2, 4, and 24 h after the repeated oral administration of silymarin (20 mg/kg as silybin, n = 20) or silymarin-SD (20 mg/kg as silybin, n = 20), according to the dosing schedule. Immediately after blood sampling, the liver was excised, rinsed in saline, and homogenized in nine volumes of saline, using a tissue homogenizer. Aliquots (50 μL) of 10% liver homogenate samples were stored at −80 °C for silybin assay.

Silybin concentrations in plasma and 10% liver homogenate samples were analyzed. Samples (100 μL) were added to 300 μL IS (naringenin, 20 ng/mL in acetonitrile) and the mixture was vigorously mixed for 10 min, followed by centrifugation at 16,000× *g* for 5 min. Supernatant aliquots (5 μL) were directly injected into an LC-MS/MS system.

2.7. LC-MS/MS Analysis of Silybin

The analysis of the silybin concentration was performed using an Agilent 6430 triple quadrupole LC/MS-MS system (Agilent, Wilmington, DE, USA) coupled to an Agilent 1290 HPLC system according to the previous method with slight modification [41]. Silybin and naringenin (IS) was separated on Synergi Polar RP column (150 × 2 mm, 5 μm particle size, Phenomenex, Torrance, CA, USA) with a mobile phase consisting of acetonitrile containing 0.1% formic acid: distilled water containing 0.1% formic acid = 85:15 (v/v) at a flow rate of 0.2 mL/min. Column oven temperature was maintained at 30 °C.

Multiple reactions monitoring conditions for silybin and naringenin (IS) in a negative ionization mode were used at m/z 481.1 → 301.0 for silybin and m/z 271.1 → 151.3 for naringenin with a collision energy of 15 eV. Quantitation was performed using the Agilent Mass Hunter Qualitative Analysis B. 04.00 software. A standard curve for silybin (2–500 ng/mL) was prepared by serially diluting silybin stock solution. The intra-day and inter-day precision and accuracy variations were within 15%.

2.8. Efficacy of Silymarin or Silymarin-SD in APAP-Induced Hepatotoxic Rats

Silymarin or silymarin-SD efficacy in APAP-induced hepatotoxic rats following repeated oral administration of silymarin or silymarin-SD for five days was measured using the same dosing schedule (Figure 1). Rats received vehicle (0.5% CMC, n = 4), TPGS (50 mg/kg suspended in 0.5% CMC, n = 4), silymarin (20 mg/kg as silybin suspended in 0.5% CMC, n = 4), and silymarin-SD (20 mg/kg as silybin, suspended in 0.5% CMC, n = 4) via oral gavage at 10 a.m. for five consecutive days. On the third and fourth day, rats received an oral APAP dose (3 g/kg dissolved in 40% PEG 400) at 4 p.m., 11 p.m., and 9 a.m. Twenty-four hours (24 h) after the last administration of vehicle, silymarin, TPGS, and silymarin-SD, blood samples were taken from the abdominal artery and centrifuged at 16,000× *g* for 1 min to collect plasma. Sample aliquots (200 μL each) were used to quantify markers of liver function, including ALT, AST, alkaline phosphatase (ALP), total cholesterol (TC), high-density lipoprotein cholesterol (HDL-C), and low-density lipoprotein cholesterol (LDL-C). Levels were measured at Seoul Clinical Laboratories (Yongin, Korea).

Immediately after blood sampling, liver tissues were excised from all rats and fixed in formalin buffer solution. Liver sections of 3 μm thick were sectioned and stained in hematoxylin and eosin (H&E). Histopathological observations were conducted by the Korea Pathology Technical Center (Cheongju, Korea).

2.9. Data Analysis

Pharmacokinetic parameters were calculated using the WinNonlin 5.1 using non-compartmental analysis. The data are expressed as the means ± standard deviation for the groups. Statistical analysis was performed using the Student t-test and one-way analysis of variance (ANOVA) test.

3. Results

3.1. Preparation of Silymarin-SD

The effect of various excipients, which have been proved for the solubility enhancement of silymarin and for the modulation of efflux transporters in the literature [29,32–34], on the silymarin solubility was measured with a silymarin to excipient ratio of 1:1 (*w*/*w*). Among the tested excipients, SDS, Tween 20, and HPC increased silymarin solubility by less than 1.5-fold. On the other hand, poloxamer 407, Tween 80, and pluronic F127 increased the silymarin solubility by 2~3-fold. Addition of PVP and TPGS showed the highest increase in silymarin solubility (Figure 2A). Finally, TPGS was selected as an excipient for silymarin formulation based on the previous results that showed TPGS inhibits the efflux transporters including P-gp [30,39,40].

To decide the ratio between silymarin and TPGS, SD of silymarin-TPGS with varying ratios of silymarin and TPGS (i.e., 1:0.001–1:5 *w*/*w*) was prepared by the freeze-drying method. Silymarin solubility, which was monitored by silybin concentration, a representative component of silymarin [41], increased sharply by the addition of TPGS up to 10 mg, and increased steadily when adding up to 50 mg TPGS (Figure 2B). Therefore, the silymarin-to-TPGS ratio was set at 1:1 for the preparation of silymarin-TPGS solid dispersion (silymarin-SD) formulations. After preparing silymarin-SD, the loading efficiency of silymarin in silymarin-SD was 50.9%.

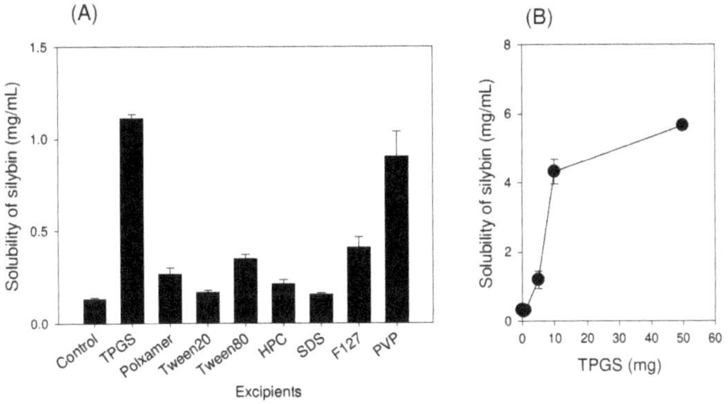

Figure 2. (**A**) Solubility of silymarin, which was monitored by silybin concentration, was measured in the presence of TPGS, Poloxamer407 (Poloxamer), Tween 20, Tween 80, hydroxypropyl cellulose (HPC), sodium dodecyl sulfate (SDS), pluronic F127 (F127), and polyvinylpyrrolidone (PVP). (**B**) Solubility of silymarin in the presence of varying amount of silymarin after preparing solid dispersion by freeze drying method. Each data represents mean ± standard deviation of triplicated determination.

3.2. Characterization of Silymarin-SD

When silymarin-SD solubility was compared with silymarin alone, a 23-fold increase in silybin solubility was observed compared with that of silymarin itself (Figure 3A). Not only was this solubility increased, but the dissolution rate of silymarin-SD was greater than silymarin alone (Figure 3B).

Silymarin, TPGS, and silymarin-SD XRD patterns are shown in Figure 3C. Silymarin and TPGS exhibited sharp peaks in a 2θ angle ranging from 10 to 30, indicating a typical crystalline structure for both. The diffraction peaks for silymarin-SD decreased markedly when compared with silymarin and TPGS, suggesting ingredients in the solid dispersion were in an amorphous state. Enhancement of silymarin solubility was 3.8-fold when the silymarin solubility of silymarin-SD prepared by the freeze-drying method was compared with that in the combined silymarin and TPGS at the same ratio (Figure 2A,B), suggesting that the 3.8-fold increase in the silymarin solubility can be explained by formulating silymarin-SD as amorphous state.

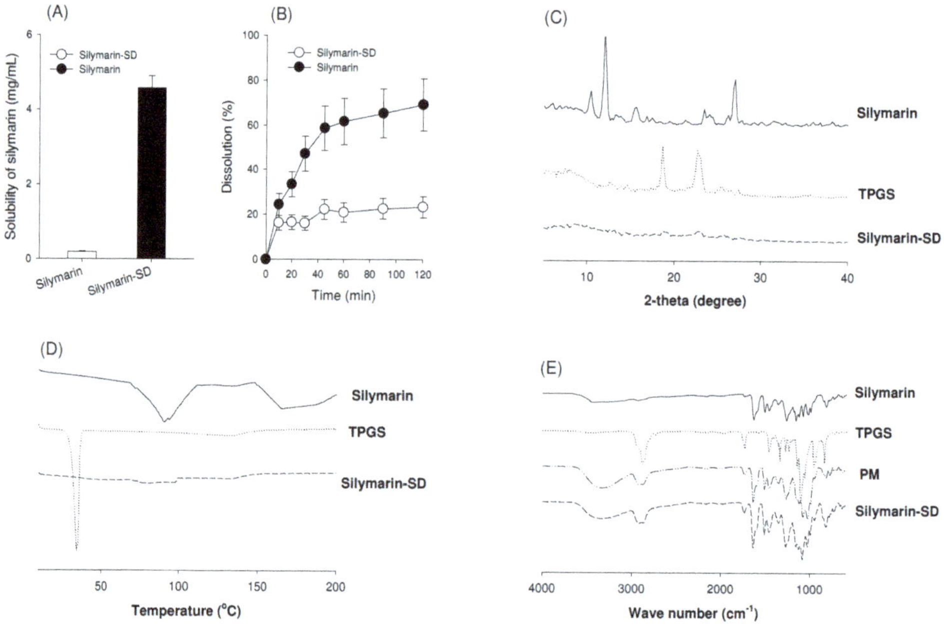

Figure 3. (**A**) Solubility and (**B**) dissolution rate of silymarin and silymarin-SD, which was monitored by silybin concentration, was measured. Each data represents mean ± standard deviation of triplicated determination. (**C**) X-ray diffraction (XRD) patterns of silymarin, TPGS, and silymarin-SD. (**D**) Differential scanning calorimetry (DSC) thermogram of silymarin, TPGS, and silymarin-SD. (**E**) Fourier-transform infrared spectroscopy (FTIR) spectrometer of silymarin, TPGS, a physical mixture of silymarin and TPGS (PM), and silymarin-SD.

The DSC results are shown in Figure 3D. Silymarin produced a wide endothermic peak at about 90 °C and glass transition temperature of 70 °C, which was consistent with previous results [33] and indicated its crystalline nature. TPGS produced a sharp endothermic peak at 33.75 °C and glass transition temperature of 30.7 °C, which was also consistent with previous results [30]. However, in the DSC thermogram of silymarin-SD, the indicative peaks for silymarin and TPGS disappeared with a slight decrease around 75 °C and an increase around 150 °C. It could be concluded that silymarin and TPGS in the silymarin-SD were in the amorphous form after the fabrication.

The FTIR pattern of silymarin, TPGS, physical mixture (PM) of silymarin and TPGS, and silymarin-SD are shown in Figure 3E. The FTIR pattern of individual silymarin and TPGS was similar to previous results [29,33]. The FTIR spectrum of PM exhibited characteristic peaks of both silymarin and TPGS and showed similar peaks to the silymarin-SD, suggesting that there was no major shift of peaks and no existence of covalent interaction between silymarin and TPGS.

3.3. Enhanced Intestinal Permeability of Silymarin-SD

To investigate transporter efflux in silymarin transport in rat intestines, we investigated the permeability of silybin, a representative component of silymarin [41], in the presence of P-gp, BCRP, and MRP inhibitors (Figure 4C). Efflux ratios, calculated by dividing B to A permeability ($P_{app,BA}$) by A to B permeability ($P_{app,AB}$) [47], of silybin was 5.8 and decreased to 1.7 and 0.7 by the presence of CsA (P-gp inhibitor) and MK571 (MRP2 inhibitor), respectively. However, FTC (BCRP inhibitor) treatment did not alter the efflux ratio of silybin (i.e., 5.5). In addition, TPGS also decreased the $P_{app,BA}$ of silybin and increased the $P_{app,AB}$ of silybin in a TPGS concentration-dependent manner (Figure 4A). In addition, efflux pump inhibitors did not alter the P_{app} of Lucifer yellow, a marker of cell integrity [45], whereas TPGS significantly increased the P_{app} of Lucifer yellow (Figure 4B). These results suggested that P-gp and MRPs were involved in silybin efflux, and TPGS increased silybin absorption by inhibiting silybin efflux. TPGS also functioned as a permeation enhancer to increase the paracellular pathway of silybin by disturbing cell integrity.

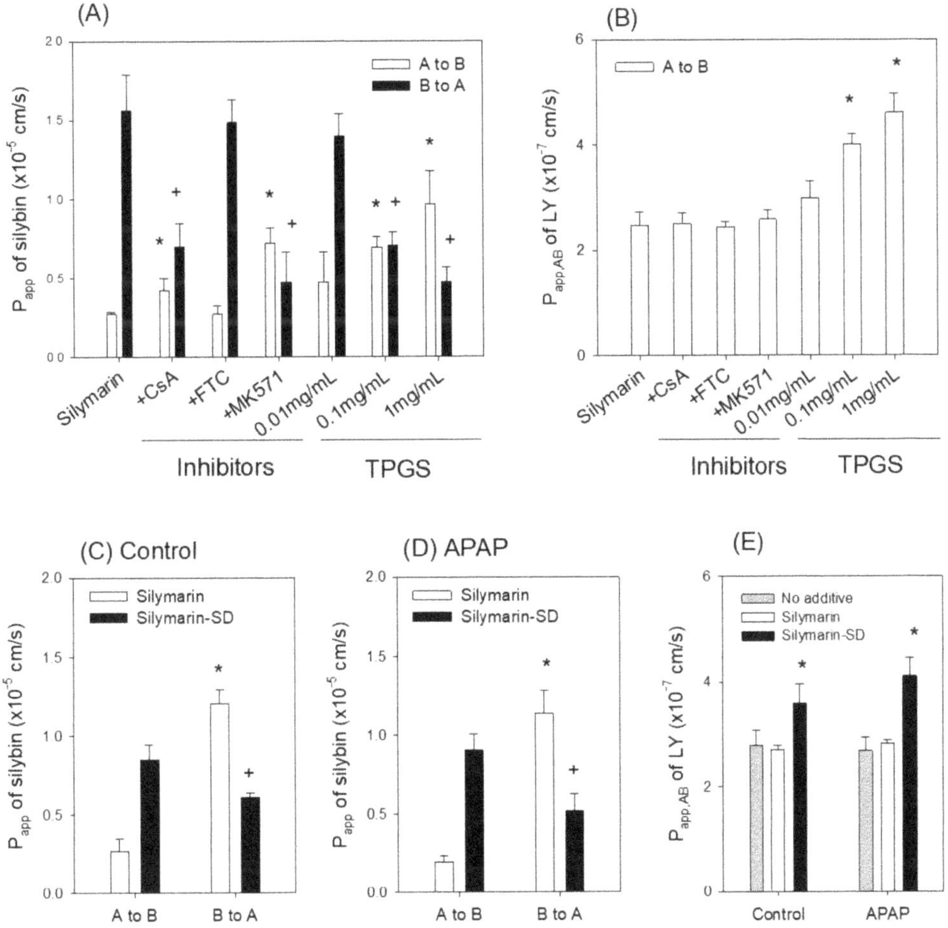

Figure 4. (**A**) The effect of efflux pump inhibitors and TPGS (0.01 mg/mL–1 mg/mL) on silybin permeability (P_{app}) in rat jejunal segments. Twenty micromole (20 μM) cyclosporine A (CsA), 20 μM fumitremorgin C (FTC), and 100 μM MK-571 were used as inhibitors of P-gp, BCRP, and MRPs, respectively. (**B**) The effects of efflux pump inhibitors and TPGS (0.01 mg/mL–1 mg/mL) on A to B permeability ($P_{app,AB}$) of Lucifer yellow (LY) in rat jejunal segments. The P_{app} of silybin in the presence of silymarin and silymarin-SD in jejunal segments from (**C**) control and (**D**) APAP-induced hepatotoxic rats. (**E**) The P_{app} of LY in the presence of silymarin and silymarin-SD in jejunal segments of control and APAP-induced hepatotoxic rats. Each data point represents the mean ± standard deviation (n = 4). * $p < 0.05$ compared with A to B P_{app} of silybin or LY. + $p < 0.05$ compared with B to A P_{app} of silybin or LY.

Next, we measured the P_{app} of silymarin and silymarin-SD in control and APAP-induced hepatotoxic rats. We observed no significant differences in Papp values between the silymarin and silymarin-SD groups (Figure 4C,D). Moreover, the $P_{app,AB}$ of Lucifer yellow in the intestinal segment of APAP-induced hepatotoxic rats was 2.8×10^{-7} cm/s, similar to control rats (Figure 4E, gray bar). This observation suggested that APAP treatment did not harm cell integrity or alter intestinal permeability [45].

However, $P_{app,BA}$ of silybin was 4.5- and 5.8-fold greater than $P_{app,AB}$ in both control and APAP rats, suggesting that the efflux pump was involved in intestinal absorption processing of silymarin; this can be a limiting factor for silymarin absorption [32]. When we compared the P_{app} of silybin in the silymarin and silymarin-SD groups (Figure 4C,D), $P_{app,AB}$ of silybin increased as silymarin-SD by 3.2- and 4.6-fold compared with silymarin itself in the control and APAP groups, respectively. $P_{app,BA}$ of silybin was decreased by the presence of silymarin-SD by 0.5- and 0.4-fold compared with silymarin itself in the control and APAP groups, respectively. The $P_{app,AB}$ of Lucifer yellow was not different in the presence of silymarin itself but significantly increased with the addition of silymarin-SD (Figure 4E). Thus, by using silymarin-SD, the efflux ratio of silybin was decreased 0.6-fold and the $P_{app,AB}$ of silybin was increased 4.6-fold, through the inhibition of efflux of silybin, and the enhancement of paracellular permeability.

3.4. Increased Bioavailability of Silymarin-SD

Plasma concentration–time silybin profiles after single and repeated oral administration of silymarin and silymarin-SD are shown (Figure 5). Pharmacokinetic parameters, as calculated from plasma concentration–time profiles, are presented in Table 1. In the single oral administration group, the maximum plasma concentration (C_{max}) and the area under the plasma concentration curve (AUC) for silybin following silymarin-SD administration were 4.0- and 1.6-fold, respectively, greater than those for silymarin only. However, the time to reach C_{max} (T_{max}) and elimination half-life ($T_{1/2}$) was not different between the silymarin and silymarin-SD groups after the single oral administration (Figure 5A and Table 1). These results suggested that increased silybin plasma concentrations in the silymarin-SD group were caused by enhanced absorption.

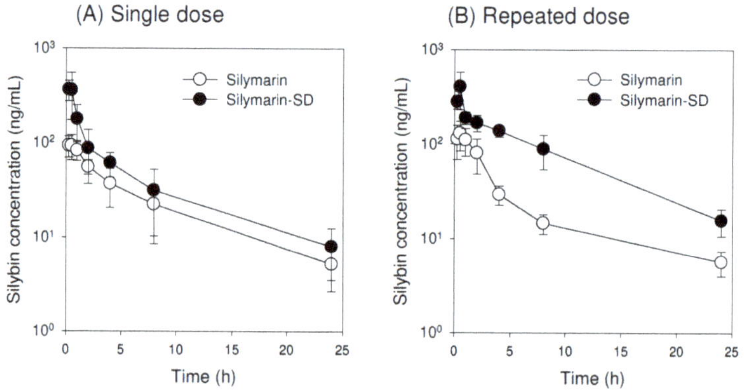

Figure 5. Plasma concentration–time profiles of silybin after (**A**) single and (**B**) repeated oral administration for five consecutive days of silymarin (20 mg/kg as silybin) and silymarin-SD (20 mg/kg as silybin) in rats with APAP-induced hepatotoxicity. Treatments followed the dosing schedule (Figure 1). Each data point represents the mean ± standard deviation of four rats per group.

Table 1. Pharmacokinetic parameters of silybin.

Parameters	Single Administration		Repeated Administration	
	Silymarin	Silymarin-SD	Silymarin	Silymarin-SD
C_{max} (ng/mL)	106 ± 14.9	427 ± 147 *	146 ± 48.1	412 ± 168 *
T_{max} (h)	0.56 ± 0.31	0.40 ± 0.14	0.45 ± 0.11	0.44 ± 0.13
AUC_{24h} (ng·h/mL)	578 ± 225	957 ± 350 *	547 ± 131	2040 ± 435 *,+
AUC_{∞} (n·h/mL)	634 ± 239	1060 ± 406 *	587 ± 138	2190 ± 374 *,+
$T_{1/2}$ (h)	6.77 ± 2.06	7.98 ± 2.80	6.74 ± 1.11	7.36 ± 1.32
MRT (h)	5.16 ± 0.47	7.66 ± 1.86 *	4.88 ± 0.72	8.32 ± 1.82 *

C_{max}, maximum plasma concentration; T_{max}: time to reach C_{max}; AUC_{24h}, area under the plasma concentration curve from zero to 24 h; AUC_{∞}, area under the plasma concentration curve from zero to infinity; $T_{1/2}$, elimination half-life; MRT, mean residence time. * $p < 0.05$, compared with silymarin itself, + $p < 0.05$, compared with a single administration.

We observed a significant increase in C_{max} and AUC of silybin after repeated oral administration of silymarin-SD for five consecutive days when compared with the repeated silymarin treatment group (Figure 5B and Table 1). However, the fold increase in the silybin AUC was greater (3.7-fold) in the repeated administration of the silymarin-SD group than silymarin itself (1.6-fold). These results suggested that the repeated silymarin-SD treatment may have increased the mean residence time (MRT) of silybin and this results in the accumulated plasma concentrations of silybin when administered repeatedly as silymarin-SD formulation.

Next, we investigated the liver distribution of silymarin-SD when compared with silymarin itself after repeated oral administration of silymarin-SD. Liver distribution is critical for the therapeutic efficacy of silymarin-SD because hepatoprotective effects of silymarin are mediated by reducing reactive oxygen species and increasing cellular glutathione and superoxide dismutase levels in the liver [8]. The liver concentrations of silybin in the silymarin-SD treatment group were significantly higher than those in the silymarin treatment group (Figure 6A). In addition, the liver silybin concentration in the silymarin group decreased sharply for 4 h, but was maintained for 24 h in the silymarin-SD group (Figure 6A). Therefore, the liver to plasma AUC ratio of silybin was significantly higher in the silymarin-SD than the silymarin group (Figure 6B).

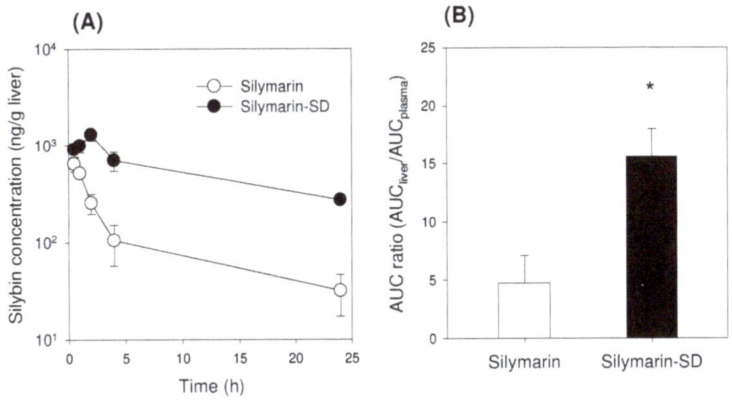

Figure 6. (**A**) Silybin concentrations in the liver. (**B**) Liver to plasma AUC ratio of silybin after the repeated oral administration for five consecutive days of silymarin (20 mg/kg as silybin) and silymarin-SD (20 mg/kg as silybin) in rats with APAP-induced hepatotoxicity. Treatment followed the dosing schedule in Figure 1. Each data represents mean ± standard deviation of four rats at individual time point per group. * $p < 0.05$, compared with silymarin group.

3.5. Effect of Silymarin-SD on the APAP-Induced Hepatotoxicity

Based on higher liver silymarin concentrations of silymarin-SD compared with silymarin only after repeated oral administration, we evaluated the therapeutic effects of silymarin-SD in study rats. As shown in Figure 7, the biochemical hepatotoxicity markers, ALT, AST, and ALP were significantly increased by APAP treatment. These were decreased by the treatment with TPGS and silymarin only (APAP + TPGS and APAP + silymarin groups). However, decreased ALT, AST, and ALP levels were greater in the silymarin-SD treatment group compared with the TPGS and silymarin groups. Alterations in TC levels were not as significant as for ALT and AST, but TPGS, silymarin, and silymarin-SD treatments decreased these levels. When HDL-C and LDL-C levels were examined, silymarin-SD treatment was effective for APAP-induced hepatotoxicity, and more effective than the TPGS and silymarin groups.

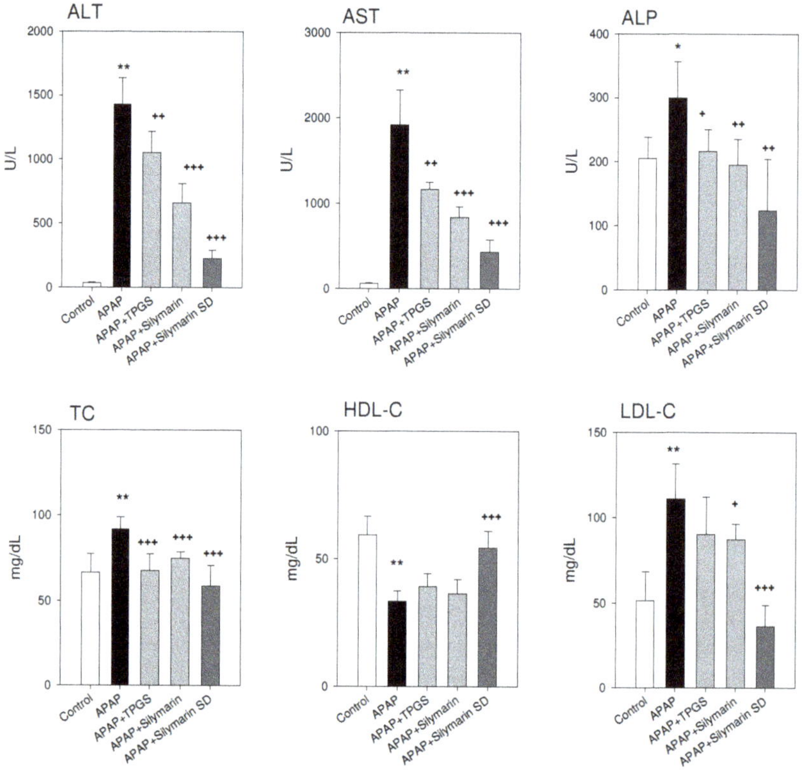

Figure 7. Alanine aminotransferase (ALT), aspartate aminotransferase (AST), alkaline phosphatase (ALP), total cholesterol (TC), high-density lipoprotein-cholesterol (HDL-C), and low-density lipoprotein-cholesterol levels (LDL-C) from control, acetaminophen (APAP)-induced hepatotoxic rat (APAP), APAP-induced hepatotoxic rats treated with TPGS 50 mg/kg (APAP+TPGS), silymarin (20 mg/kg as silybin) (APAP+Silymarin), and silymarin-SD (20 mg/kg as silybin) (APAP+Silymarin-SD). Treatment followed the dosing schedule in Figure 1. Each data represents mean ± standard deviation of four rats per group. * $p < 0.05$, and ** $p < 0.01$, compared with silymarin group; $^{+}$ $p < 0.05$, $^{++}$ $p < 0.01$, and $^{+++}$ $p < 0.001$, compared with APAP group.

Histopathology images from liver sections near the central vein are shown in Figure 8. APAP-toxicity sections showed inflammatory cell infiltration and disarranged hepatic cells (Figure 8B) compared to controls (Figure 8A). TPGS, silymarin, and silymarin-SD treatment groups showed less inflammatory cell infiltration compared with the APAP group (Figure 8C–E). When biochemical and histological results were combined, silymarin-SD treatment indicated superior protective effects toward liver tissue when compared with the TPGS only or silymarin only groups.

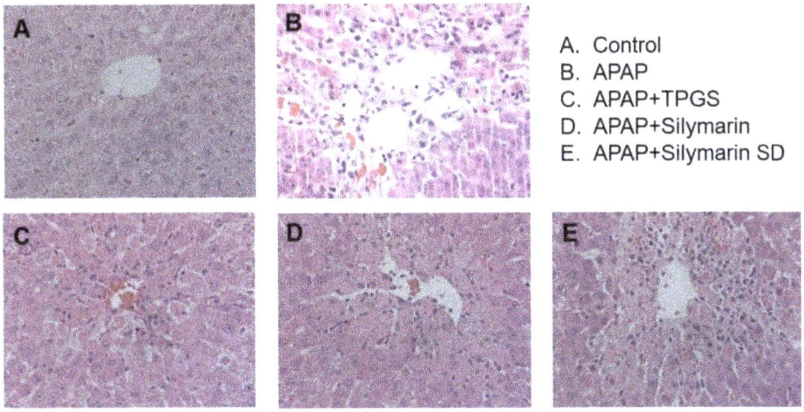

Figure 8. Representative liver histopathology hematoxylin and eosin (400×) images. The effect of silymarin-TPGS on APAP-induced hepatotoxicity in rats. (**A**) Control rats, (**B**) acetaminophen (APAP)-induced hepatotoxic rats, (**C**) APAP-induced hepatotoxic rats treated with TPGS (50 mg/kg) (APAP + TPGS), (**D**) APAP-induced hepatotoxic rats treated with silymarin (20 mg/kg as silybin) (APAP + silymarin), and (**E**) APAP-induced hepatotoxic rats treated with silymarin-SD (20 mg/kg as silybin) (APAP + silymarin-SD). Treatments followed the dosing schedule (Figure 1).

4. Discussion

Herbal based-dietary supplements are increasingly popular with more than 60% of adults taking these herbal supplements [48]. Silymarin, the concentrated extract of milk thistle, is one of the six best-selling herbal supplements and has long been used as a treatment for liver disease [12]. Despite the popularity of silymarin and its poor chemical properties and limited bioavailability, studies have attempted to enhance this bioavailability [37], which is limited by low solubility and efflux pump-mediated low intestinal permeability [13,26]. In recent years, several pharmaceutical excipients have emerged, not only as solubilizing agents, but also as potential inhibitors of intestinal first pass effect [32]. TPGS has been used as a solubilizer, stabilizer, permeation enhancer, and absorption enhancer, and P-gp inhibitors in a wide range of nanoliposomes, emulsions, micelles, and solid dispersions [30,38].

By formulating amorphous solid dispersions with silymarin and TPGS using freeze-drying methods, silybin solubility was increased 23-fold and intestinal permeability increased 4.6-fold (Figures 2 and 4). In addition, the efflux ratio of silybin was decreased from 5.8 to 0.6 (Figure 4). Considering the efflux ratio of silybin was decreased by the presence of P-gp and MRP2 inhibitors and Lucifer yellow permeability was also enhanced by the presence of silymarin-SD, the increased intestinal permeability of silybin could be attributed to the permeation-enhancing effect and inhibition of P-gp- and MRP2-mediated silybin efflux. This enhanced permeation and dissolution rate of silybin in a silymarin-SD formulation generated increased silybin plasma concentrations. The AUC of silybin was increased 1.6-fold by the single oral administration of silymarin-SD when compared with silymarin administration (Figure 5A, Table 1). From the repeated administration of silymarin-SD for five days, plasma AUC was increased 2.1-fold when compared to the single administration of silymarin-SD and increased 3.7-fold when compared to the repeated administrations of silymarin itself (Figure 5B, Table 1). Moreover, silybin liver distribution was increased 3.3-fold when compared to the repeated administration of silymarin alone

(Figure 6). Increased silybin accumulation by repeated administration of silymarin-SD may be attributed to decreased silybin elimination, consistent with increased MRT of silybin in the silymarin-SD group.

This increased liver distribution may result in enhanced therapeutic efficacy of silymarin-SD. The pre-treatment and co-treatment of silymarin-SD during APAP-induced hepatotoxicity showed superior effects in reducing hepatotoxic biomarkers, such as ALT, AST, and ALP compared with pre-treatment and co-treatment with silymarin itself. Since TPGS also reduces oxidative stress [38], we investigated the effects of TPGS on APAP-induced hepatotoxicity. As shown in Figure 7, TPGS exhibited partial activity on APAP-induced hepatotoxicity. Therefore, the superior effects of silymarin-SD increased liver concentrations of silybin and the resultant hepatoprotective effect could be attributed to the partial effect of TPGS. Taken together, the solid dispersion formulation of silymarin with TPGS not only enhanced bioavailability and increased distribution to target tissues, but also reinforced the practicality of functional excipient like TPGS (i.e., solubilizing effects, permeation enhancer, efflux pump modulation, and antioxidative effects) [38,40,49].

In conclusion, the solid dispersion formulation of silymarin-TPGS may be used to increase solubility and intestinal permeability; therefore, multiple silymarin-SD treatment (at a dose of 20 mg/kg as silybin) exhibited higher plasma concentrations and better hepatoprotective properties than the treatment of silymarin alone in APAP-induced hepatotoxic rats.

Author Contributions: Conceptualization, I.-S.S.; methodology, M.-K.C.; investigation, I.-S.S., S.-J.N., S.-J.P. and J.-H.J.; analysis and interpretation of data, S.-J.N., J.-H.J. and S.-J.P.; writing—original draft preparation, I.-S.S.; writing—review and editing, I.-S.S. and M.-K.C.; supervision, I.-S.S. and M.-K.C.; grant acquisition, I.-S.S. All authors have read and agreed to the published version of the manuscript.

Funding: This work was supported, in part, by the National Research Foundation of Korea (NRF) grant funded by the Korea government (MSIT) (Nos. NRF-2020R1I1A3074384 and NRF-2020R1A5A2017323).

Institutional Review Board Statement: All animal procedures were approved by the Animal Care and Use Committee of Kyungpook National University (Protocol code: 2015-0067, date of approval: 18 May 2015; Protocol code: 2019-0004, date of approval: 7 January 2019).

Informed Consent Statement: Not applicable.

Data Availability Statement: The data presented in this study are available upon request.

Conflicts of Interest: The authors declare no conflict of interest.

References

1. Schuppan, D.; Jia, J.D.; Brinkhaus, B.; Hahn, E.G. Herbal products for liver diseases: A therapeutic challenge for the new millennium. *Hepatology* **1999**, *30*, 1099–1104. [CrossRef]
2. Flora, K.; Hahn, M.; Rosen, H.; Benner, K. Milk thistle (*Silybum marianum*) for the therapy of liver disease. *Am. J. Gastroenterol.* **1998**, *93*, 139–143. [CrossRef]
3. Brinda, B.J.; Zhu, H.J.; Markowitz, J.S. A sensitive LC-MS/MS assay for the simultaneous analysis of the major active components of silymarin in human plasma. *J. Chromatogr. B Analyt. Technol. Biomed. Life Sci.* **2012**, *902*, 1–9. [CrossRef] [PubMed]
4. Saller, R.; Meier, R.; Brignoli, R. The use of silymarin in the treatment of liver diseases. *Drugs* **2001**, *61*, 2035–2063. [CrossRef]
5. Dixit, N.; Baboota, S.; Kohli, K.; Ahmad, S.; Ali, J. Silymarin: A review of pharmacological aspects and bioavailability enhancement approaches. *Indian J. Pharmacol.* **2007**, *39*, 172–179. [CrossRef]
6. Deng, J.W.; Shon, J.H.; Shin, H.J.; Park, S.J.; Yeo, C.W.; Zhou, H.H.; Song, I.S.; Shin, J.G. Effect of silymarin supplement on the pharmacokinetics of rosuvastatin. *Pharm. Res.* **2008**, *25*, 1807–1814. [CrossRef]
7. Abenavoli, L.; Izzo, A.A.; Milic, N.; Cicala, C.; Santini, A.; Capasso, R. Milk thistle (*Silybum marianum*): A concise overview on its chemistry, pharmacological, and nutraceutical uses in liver diseases. *Phytother. Res.* **2018**, *32*, 2202–2213. [CrossRef] [PubMed]
8. Raskovic, A.; Stilinovic, N.; Kolarovic, J.; Vasovic, V.; Vukmirovic, S.; Mikov, M. The protective effects of silymarin against doxorubicin-induced cardiotoxicity and hepatotoxicity in rats. *Molecules* **2011**, *16*, 8601–8613. [CrossRef] [PubMed]
9. Javed, S.; Kohli, K.; Ali, M. Reassessing bioavailability of silymarin. *Altern. Med. Rev.* **2011**, *16*, 239–249. [PubMed]
10. Schulz, H.U.; Schurer, M.; Krumbiegel, G.; Wachter, W.; Weyhenmeyer, R.; Seidel, G. The solubility and bioequivalence of silymarin preparations. *Arzneimittelforschung* **1995**, *45*, 61–64. [PubMed]
11. Morazzoni, P.; Montalbetti, A.; Malandrino, S.; Pifferi, G. Comparative pharmacokinetics of silipide and silymarin in rats. *Eur. J. Drug Metab. Pharmacokinet.* **1993**, *18*, 289–297. [CrossRef]

12. Fenclova, M.; Novakova, A.; Viktorova, J.; Jonatova, P.; Dzuman, Z.; Ruml, T.; Kren, V.; Hajslova, J.; Vitek, L.; Stranska-Zachariasova, M. Poor chemical and microbiological quality of the commercial milk thistle-based dietary supplements may account for their reported unsatisfactory and non-reproducible clinical outcomes. *Sci. Rep.* **2019**, *9*, 11118. [CrossRef]
13. Xie, Y.; Zhang, D.Q.; Zhang, J.; Yuan, J.L. Metabolism, transport and drug-drug interactions of silymarin. *Molecules* **2019**, *24*, 3693. [CrossRef] [PubMed]
14. Di Costanzo, A.; Angelico, R. Formulation Strategies for Enhancing the Bioavailability of Silymarin: The State of the Art. *Molecules* **2019**, *24*, 2155. [CrossRef] [PubMed]
15. Abrol, S.; Trehan, A.; Katare, O.P. Formulation, characterization, and in vitro evaluation of silymarin-loaded lipid microspheres. *Drug Deliv.* **2004**, *11*, 185–191. [CrossRef] [PubMed]
16. Woo, J.S.; Kim, T.S.; Park, J.H.; Chi, S.C. Formulation and biopharmaceutical evaluation of silymarin using SMEDDS. *Arch. Pharm. Res.* **2007**, *30*, 82–89. [CrossRef] [PubMed]
17. Li, X.; Yuan, Q.; Huang, Y.; Zhou, Y.; Liu, Y. Development of silymarin self-microemulsifying drug delivery system with enhanced oral bioavailability. *AAPS PharmSciTech* **2010**, *11*, 672–678. [CrossRef]
18. Yang, K.Y.; Hwang du, H.; Yousaf, A.M.; Kim, D.W.; Shin, Y.J.; Bae, O.N.; Kim, Y.I.; Kim, J.O.; Yong, C.S.; Choi, H.G. Silymarin-loaded solid nanoparticles provide excellent hepatic protection: Physicochemical characterization and in vivo evaluation. *Int. J. Nanomed.* **2013**, *8*, 3333–3343.
19. Calligaris, S.; Comuzzo, P.; Bot, F.; Lippe, G.; Zironi, R.; Anese, M.; Nicoli, M.C. Nanoemulsions as delivery systems of hydrophobic silybin from silymarin extract: Effect of oil type on silybin solubility, in vitro bioaccessibility and stability. *LWT Food Sci. Technol.* **2015**, *63*, 77–84. [CrossRef]
20. Nagi, A.; Iqbal, B.; Kumar, S.; Sharma, S.; Ali, J.; Baboota, S. Quality by design based silymarin nanoemulsion for enhancement of oral bioavailability. *J. Drug Del. Sci. Technol.* **2017**, *40*, 35–44. [CrossRef]
21. Xiao, Y.Y.; Song, Y.M.; Chen, Z.P.; Ping, Q.N. Preparation of silymarin proliposome: A new way to increase oral bioavailability of silymarin in beagle dogs. *Int. J. Pharm.* **2006**, *319*, 162–168.
22. Chu, C.; Tong, S.-S.; Xu, Y.; Wang, L.; Fu, M.; Ge, Y.-R.; Yu, J.-N.; Xu, X.-M. Proliposomes for oral delivery of dehydrosilymarin: Preparation and evaluation in vitro and in vivo. *Acta Pharmacol. Sin.* **2011**, *32*, 973–980. [CrossRef]
23. Elmowafy, M.; Viitala, T.; Ibrahim, H.M.; Abu-Elyazid, S.K.; Samy, A.; Kassem, A.; Yliperttula, M. Silymarin loaded liposomes for hepatic targeting: In vitro evaluation and HepG2 drug uptake. *Eur. J. Pharm. Sci.* **2013**, *50*, 161–171. [CrossRef]
24. He, J.; Hou, S.X.; Lu, W.G.; Zhu, L.; Feng, J.F. Preparation, pharmacokinetics and body distribution of silymarin-loaded solid lipid nanoparticles after oral administration. *J. Biomed. Nanotechnol.* **2007**, *3*, 195–202. [CrossRef]
25. Saller, R.; Melzer, J.; Reichling, J.; Brignoli, R.; Meier, R. An updated systematic review of the pharmacology of silymarin. *Forsch Komplementmed.* **2007**, *14*, 70–80. [CrossRef] [PubMed]
26. Yuan, Z.W.; Li, Y.Z.; Liu, Z.Q.; Feng, S.L.; Zhou, H.; Liu, C.X.; Liu, L.; Xie, Y. Role of tangeretin as a potential bioavailability enhancer for silybin: Pharmacokinetic and pharmacological studies. *Pharmacol. Res.* **2018**, *128*, 153–166. [CrossRef] [PubMed]
27. Pérez-Sánchez, A.; Cuyàs, E.; Ruiz-Torres, V.; Agulló-Chazarra, L.; Verdura, S.; González-Álvarez, I.; Bermejo, M.; Joven, J.; Micol, V.; Bosch-Barrera, J.; et al. Intestinal permeability study of clinically relevant formulations of silibinin in Caco-2 cell monolayers. *Int. J. Mol. Sci.* **2019**, *20*, 1606. [CrossRef]
28. Sahibzada, M.U.K.; Sadiq, A.; Khan, S.; Faidah, H.S.; Naseemullah; Khurram, M.; Amin, M.U.; Haseeb, A. Fabrication, characterization and in vitro evaluation of silibinin nanoparticles: An attempt to enhance its oral bioavailability. *Drug Des. Dev. Ther.* **2017**, *11*, 1453–1464. [CrossRef] [PubMed]
29. Yousaf, A.M.; Malik, U.R.; Shahzad, Y.; Hussain, T.; Khan, I.U.; Din, F.U.; Mahmood, T.; Ahsan, H.M.; Syed, A.S.; Akram, M.R. Silymarin-laden PVP-nanocontainers prepared via the electrospraying technique for improved aqueous solubility and dissolution rate. *Braz. Arch. Biol. Technol.* **2019**, *62*, e19170754. [CrossRef]
30. Song, I.S.; Cha, J.S.; Choi, M.K. Characterization, in vivo and in vitro evaluation of solid dispersion of curcumin containing d-alpha-tocopheryl polyethylene glycol 1000 succinate and mannitol. *Molecules* **2016**, *21*, 1386. [CrossRef]
31. Choi, Y.A.; Yoon, Y.H.; Choi, K.; Kwon, M.; Goo, S.H.; Cha, J.S.; Choi, M.K.; Lee, H.S.; Song, I.S. Enhanced oral bioavailability of morin administered in mixed micelle formulation with PluronicF127 and Tween80 in rats. *Biol. Pharm. Bull.* **2015**, *38*, 208–217. [CrossRef]
32. Kwon, M.; Lim, D.Y.; Lee, C.H.; Jeon, J.H.; Choi, M.K.; Song, I.S. Enhanced intestinal absorption and pharmacokinetic modulation of berberine and its metabolites through the inhibition of P-glycoprotein and intestinal metabolism in rats using a berberine mixed micelle formulation. *Pharmaceutics* **2020**, *12*, 882. [CrossRef]
33. Hwang, D.H.; Kim, Y.-I.; Cho, K.H.; Poudel, B.K.; Choi, J.Y.; Kim, D.-W.; Shin, Y.-J.; Bae, O.-N.; Yousaf, A.M.; Yong, C.S.; et al. A novel solid dispersion system for natural product-loaded medicine: Silymarin-loaded solid dispersion with enhanced oral bioavailability and hepatoprotective activity. *J. Microencapsul.* **2014**, *31*, 619–626. [CrossRef]
34. Johnson, B.M.; Charman, W.N.; Porter, C.J. An in vitro examination of the impact of polyethylene glycol 400, Pluronic P85, and vitamin E d-alpha-tocopheryl polyethylene glycol 1000 succinate on P-glycoprotein efflux and enterocyte-based metabolism in excised rat intestine. *AAPS PharmSci* **2002**, *4*, E40. [CrossRef]
35. Guan, Y.; Wang, L.Y.; Wang, B.; Ding, M.H.; Bao, Y.L.; Tan, S.W. Recent advances of D-alpha-tocopherol polyethylene glycol 1000 succinate based stimuli-responsive nanomedicine for cancer treatment. *Curr. Med. Sci.* **2020**, *40*, 218–231. [CrossRef]

36. Zhang, Z.; Tan, S.; Feng, S.S. Vitamin E TPGS as a molecular biomaterial for drug delivery. *Biomaterials* **2012**, *33*, 4889–4906. [CrossRef] [PubMed]
37. Yu, L.; Bridgers, A.; Polli, J.; Vickers, A.; Long, S.; Roy, A.; Winnike, R.; Coffin, M. Vitamin E-TPGS increases absorption flux of an HIV protease inhibitor by enhancing its solubility and permeability. *Pharm. Res.* **1999**, *16*, 1812–1817. [CrossRef] [PubMed]
38. Luiz, M.T.; Di Filippo, L.D.; Alves, R.C.; Araujo, V.H.S.; Duarte, J.L.; Marchetti, J.M.; Chorilli, M. The use of TPGS in drug delivery systems to overcome biological barriers. *Eur. Polym. J.* **2021**, *142*, 110129. [CrossRef]
39. Collnot, E.M.; Baldes, C.; Schaefer, U.F.; Edgar, K.J.; Wempe, M.F.; Lehr, C.M. Vitamin E TPGS P-glycoprotein inhibition mechanism: Influence on conformational flexibility, intracellular ATP levels, and role of time and site of access. *Mol. Pharm.* **2010**, *7*, 642–651. [CrossRef] [PubMed]
40. Collnot, E.M.; Baldes, C.; Wempe, M.F.; Kappl, R.; Huttermann, J.; Hyatt, J.A.; Edgar, K.J.; Schaefer, U.F.; Lehr, C.M. Mechanism of inhibition of P-glycoprotein mediated efflux by vitamin E TPGS: Influence on ATPase activity and membrane fluidity. *Mol. Pharm.* **2007**, *4*, 465–474. [CrossRef] [PubMed]
41. Wen, Z.; Dumas, T.E.; Schrieber, S.J.; Hawke, R.L.; Fried, M.W.; Smith, P.C. Pharmacokinetics and metabolic profile of free, conjugated, and total silymarin flavonolignans in human plasma after oral administration of milk thistle extract. *Drug Metab. Dispos.* **2008**, *36*, 65–72. [CrossRef] [PubMed]
42. Larson, A.M. Acetaminophen hepatotoxicity. *Clin. Liver Dis.* **2007**, *11*, 525–548, vi. [CrossRef] [PubMed]
43. Knight, T.R.; Kurtz, A.; Bajt, M.L.; Hinson, J.A.; Jaeschke, H. Vascular and hepatocellular peroxynitrite formation during acetaminophen toxicity: Role of mitochondrial oxidant stress. *Toxicol. Sci.* **2001**, *62*, 212–220. [CrossRef] [PubMed]
44. El-Shafey, M.M.; Abd-Allah, G.M.; Mohamadin, A.M.; Harisa, G.I.; Mariee, A.D. Quercetin protects against acetaminophen-induced hepatorenal toxicity by reducing reactive oxygen and nitrogen species. *Pathophysiology* **2015**, *22*, 49–55. [CrossRef]
45. Kwon, M.; Ji, H.K.; Goo, S.H.; Nam, S.J.; Kang, Y.J.; Lee, E.; Liu, K.H.; Choi, M.K.; Song, I.S. Involvement of intestinal efflux and metabolic instability in the pharmacokinetics of platycodin D in rats. *Drug Metab. Pharmacokinet.* **2017**, *32*, 248–254. [CrossRef]
46. Choi, M.K.; Kwon, M.; Ahn, J.H.; Kim, N.J.; Bae, M.A.; Song, I.S. Transport characteristics and transporter-based drug-drug interactions of TM-25659, a novel TAZ modulator. *Biopharm. Drug Dispos.* **2014**, *35*, 183–194. [CrossRef]
47. Song, I.S.; Jeong, H.U.; Choi, M.K.; Kwon, M.; Shin, Y.; Kim, J.H.; Lee, H.S. Interactions between cyazofamid and human drug transporters. *J. Biochem. Mol. Toxic.* **2020**, *34*, e22459. [CrossRef]
48. Choi, M.K.; Song, I.S. Interactions of ginseng with therapeutic drugs. *Arch. Pharm. Res.* **2019**, *42*, 862–878. [CrossRef]
49. Guo, Y.; Luo, J.; Tan, S.; Otieno, B.O.; Zhang, Z. The applications of Vitamin E TPGS in drug delivery. *Eur. J. Pharm. Sci.* **2013**, *49*, 175–186. [CrossRef]

pharmaceutics

Article

Characterization of P-Glycoprotein Inhibitors for Evaluating the Effect of P-Glycoprotein on the Intestinal Absorption of Drugs

Yusuke Kono [1], Iichiro Kawahara [2,†], Kohei Shinozaki [2], Ikuo Nomura [2], Honoka Marutani [1], Akira Yamamoto [2] and Takuya Fujita [1,*]

1 Laboratory of Molecular Pharmacokinetics, Graduate School of Pharmaceutical Sciences, Ritsumeikan University, 1-1-1 Noji-Higashi, Kusatsu 525-8577, Japan; y-kono@fc.ritsumei.ac.jp (Y.K.); ph0107ih@ed.ritsumei.ac.jp (H.M.)
2 Department of Biopharmaceutics, Kyoto Pharmaceutical University, 5 Misasagi Nakauchi-cho, Yamashina, Kyoto 607-8412, Japan; iichiro.kawahara@jt.com (I.K.); ky02315@poppy.kyoto-phu.ac.jp (K.S.); ky03243@poppy.kyoto-phu.ac.jp (I.N.); yamamoto@mb.kyoto-phu.ac.jp (A.Y.)
* Correspondence: fujita-t@ph.ritsumei.ac.jp; Tel.: +81-77-561-5974
† Current Affiliations: Japan Tobacco Inc., 2-chōme-2-1 Toranomon, Tokyo 105-0001, Japan.

Abstract: For developing oral drugs, it is necessary to predict the oral absorption of new chemical entities accurately. However, it is difficult because of the involvement of efflux transporters, including P-glycoprotein (P-gp), in their absorption process. In this study, we conducted a comparative analysis on the inhibitory activities of seven P-gp inhibitors (cyclosporin A, GF120918, LY335979, XR9576, WK-X-34, VX-710, and OC144-093) to evaluate the effect of P-gp on drug absorption. GF120918, LY335979, and XR9576 significantly decreased the basal-to-apical transport of paclitaxel, a P-gp substrate, across Caco-2 cell monolayers. GF120918 also inhibited the basal-to-apical transport of mitoxantrone, a breast cancer resistance protein (BCRP) substrate, in Caco-2 cells, whereas LY335979 hardly affected the mitoxantrone transport. In addition, the absorption rate of paclitaxel after oral administration in wild-type mice was significantly increased by pretreatment with LY335979, and it was similar to that in *mdr1a/1b* knockout mice. Moreover, the absorption rate of topotecan, a BCRP substrate, in wild-type mice pretreated with LY335979 was similar to that in *mdr1a/1b* knockout mice but significantly lower than that in *bcrp* knockout mice. These results indicate that LY335979 has a selective inhibitory activity for P-gp, and would be useful for evaluating the contribution of P-gp to drug absorption.

Keywords: intestinal absorption; P-glycoprotein; breast cancer resistance protein; LY335979; WK-X-34

Citation: Kono, Y.; Kawahara, I.; Shinozaki, K.; Nomura, I.; Marutani, H.; Yamamoto, A.; Fujita, T. Characterization of P-Glycoprotein Inhibitors for Evaluating the Effect of P-Glycoprotein on the Intestinal Absorption of Drugs. *Pharmaceutics* **2021**, *13*, 388. https://doi.org/10.3390/pharmaceutics13030388

Academic Editor: Im-Sook Song

Received: 10 February 2021
Accepted: 5 March 2021
Published: 15 March 2021

1. Introduction

Most new chemical entities (NCEs) are developed as oral drug formulations because the oral route has several advantages, such as its convenience, non-invasiveness, and good patient adherence [1]. However, a lot of NCEs suffer from poor intestinal permeability because they are recognized and transported by efflux transporters, such as P-glycoprotein (P-gp) and breast cancer resistant protein (BCRP), expressed on the apical membrane of small intestinal epithelial cells [2].

P-glycoprotein (P-gp) is a member of the ATP-binding cassette (ABC) transporter family and exhibits broad substrate specificity. P-gp substrates tend to have a large molecular volume, electronegative groups, and hydrogen bonding groups [3], and a large number of drugs, including anti-cancer drugs and steroids, have been identified as substrates for P-gp [4]. The intestinal permeability of P-gp substrates is known to be lower than that estimated from their lipophilicity [5]. On the other hand, several drugs, such as verapamil and quinidine, are efficiently absorbed from the small intestine, although they are typical substrates for P-gp [6]. Therefore, it is important to appropriately assess the contribution of P-gp to the intestinal permeability of NCEs in order to evaluate their oral absorption.

For evaluating the effect of P-gp on the intestinal absorption of drugs, Caco-2 cells, a human colorectal adenocarcinoma cell line, are widely used in vitro studies because Caco-2 cells express several solute carrier (SLC) transporters, ABC transporters, and metabolic enzymes [7–9]. On the other hand, *mdr1a/1b* knockout (KO) mice are often used for in vivo investigations of P-gp function [10–12]. However, there is little evidence that the physiological function of the gastrointestinal tract in *mdr1a/1b* KO mice is as same as that in wild-type (WT) mice. Therefore, it is necessary to develop a new approach to assess the in vivo contribution of P-gp to drug absorption correctly and conveniently, instead of using *mdr1a/1b* KO mice.

Previous reports have demonstrated that the effect of P-gp on in vivo drug absorption could evaluate in WT animals by using P-gp inhibitors, such as cyclosporin A (CsA) and verapamil [13,14]. However, other efflux transporters such as BCRP are expressed in the intestinal epithelial cells [15]. Moreover, the substrate specificity of P-gp extensively overlaps with that of cytochrome P450 (CYP) 3A [16], and the metabolism and elimination of these substrates have been reported to be conducted concertedly [17]. Taking the above into consideration, P-gp inhibitors would inhibit the function of not only P-gp but other efflux transporters and metabolic enzymes, and therefore P-gp inhibitors require the excellent affinity and selectivity for P-gp.

So far, various P-gp inhibitors have been developed for overcoming multidrug resistance of cancer [18–20]. First-generation P-gp inhibitors, CsA and verapamil, have pharmacological activities with low affinity and low transporter selectivity [18,19]. Since verapamil is a well-known substrate for P-gp, verapamil inhibits the function of P-gp in a competitive manner [21]. Second-generation P-gp inhibitors, including VX-710 (biricodar), lack the same pharmacological activity, and they have relatively high and selective inhibitory activity on P-gp. However, these inhibitors also inhibit CYP3A4 [18,19]. Third-generation P-gp inhibitors, including GF120918 (elacridar), LY335979 (zosuquidar), XR9576 (tariquidar), WK-X-34, and OC144-093 (ontogen), are capable of inhibiting P-gp function at a lower concentration compared with first- and second-generation P-gp inhibitors. In addition, their affinity for CYP3A4 is lower than second-generation inhibitors [18–20]. These inhibitors have been reported to improve the oral bioavailability (BA) and area under the curve (*AUC*) for plasma concentration-time of P-gp substrates [22–24]. However, there are few reports performing the comparative analysis of these P-gp inhibitors to select suitable ones for evaluating the effect of P-gp on intestinal drug absorption.

In this study, we selected seven P-gp inhibitors, CsA, GF120918, XR9576, LY335979, WK-X-34, VX-710, and OC144-093 (Figure 1), and comparatively evaluated their inhibitory activity and selectivity for P-gp both in vitro and in vivo. Here, we used paclitaxel as a well-known P-gp substrate with no affinity for BCRP for both in vitro and in vivo studies [25]. We also used mitoxantrone as a typical substrate for BCRP with a lower affinity for P-gp for in vitro studies [26]. For in vivo studies, topotecan, which we have used in pharmacokinetic studies in mice, was selected as a typical BCRP substrate [12,27].

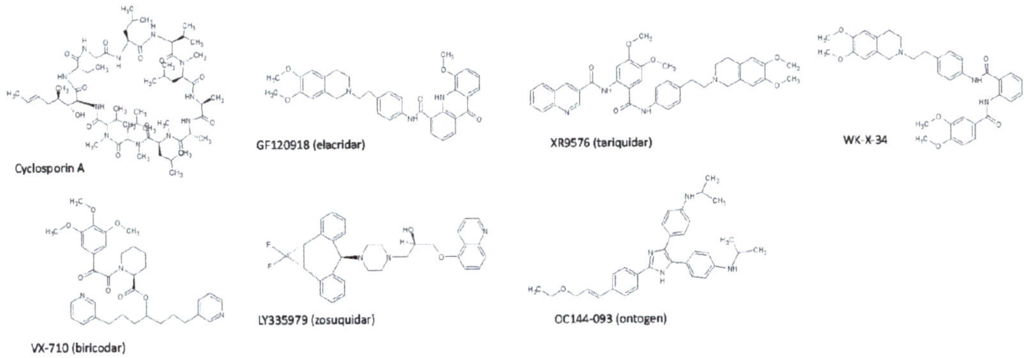

Figure 1. Chemical structures of cyclosporin A and P-glycoprotein P-gp inhibitors used in this study [20,28,29].

2. Materials and Methods

2.1. Chemicals

N-(4-(2-(6,7-Dimethoxy-3,4-dihydroisoquinolin-2(1*H*)-yl)ethyl)phenyl)-5-methoxy-9-oxo-9,10-dihydroacridine-4-carboxamide (GF120918), *N*-(2-([(4-(2-[3,4-Dihydro-6,7-dimethoxy-2(1H)-isoquinolinyl]ethyl)phenyl)amino]carbonyl)-4,5-dimethoxyphenyl)-3-quinolinecarboxamide (XR9576), paclitaxel, mitoxantrone, Hank's Balanced Salt (HBS) without phenol red and sodium bicarbonate, and solutol were obtained from Sigma-Aldrich (St. Louis, MO, USA). (*R*)-1-(4-([1a*R*,6s,10b*S*]-1,1-difluoro-1,1a,6,10b-tetrahydrodibenzo[a,e] cyclopropa(c)(7)annulen-6-yl)piperazin-1-yl)-3-(quinolin-5-yloxy)propan-2-ol trihydrochloride (LY335979) was purchased from Funakoshi (Tokyo, Japan). *N*-(2-(4-[2-(6,7-Dimethoxy-3,4-dihydro-1*H*-isochinolin-2-yl)-ethyl]phenylcarbamoyl)phenyl)-3,4-dimethoxybenzamide (WK-X-34) was purchased from Cosmo Bio Co. Ltd. (Tokyo, Japan). (*S*)-*N*-(2-Oxo-2-(3,4,5-trimethoxyphenyl)-acetyl)piperidine-2-carboxylic acid 1,7-bis(3-pyridyl)-4-heptyl ester (VX-710) was obtained from Namiki Shoji Co. Ltd. (Tokyo, Japan). (*E*)-4,4′-(2-(4-[3-ethoxyprop-1-en-1-yl]phenyl)-1H-imidazole-4,5-diyl)bis(*N*-isopropylaniline) (OC144-093) was purchased from MedKoo Biosciences, Inc. (Morrisville, NC, USA). Dulbecco's Modified Eagles Medium (DMEM), antibiotic-antimycotic mixed stock solution (×100), 0.25% trypsin/1 mM EDTA solution, nonessential amino acids, and L-glutamine were purchased from Nacalai Tesque (Kyoto, Japan). Fetal bovine serum was purchased from Thermo Fisher Scientific (Waltham, MA, USA). CsA was purchased from Tokyo Chemical Industry Co., Ltd. (Tokyo, Japan). [^{3}H]Taxol (identical to paclitaxel, specific radioactivity: 12.9 Ci/mmol) was purchased from Moravek Biochemicals (Brea, CA, USA). Transwell® was purchased from Corning (Corning, NY, USA). Topotecan HCl was purchased from ALEXIS CORPORATION (Lausen, Switzerland). WellSolve, a water-soluble solubilizing agent [30], was kindly supplied from Celeste Corporation (Tokyo, Japan). Other chemicals were all of guaranteed reagent grade and were obtained commercially.

2.2. Cell Culture

Caco-2 cells from Dainippon Sumitomo Pharma (Osaka, Japan) were cultured in DMEM supplemented with 10% heat-inactivated fetal bovine serum, 1% antibiotic-antimycotic, 1% nonessential amino acids, and 2 mM L-glutamine [31]. Cells were maintained at 37 °C in 5% CO_2/95% air and passaged upon reaching approximately 80% confluence using 0.25% trypsin/1 mM EDTA solution. For transport experiments, Caco-2 cells were grown on a polyethylene terephthalate insert (0.4 μm pore size, 12 mm diameter) at 1.0×10^5 cells/well, and cultured for 14–21 days with the replacement of the medium once every 2 days. Caco-2 cells used in this study were within the passage range of 55 through 70.

2.3. Animals

Male WT FVB mice (20–30 g, 8 weeks old), and *mdr1a/1b*$^{-/-}$ (mdr1a/1b KO) and *bcrp*$^{-/-}$ (bcrp KO) mice of the same genetic background (FVB) mice (20–30 g, 8 weeks old) were obtained from Taconic Farms (Germantown, NY, USA). Animals were maintained under standard conditions (temperature at 23 ± 1 °C with a relative humidity between 40% and 60%) with a 12 h light/dark cycle. Food and water were available *ad libitum*. All animal experiments were carried out in accordance with principles and procedures outlined in the National Institutes of Health Guide for the Care and Use of Laboratory. All experimental animal procedures were reviewed and approved by the Animal Care and Use Committee of the Kyoto Pharmaceutical University (2005-239) and Ritsumeikan University (BKC2010-27).

2.4. Transport/Inhibition Experiments

Each P-gp inhibitor was dissolved in dimethylsulfoxide (DMSO) at concentrations of 0.002, 0.006, 0.02, 0.06, 0.2, 0.6, and 2 mM, and diluted 200 times with HBS solution (HBSS) at pH 6.5 or pH 7.4. The final % of DMSO in HBSS was 0.5%. The confluent Caco-2 cells were washed with HBSS, and the transepithelial electrical resistance (TEER) values of the cell monolayer were measured using a Millicell-ERS volt-ohm meter (EMD Millipore Co., MA, USA). Then, 0.5 mL of HBSS at pH 6.5 with 0.5% DMSO in the presence or absence of each P-gp inhibitor (0.01, 0.03, 0.1, 0.3, 1, 3, and 10 μM) was added to the apical (AP) side of the cell monolayer. Similarly, 1.5 mL of HBSS at pH 7.4 with 0.5% DMSO in the presence or absence of each P-gp inhibitor was added to the basal (BL) side of the cell monolayer. After preincubating for 10 min, either AP or BL side of the cell monolayer was replaced with HBSS at pH 6.5 or pH 7.4, containing each inhibitor and paclitaxel (5 μM) or mitoxantrone (5 μM) [32,33]. Small amounts of paclitaxel and mitoxantrone were replaced with [^{3}H]taxol and [^{3}H]mitoxantrone, respectively. Lucifer yellow (100 μM) was also added to either the AP or BL side as a paracellular marker. The cells were incubated at 37 °C, and 100 μL of the medium was collected from each compartment at specified times. After the sample collection, an equal volume of fresh HBSS at pH 6.5 or pH 7.4 with 0.5% DMSO containing each inhibitor was immediately added to each compartment. After the transport experiments, the medium was collected from the donor side for measuring the drug recovery, and the TEER values of the cell monolayer were measured again.

2.5. Preparation of Drug Solution for In Vivo Study

For oral administration, paclitaxel was dissolved at a concentration of 2 mg/mL in water with 1% DMSO and 20% WellSolve. Topotecan was dissolved at a concentration of 2.5 mg/mL in water with 1% DMSO and 10% Solutol. For intravenous injection, paclitaxel was dissolved at a concentration of 1 mg/mL in water with 1% DMSO and 20% WellSolve. The solution was filtrated through a 0.22 μm sterile membrane filter (EMD Millipore Co., Tokyo, Japan).

The in vivo pharmacokinetic studies were carried out according to the portal-systemic blood concentration (P-S) difference method [12,34,35]. The mice (n = 3) were orally administered with WK-X-34 or LY335979 at a dose of 40 mg/kg or 60 mg/kg, respectively. At 10 min after the administration of P-gp inhibitors, paclitaxel was orally administered at a dose of 20 mg/kg. In another experiment, the mice (n = 3) were intravenously administered with PTX via the tail vein at a dose of 5 mg/kg. These doses of PTX are less than those used in the previous reports [36,37]. After the administration, 300 μL of blood samples were collected from the portal and abdominal veins, respectively, of the mice under isoflurane anesthesia at 0.083, 0.17, 0.5, 1, 2, 4, and 8 h. Three mice per group were used at each time point, and the mice were euthanized after the sample collection. For evaluating the absorption rate, the mice (n = 2–6) were orally administered with CsA, WK-X-34, or LY335979 at a dose of 15–30 mg/kg. Then, paclitaxel or topotecan was orally administered at a dose of 10 mg/kg or 2 mg/kg, respectively [36,38]. After the administration, 300 μL of blood samples were collected from the portal and abdominal veins, respectively, of the mice under isoflurane anesthesia at 10 or 30 min. Two to six mice per group were used at each time point, and the mice were euthanized after the sample collection. The collected blood samples were immediately centrifuged at 14,000 g for 10 min at 4 °C, and the plasma samples were obtained. The plasma samples were kept at −80 °C until sample analysis.

2.6. Analytical Methods

The radiolabeled compounds ([^{3}H]taxol and [^{3}H]mitoxantrone) were measured by mixing the samples with a scintillation cocktail (Clearsol I; Nacalai Tesque) in counting vials, followed by placing them in a liquid scintillation counter (LS-6500; Beckman Instruments, Fullerton, CA, USA). The concentration of lucifer yellow was determined by measuring fluorescent intensity at a wavelength of 428 nm (Excitation (Ex))/540 nm (Emission (EM)) using an Infinite F200 microplate reader (Tecan Japan Co. Ltd. Kanagawa, Japan).

In animal studies, 0.1 mL of plasma samples were mixed with 0.9 mL of ultra-pure water and 6 mL of ethyl acetate for extracting paclitaxel. For extracting topotecan, 0.1 mL of the samples were mixed with 0.1 mL of 0.85% phosphoric acid and 1 mL of acetonitrile. The mixture was centrifuged at 750 g for 10 min at 4 °C, and the supernatants were collected. After the evaporation of the supernatants, the residues were dissolved in the high-performance liquid chromatography (HPLC) mobile phase. Paclitaxel and topotecan were measured using HPLC (Shimadzu LC-10AS pump, SIL-10A autosampler; Shimadzu) equipped with a reverse-phase column (COSMOSIL 5C_{18}-AR-II, 3.5 μm inner diameter, 4.6 × 100 mm). The composition of the mobile phase for paclitaxel was 20 mM potassium phosphate buffer (pH 3.0) with acetonitrile, according to the following gradient program:

- 0–15.0 min, 45% acetonitrile
- 15.0–25.0 min, 45–70% acetonitrile
- 25.0–30.0 min, 70% acetonitrile
- 30.0–40.0 min, 70–45% acetonitrile
- 40.0–50.0 min, 45% acetonitrile

The composition of the mobile phase for topotecan was 10 mM phosphate buffer (pH 3.74) with methanol (76:24, *v*/*v*). The flow rate was 1.0 mL/min. Paclitaxel was detected by absorbance at 227 nm using Shimadzu SPD-20A UV spectrophotometric detector. Topotecan was analyzed by measuring fluorescence (Excitation: 361 nm, Emission: 527 nm) with a Shimadzu RF-10A XL fluorescence detector.

2.7. Data Analysis

Pharmacokinetic data analysis was performed using SigmaPlot software (HULINKS Inc., Tokyo, Japan).

For in vitro transport studies, mass balance (% recovery) was calculated using Equation (1)

$$\% \text{ recovery} = (C_{D,4\,h} \times V_D + C_{R,4\,h} \times V_R)/C_{D,0\,h} \times V_D \quad (1)$$

where $C_{D,0\,h}$ is the initial drug concentration at the donor side, $C_{D,4\,h}$ and $C_{R,4\,h}$ are the drug concentration at the donor and receiver side, respectively, at 4 h; V_D and V_R are the solution volumes at the donor and receiver side, respectively.

The apparent permeability coefficient (P_{app}) was calculated using Equation (2)

$$P_{app} = \Delta Q/\Delta t \times 1/(A \times C_0) \quad (2)$$

where $\Delta Q/\Delta t$ is the transported flux of paclitaxel or mitoxantrone, A is the surface area of the porous membrane (1.13 cm^2), and C_0 is the initial concentration of paclitaxel or mitoxantrone added to the donor compartment.

The efflux ratio (*ER*) was calculated using Equation (3)

$$ER = P_{app,BA}/P_{app,AB} \quad (3)$$

where $P_{app,AB}$ and $P_{app,BA}$ are the P_{app} values for AP-to-BL and BL-to-AP transport, respectively.

The inhibitor concentration to achieve 50% increase of $P_{app,AB}$ of paclitaxel or mitoxantrone (IC_{50}) was obtained by fitting the collected permeability data to the Equation (4)

$$P_{app,AB} = \text{Range}/[1 + (C/IC_{50})^{\gamma}] + \text{Background} \quad (4)$$

where C is the concentration of an inhibitor, γ is the Hill coefficient, Range is the arithmetic difference of $P_{app,AB}$ value between on complete inhibition and in the absence of an inhibitor; Background is the $P_{app,AB}$ in the absence of inhibitors. IC_{50} values of $P_{app,BA}$ and ER were also determined using Equation (4).

For in vivo pharmacokinetic studies, apparent F_aF_g (F_a, absorption ratio; F_g, intestinal availability) in the P-S difference method was calculated by Equation (5)

$$F_aF_g = Q_{pv} \times R_b \times (AUC_{pv} - AUC_{sys})/Dose \quad (5)$$

where Q_{pv} is the portal blood flow (72.5 mL/min/kg) [39], R_b is the blood/plasma concentration ratio, AUC_{pv} and AUC_{sys} are the AUC in the portal vein, and systemic circulation after oral administration, respectively.

The apparent absorption rate (V) was estimated using Equation (6)

$$V = Q_{pv} \times R_b \times (C_{pv} - C_{sys}) \quad (6)$$

where C_{pv} and C_{sys} are the drug concentrations in the portal vein and systemic circulation, respectively.

The elimination rate constant (k_e) was determined by using least-squares regression analysis of plasma concentration versus time curve. Elimination half-life ($t_{1/2}$) was calculated using Equation (7):

$$t_{1/2} = \ln 2/k_e \quad (7)$$

AUC and area under the first moment curve ($AUMC$) from time 0 to infinity were calculated using the trapezoidal rule. Mean residence time (MRT), total body clearance (CL_{tot}), and distribution volume at the steady state (Vd_{ss}) were calculated using the following equations:

$$MRT = AUMC/AUC \quad (8)$$

$$CL_{tot} = Dose/AUC \quad (9)$$

$$Vd_{ss} = MRT \times CL_{tot} \quad (10)$$

Mean absorption time (MAT) and absorption constant (k_a) after oral administration were calculated using the following equations

$$MAT = MRT_{oral} - MRT_{iv} \quad (11)$$

$$k_a = 1/MAT \quad (12)$$

where MRT_{oral} and MRT_{iv} are the MRT after oral and intravenous administration, respectively.

BA was calculated by Equation (13)

$$BA = AUC_{sys}/AUC_{iv} \times Dose_{iv}/Dose_{oral} \times 100 \quad (13)$$

where AUC_{iv} is the AUC after intravenous administration. $Dose_{iv}$ and $Dose_{oral}$ are administered doses in the intravenous and oral administration study, respectively.

Hepatic availability (F_h) was calculated by Equation (14):

$$F_h = BA/(F_a \times F_g) \quad (14)$$

2.8. Statistical Analysis

In vitro transport experiments were carried out in 3 independent cell passages, ranging from 55 to 70. Here, data about in vitro transport experiments are represented as the mean ± standard deviation (S.D.) for 3 experiments using Caco-2 cells with different passages with 3 replicates per *n*. For the in vivo study, 2–6 mice were used in each group, and data obtained from more than 3 mice were represented as the mean ± S.D.

3. Results

3.1. Inhibitory Effect of P-gp Inhibitors on the Transport of Paclitaxel in Caco-2 Cells

Prior to the transport study, we measured the mRNA expression levels of efflux transporters in Caco-2 cells. We could detect the mRNA expression of MDR1 and BCRP in Caco-2 cells, although their expression levels were lower than those in human small intestine cells (Figure S1). We also confirmed the barrier properties of Caco-2 cell monolayers. The transepithelial electrical resistance value of the monolayer was more than 500 $\Omega \cdot cm^2$, and it was maintained during the transport study. In addition, the $P_{app,AB}$ value of lucifer yellow, a robust paracellular permeability marker, was very low (0.10×10^{-6} cm/s). These results indicate that the tight junction in Caco-2 cell monolayers was effectively formed and maintained during the experiments. In addition, the recovery of paclitaxel in all transport studies was 85–105%. Then, we evaluated the inhibitory effects of P-gp inhibitors on the P-gp-mediated efflux of paclitaxel across Caco-2 cells. The seven P-gp inhibitors used in this study are listed in Figure 1. We observed that the AP-to-BL transport of paclitaxel was increased by the presence of P-gp inhibitors, except for OC144-093, in a concentration-dependent manner (Figure 2, Figure S2). On the other hand, the BL-to-AP transport of paclitaxel was significantly decreased by increasing inhibitor concentrations. Table 1 summarizes the IC_{50} values and Hill coefficients of each inhibitor for both AP-to-BL and BL-to-AP transport of paclitaxel across Caco-2 cell monolayers. GF120918, XR9576, LY335979, and WK-X-34 had much lower IC_{50} values than CsA. These results indicate that GF120918, XR9576, and LY335979 have potent inhibitory activities on P-gp. On the other hand, the IC_{50} value of VX-710 was higher than that of CsA. In the case of OC144-093, the transport of paclitaxel in Caco-2 cells was not changed by its addition, indicating that OC144-093 is not a suitable P-gp inhibitor.

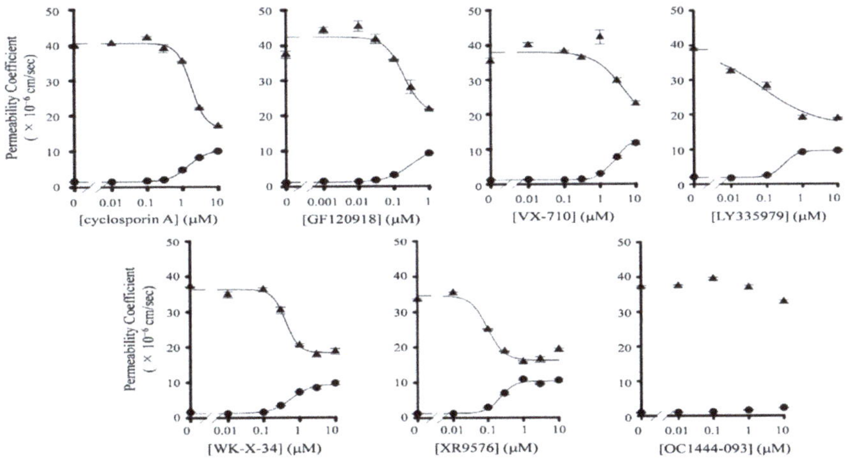

Figure 2. Inhibitory effect of P-gp inhibitors on P-gp-mediated efflux of paclitaxel in Caco-2 cells. The apical-to-basal (AP-to-BL) P_{app} value ($P_{app,AB}$) (●), and basal-to-apical (BL-to-AP) P_{app} value ($P_{app,BA}$) (▲) values were determined by the AP-to-BL and BL-to-AP transport of paclitaxel in Caco-2 cells in the presence or absence of various concentrations of P-gp inhibitors. The $P_{app,BA}$ values of paclitaxel in the presence of GF120918, LY335979, and WK-X-34 were cited from our previous report [31]. Data are represented as mean ± S.D. for three experiments using different wells from a single passage of Caco-2 cells.

Table 1. Fifty percent inhibitory concentration (IC_{50}) values and Hill coefficient of selected inhibitors on apparent AP-to-BL and BL-to-AP permeability, and efflux ratio (*ER*) of paclitaxel in Caco-2 cell monolayers.

Inhibitor	IC_{50} (nM)			Hill Coefficient		
	$P_{app,AB}$	$P_{app,BA}$	*ER*	$P_{app,AB}$	$P_{app,BA}$	*ER*
Cyclosporin A	1973 ± 21	1820 ± 126	502 ± 126	−1.63 ± 0.09	2.18 ± 0.39	1.63 ± 0.20
GF120918	319 ± 30	239 ± 97 [a]	60 ± 21	−1.28 ± 0.09	1.63 ± 1.28	1.66 ± 0.51
XR9576	234 ± 61	64 ± 40	46 ± 19	−2.10 ± 0.64	18.4 ± 4.76	3.41 ± 0.28
LY335979	427 ± 52	107 ± 59 [a]	115 ± 22	−2.23 ± 0.31	0.57 ± 0.35	1.71 ± 0.41
WK-X-34	935 ± 33	501 ± 132 [a]	214 ± 113	−10.7 ± 6.00	1.29 ± 0.42	2.07 ± 1.22
VX-710	2680 ± 53	4496 ± 84	871 ± 277	−1.84 ± 0.07	1.08 ± 0.60	1.68 ± 0.38
OC144-093	n.c.	n.c.	n.c.	n.c.	n.c.	n.c.

[a] Data from our previous report [31]. n.c., not calculated. IC_{50} on $P_{app,AB}$: the inhibitor concentration to achieve 50% increase of $P_{app,AB}$ of paclitaxel. IC_{50} on $P_{app,BA}$: the inhibitor concentration to achieve 50% decrease of $P_{app,BA}$ of paclitaxel. IC_{50} on *ER*: the inhibitor concentration to achieve 50% decrease of *ER* of paclitaxel (Figure S3). Data are represented as mean ± S.D. for three experiments using different wells from a single passage of Caco-2 cells.

3.2. Effect of P-gp Inhibitors on BCRP-Mediated Drug Efflux in Caco-2 Cells

In order to determine the selectivity of P-gp inhibitors, we investigated the effect of P-gp inhibitors on the transport of mitoxantrone, a typical BCRP substrate, across Caco-2 cells monolayers. The recovery of mitoxantrone in all transport studies was 80–85%. The AP-to-BL transport of mitoxantrone was hardly affected by increasing the concentration of P-gp inhibitors (Figure 3 and Figure S4). On the contrary, six P-gp inhibitors (not LY335979) significantly decreased the BL-to-AP transport of mitoxantrone across Caco-2 cell monolayers (Figure 3 and Figure S4). The IC_{50} value and Hill coefficients of these compounds are summarized in Table 2. The IC_{50} values of GF120918, WK-X-34, and VX-710 were similar to those cases in paclitaxel (239 nM, 501 nM, and 4496 nM, respectively), indicating that these compounds seem to act as dual inhibitors for P-gp and BCRP. On the other hand, the inhibitory activity of XR9576 and LY335979 on the BL-to-AP transport of mitoxantrone values were lower than those of paclitaxel (Table 2). These results indicate that XR9576 and LY335979, particularly LY335979, seem to be selective inhibitors for P-gp.

Table 2. IC_{50} values and Hill coefficient of selected inhibitors on apparent AP-to-BL and BL-to-AP permeability, and *ER* of mitoxantrone in Caco-2 cell monolayers.

Inhibitor	IC_{50} (nM)			Hill Coefficient		
	$P_{app,AB}$	$P_{app,BA}$	*ER*	$P_{app,AB}$	$P_{app,BA}$	*ER*
Cyclosporin A	n.c.	2038 ± 13	1708 ± 248	n.c.	1.25 ± 0.17	1.33 ± 0.25
GF120918	n.c.	298 ± 13 [a]	307 ± 23	n.c.	0.93 ± 0.41	0.92 ± 0.15
XR9576	n.c.	1000 ± 45	531 ± 162	n.c.	0.41 ± 0.08	0.44 ± 0.05
LY335979	n.c.	>10 µM [a]	>10 µM	n.c.	n.c.	n.c.
WK-X-34	n.c.	370 ± 38 [a]	328 ± 96	n.c.	1.56 ± 0.53	1.51 ± 0.41
VX-710	n.c.	2675 ± 31	1638 ± 520	n.c.	1.04 ± 0.40	0.46 ± 0.12
OC144-093	n.c.	n.c.	n.c.	n.c.	1.83 ± 0.59	3.61 ± 0.41

[a] Data from our previous report [31]. n.c., not calculated. IC_{50} on $P_{app,AB}$: the inhibitor concentration to achieve 50% increase of $P_{app,AB}$ of mitoxantrone. IC_{50} on $P_{app,BA}$: the inhibitor concentration to achieve 50% decrease of $P_{app,BA}$ of mitoxantrone. IC_{50} on *ER*: the inhibitor concentration to achieve 50% decrease of *ER* of mitoxantrone (Figure S3). Data are represented as mean ± S.D. for three experiments using different wells from a single passage of Caco-2 cells.

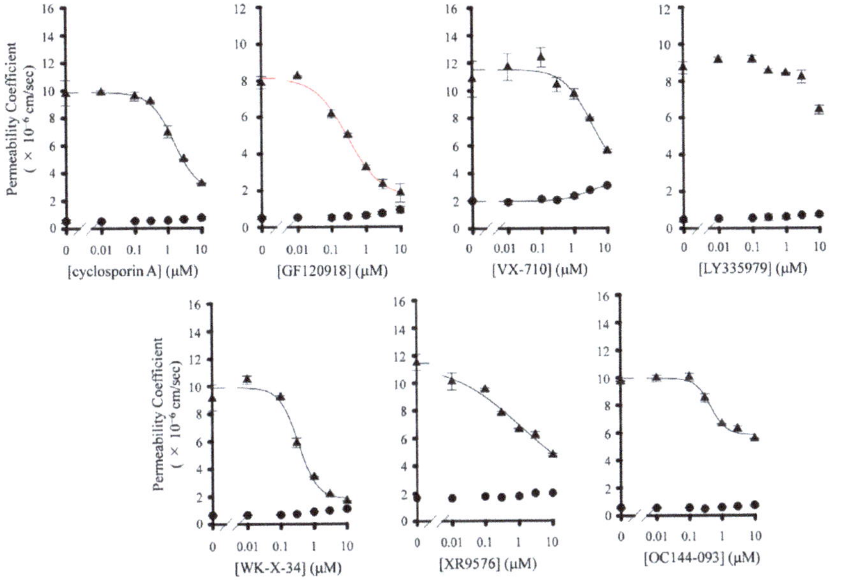

Figure 3. Inhibitory effects of P-gp inhibitors on BCRP-mediated efflux of mitoxantrone in Caco-2 cells. The $P_{app,AB}$ (•), and $P_{app,BA}$ (▲) values were determined by the AP-to-BL and BL-to-AP transport of mitoxantrone in Caco-2 cells in the presence or absence of various concentrations of P-gp inhibitors. The $P_{app,BA}$ values of mitoxantrone in the presence of GF120918, LY335979, and WK-X-34 were cited from our previous report [31]. Data are represented as mean ± S.D. for three experiments using different wells from a single passage of Caco-2 cells.

3.3. *In Vivo Inhibitory Effect of LY335979 and WK-X-34 on P-gp- and BCRP-Mediated Drug Efflux*

Since LY335979 is shown to be a potent and selective inhibitor for P-gp, we next evaluated the in vivo effect of LY335979 on the intestinal absorption of paclitaxel in mice by using the P-S difference method. In addition to LY335979, we also investigated the effect of WK-X-34 as a dual inhibitor for P-gp and BCRP.

Initially, we investigated the contribution of P-gp to the intestinal absorption of paclitaxel in mice. As shown in Figure 4A,B and Table 3, the AUC_{sys} value of paclitaxel after oral administration in *mdr1a/1b* KO mice was 3086 nM·h, which was approximately 2.8-fold higher than that in WT mice (1089 nM·h). Moreover, the AUC_{pv} value in *mdr1a/1b* KO mice was 3.3-fold as high as that in WT mice. The maximum plasma concentration (C_{max}) value of paclitaxel in systemic circulation and portal vein after oral administration in *mdr1a/1b* KO mice was 1179 nM and 2523 nM, respectively, and each value was 2.7- and 3.5-fold higher than that in WT mice (442 nM and 730 nM, respectively). On the other hand, the AUC_{iv}, Vd_{ss}, and the CL_{tot} of paclitaxel after intravenous injection were not significantly different between WT mice and *mdr1a/1b* KO mice. Based on these results, we calculated the *BA* and F_aF_g values of paclitaxel in *mdr1a/1b* KO mice (29.0% and 66.3%, respectively), and these values were 2.5- and 4.0-fold as high as those in WT mice (11.7% and 16.6%, respectively). These results indicate that the intestinal absorption of paclitaxel is restricted by P-gp expressed in the intestinal epithelium.

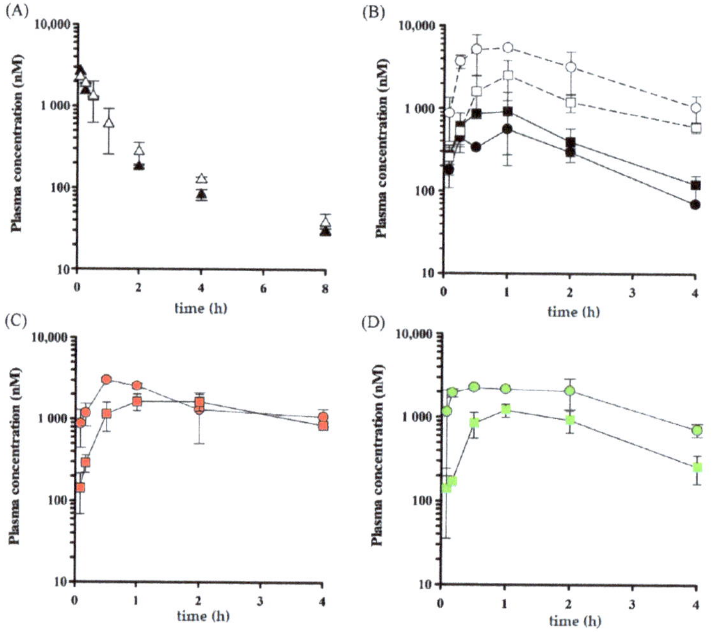

Figure 4. Plasma concentration-time profiles of paclitaxel after intravenous and oral administration with or without WK-X-34 and LY335979 pretreatment in mice. (**A**) Paclitaxel was intravenously injected into WT mice (▲) and mdr1a/1b KO mice (▵) at a dose of 5 mg/kg. (**B**) Paclitaxel was orally administered into WT mice and mdr1a/1b KO mice at a dose of 20 mg/kg. •: portal plasma concentration in WT mice, ■: systemic plasma concentration in WT mice, ○: portal plasma concentration in mdr1a/1b KO mice, and □: systemic plasma concentration in mdr1a/1b KO mice. (**C**,**D**) Paclitaxel was orally administered into WT mice at a dose of 20 mg/kg, pretreated with 40 mg/kg WK-X-34 (**C**) or 60 mg/kg LY335979 (**D**). •: portal plasma concentration, ■: systemic plasma concentration. Data are represented as mean ± S.D. (n = 3).

Table 3. Pharmacokinetic parameters of paclitaxel after intravenous and oral administration to wild type (WT) and *mdr1a/1b* knockout (KO) mice.

		WT			*mdr1a/1b* KO			WT + WK-X-34		WT + LY335979	
		IV	po		IV	po		po		po	
			pv	sys		pv	sys	pv	sys	pv	sys
Dose	(mg/kg)	5	20		5	20		20		20	
C_{max}	(nM)	—	730	442	—	2523	1179	3018	1631	2258	1208
T_{max}	(h)	—	1	1	—	1	1	0.5	2	0.5	1
AUC	(nM·hr)	2320	2002	1089	2661	6575	3086	10,615	8636	7970	3201
k_e	(h^{-1})		0.43	0.50		0.55	0.35	0.26	0.23	0.53	0.64
$t_{1/2}$	(h)	2.38	1.62	1.37	2.12	1.25	2.00	2.69	2.98	1.30	1.09
MRT	(h)	1.71	2.51	2.29	1.47	2.16	3.09	4.15	4.67	2.42	2.25
CL_{tot}	(L/h/kg)	2.52			2.20						
Vd_{ss}	(L/kg)	4.32			4.15						
BA			11.7			29.0					
F_aF_g			16.6			66.3		36.0		86.8	
F_h			70.6			45.7					

C_{max}: maximum plasma concentration; T_{max}: time to maximum plasma concentration; k_e: elimination rate constant; $t_{1/2}$: elimination half-life; *MRT*: mean residence time; F_aF_g: apparent absorption ratio (F_a) intestinal availability (F_g); F_h: hepatic availability.

We next evaluated the effect of P-gp inhibitors on the oral absorption of paclitaxel in mice. Figure 4C illustrates the plasma concentration profile of paclitaxel (20 mg/kg) after oral administration in WT mice pretreated with WK-X-34 (40 mg/kg). The calculated pharmacokinetic parameters are listed in Table 3. The k_e value of paclitaxel in systemic circulation after oral administration in WT mice pretreated with WK-X-34 (0.23 h^{-1}) was much lower than that in non-treated WT mice (0.50 h^{-1}). Moreover, it was also lower than that in non-treated *mdr1a/1b* KO mice (0.35 h^{-1}). In addition, the AUC_{sys} value of paclitaxel in WT mice pretreated with WK-X-34 was 8636 nM·h, which was approximately three times higher than that in non-treated *mdr1a/1b* KO mice (3086 nM·h). These results suggest that WK-X-34 inhibits transporters, apart from P-gp, or metabolic enzymes involved in the elimination process of paclitaxel.

We also assessed the pharmacokinetic profile of paclitaxel (20 mg/kg) after oral administration in WT or *mdr1a/1b* KO mice with or without LY335979 pretreatment (60 mg/kg). We preliminarily confirmed that this dose of LY335979 is enough to potently inhibit P-gp in the murine small intestine, and this dose is reasonable because the previous report used LY335979 at a dose of 25–80 mg/kg [40]. The C_{max} value of paclitaxel in systemic circulation after oral administration in WT mice pretreated with LY335979 was 1208 nM, which was approximately 2.7-fold higher than that in non-treated WT mice (442 nM) and as same as that in non-treated *mdr1a/1b* KO mice (1179 nM) (Figure 4D, Table 3). The C_{max} value of paclitaxel in portal vein in LY335979-pretreated WT mice was also similar to that in non-treated *mdr1a/1b* KO mice. However, the AUC_{sys} and AUC_{pv} values of paclitaxel after oral administration in WT mice pretreated with LY335979 were 3201 nM·h and 7970 nM·h, respectively, and these were slightly higher than those in *mdr1a/1b* KO mice (3086 nM·h and 6575 nM·h, respectively). Furthermore, the F_aF_g value in WT mice pretreated with LY335979 was 86.8%, which was approximately 5.2- and 1.3-fold higher than that in non-treated WT mice and *mdr1a/1b* KO mice, respectively (16.6% and 66.3%, respectively). These results suggest that LY335979 has the potential to inhibit the metabolic enzymes in intestinal epithelial cells. On the other hand, the k_e value of paclitaxel in systemic circulation after oral administration in WT mice pretreated with LY335979 (0.64 h^{-1}) was not lower than that in non-treated WT mice and *mdr1a/1b* KO mice (0.50 and 0.35 h^{-1}). These results suggest that LY335979 hardly affects the metabolic enzymes involved in the elimination process of paclitaxel.

3.4. Effect of P-gp Inhibitors on the Absorption Rate of Paclitaxel

We have evaluated the effect of P-gp inhibitors on the intestinal absorption of paclitaxel in mice by using P-S difference method; however, there was a risk of overestimation or underestimation of the pharmacokinetics of paclitaxel because of the duration of P-gp inhibitors and the effect of inhibitors on metabolic enzymes involved in absorptive and/or elimination process of paclitaxel. Therefore, in order to minimize the effect of P-gp inhibitors on factors except for P-gp, we next investigated the absorption rate (V) of paclitaxel in mice by P-S difference method with two improvements; to decrease a dose of P-gp inhibitors and to carry out the blood sampling at early time points. In this experiment, a dose of paclitaxel was also decreased to 10 mg/kg, along with the reduction in a dose of P-gp inhibitors.

Table 4 shows the plasma concentration of paclitaxel (10 mg/kg) in systemic circulation and portal vein at 10 min after oral absorption in mice pretreated with P-gp inhibitors, and the absorption rates were also calculated. The C_{sys} value was not significantly different between WT mice and *mdr1a/1b* KO mice. However, the C_{pv} value in *mdr1a/1b* KO mice was 967 nM, which was higher than that in WT mice (439 nM). Moreover, the V value in mdr1a/1b mice (54.3 nmol/min/kg) was approximately 3.5-fold higher than that in WT mice (15.7 nmol/min/kg). When WT mice were pretreated with CsA and WK-X-34, the V value of paclitaxel was increased to 38.7 nmol/min/kg and 39.8 nmol/min/kg, respectively, which were slightly lower than that in *mdr1a/1b* KO mice. On the other hand, the V value in WT mice was significantly increased by the pretreatment with LY335979

(60.2 nmol/min/kg). This *V* value was as same as that in WT mice. In addition, the C_{sys} value in WT mice pretreated with CsA, LY335979, and WK-X-34 was similar to that in *mdr1a/1b* KO mice. Thus, we succeeded in evaluating the effect of P-gp inhibitors on the absorption of paclitaxel with minimizing their influence on the metabolism.

Table 4. Absorption rate of paclitaxel (10 mg/kg) at 10 min after its oral administration with or without P-gp inhibitors in WT and *mdr1a/1b* KO mice.

	n	+Inhibitor (mg/kg)	C_{pv} (nM)	C_{sys} (nM)	$C_{pv} - C_{sys}$ (nM)	Absorption Rate (*V*) (nmol/min/kg)
WT mice	3		439 ± 98	223 ± 76	216 ± 80	15.7
+Cyclosporin A	5	30	708 ± 77	263 ± 168	534 ± 102	38.7
+LY335979	6	30	1009 ± 149	202 ± 52	830 ± 140	60.2
+WK-X-34	3	30	746 ± 57	196 ± 64	549 ± 7.5	39.8
mdr1a/1b KO mice	6		967 ± 191	218 ± 100	749 ± 165	54.3

Data are represented as mean ± S.D. C_{pv}: portal vein concentration; C_{sys}: systemic circulation concentration.

We also assessed the plasma concentration of paclitaxel (10 mg/kg) in systemic circulation and in the portal vein and its absorption rate at 30 min after oral absorption in mice pretreated with P-gp inhibitors (Table 5). The C_{sys} value in *mdr1a/1b* KO mice was slightly higher than that in WT mice, whereas the C_{pv} value in *mdr1a/1b* KO mice was significantly higher than that in WT mice. Consequently, the *V* value in *mdr1a/1b* KO mice was 63.7 nmol/min/kg, which was approximately 5.1-fold higher than that in WT mice (12.4 nmol/min/kg). Although the C_{sys} and C_{pv} values in WT mice were increased by the pretreatment with P-gp inhibitors at a concentration of 15 mg/kg, the differences were not remarkable. On the other hand, the C_{sys}, C_{pv}, and *V* values in WT mice were all increased significantly when the mice were pretreated with 30 mg/kg of P-gp inhibitors. In particular, the *V* values in WT mice were increased to 66.4 nmol/min/kg by the pretreatment with LY335979, which was almost as same as that in *mdr1a/1b* KO mice. Meanwhile, the *V* values in CsA-pretreated WT mice were lower than that in *mdr1a/1b* KO mice. Although the C_{sys} value of paclitaxel in WT mice pretreated with 30 mg/kg of P-gp inhibitors was higher than that in non-treated WT mice and *mdr1a/1b* KO mice, LY335979 exhibited the least effect on the C_{sys}. These results suggest that LY335979 has the least effect on the metabolic enzymes for paclitaxel even at 30 min after oral administration of paclitaxel. On the other hand, the *V* and C_{sys} values in WK-X-34-pretreated WT mice were higher than that in *mdr1a/1b* KO mice, suggesting that WK-X-34 greatly affects the metabolic process of paclitaxel.

Table 5. Absorption rate of paclitaxel (10 mg/kg) at 30 min after its oral administration with or without P-gp inhibitor in WT and *mdr1a/1b* KO mice.

	n	+Inhibitor (mg/kg)	C_{pv} (nM)	C_{sys} (nM)	$C_{pv} - C_{sys}$ (nM)	Absorption Rate V (nmol/min/kg)
WT mice	3		328 ± 41	135 ± 41	165 ± 61	12.4
+Cyclosporin A	2	15	540	315	225	16.9
+LY335979	3	15	626 ± 82	368 ± 30	259 ± 45	19.5
+WK-X-34	3	15	674 ± 139	238 ± 63	437 ± 127	32.9
+Cyclosoprin A	3	30	1488 ± 146	829 ± 166	657 ± 38	49.4
+LY335979	3	30	1407 ± 70	524 ± 58	883 ± 59	66.4
+WK-X-34	3	30	2069 ± 204	757 ± 100	1311 ± 87	98.6
mdr1a/1b KO mice	3		1092 ± 118	245 ± 69	847 ± 144	63.7

Data are represented as mean ± S.D.

3.5. Effect of P-gp Inhibitors on BCRP-Mediated Efflux In Vivo

In order to determine the selectivity of P-gp inhibitors for p-gp in vivo, we also assessed the effect of P-gp inhibitors on the C_{sys}, C_{pv}, and V values of topotecan, a substrate for BCRP, at 30 min after oral administration in mice. As shown in Table 6, the C_{sys} value of topotecan in *mdr1a/1b* KO mice was similar to that in WT mice, whereas the C_{sys} value in *bcrp* KO mice was higher than that in WT mice and *mdr1a/1b* KO mice. Moreover, the C_{pv} value in *bcrp* KO mice was 469 nM, and it was approximately twice as high as that in WT mice and *mdr1a/1b* KO mice. Furthermore, the V value of topotecan in *bcrp* KO mice was 5.30 nmol/min/kg, which was approximately 4.1-fold and 2.4-fold higher than that in WT mice and *mdr1a/1b* KO mice, respectively. These results indicate that BCRP greatly influences the intestinal absorption of topotecan. We also observed that the V value of topotecan in WT mice was significantly increased by the pretreatment with 30 mg/kg of WK-X-34, and reached the same level as in *bcrp* KO mice. On the other hand, LY335979 showed little effect on the V value of topotecan in WT mice, and this value was as same as that in *mdr1a/1b* KO mice. These results suggest that WK-X 34 has a potent inhibitory activity for BCRP, whereas LY335979 has little affinity for BCRP.

Table 6. Absorption rate of topotecan (2 mg/kg) at 30 min after its oral administration with or without P-gp inhibitor in WT, *mdr1a/1b* KO and *bcrp* KO mice.

	n	+Inhibitor (mg/kg)	C_{pv} (nM)	C_{sys} (nM)	$C_{pv} - C_{sys}$ (nM)	Absorption Rate V (nmol/min/kg)
WT mice	3		196 ± 29	179 ± 25	17.1 ± 5.7	1.29
+Cyclosporin A	2	30	298	240	58.5	4.40
+LY335979	3	30	249 ± 26	228 ± 22.3	20.5 ± 9.7	1.54
+WK-X-34	3	30	464 ± 53	388 ± 19	76.6 ± 27	5.76
mdr1a/1b KO mice	3		236 ± 30	207 ± 28	28.9 ± 8.4	2.17
bcrp KO mice	3		469 ± 64	398 ± 88	70.5 ± 20	5.30

Data are represented as mean ± S.D. *bcrp*: breast cancer resistance protein.

4. Discussion

In this study, we assessed the usability of P-gp inhibitors for evaluating the influence of P-gp on intestinal absorption of drugs both in vitro and in vivo.

In vitro transport studies, we determined the $P_{app,AB}$, and $P_{app,BA}$ of paclitaxel and mitoxantrone in Caco-2 cells with or without P-gp inhibitors. We observed that the IC_{50} value of each P-gp inhibitor for $P_{app,AB}$ of paclitaxel was higher than that for $P_{app,BA}$ of paclitaxel. In addition, the increase in the $P_{app,AB}$ of mitoxantrone by the presence of P-gp inhibitors was hardly observed, and consequently, the IC_{50} of P-gp inhibitors for $P_{app,AB}$ of mitoxantrone could not be determined. These results suggest that the inhibitory efficiency of P-gp inhibitors against P-gp- and BCRP-mediated drug transport is lower in absorptive direction than in secretory direction. Troutman et al. have demonstrated that apparent K_m for P-gp-mediated efflux of P-gp substrates in Caco-2 cells was much larger in absorptive direction than in secretory direction [41]. This finding is in accordance with our present observation. In addition, we also considered that the difference in the inhibitory activity of P-gp inhibitors between absorptive direction and secretory direction would be responsible for the inaccurate ER values (Figure S3). Therefore, we decided to evaluate the inhibitory effects of P-gp inhibitors on P-gp and BCRP based on the IC_{50} for $P_{app,BA}$ of paclitaxel, and mitoxantrone.

In Caco-2 transport studies, we observed that GF120918, WK-X-34, and VX-710 had the inhibitory effect for both P-gp and BCRP. Jonker et al. demonstrated that the AUC of topotecan after oral administration in *mdr1a/1b* KO mice treated with GF120918 was approximately six-fold higher than that in non-treated mice [42]. Other studies have also reported that GF120918 significantly increases the plasma and brain concentration of dasatinib and crizotinib, which is a substrate for P-gp and BCRP, respectively, in WT mice up to the equal level in *mdr1a/1b* or *bcrp* KO mice [43,44]. These findings indicate that GF120918 is a potent dual inhibitor for P-gp and BCRP. WK-X-34 has also been reported to significantly inhibit the cellular uptake of mitoxantrone in BCRP-overexpressing MCF7 cells [20]. Since GF120918 and WK-X-34 have similar chemical structures, including N-ethyl-tetrahydroisoquinoline, which frequently appears in potent P-gp inhibitors [45], this structure would have the potential to be recognized by BCRP. VX-710 has also been shown to be capable of inhibiting the uptake of mitoxantrone and SN-38 into BCRP-overexpressing MCF7 AdVp3000 cells [46]. These findings support the present results. Taken together, these three P-gp inhibitors, especially GF120918 and WK-X-34, would be useful for evaluating the pharmacokinetics of drugs under conditions of inhibiting the efflux transporters.

We also revealed that XR9576 and LY335979 strongly inhibited P-gp whereas their affinity for BCRP was relatively low in Caco-2 permeation studies. In particular, the IC_{50} value of LY335979 for $P_{\mathrm{app,BA}}$ of paclitaxel was less than one hundredth lower than that of mitoxantrone. These results agree with the report of Shepard et al., demonstrating that the affinity of LY335979 for P-gp is 100-fold higher than that for BCRP [47]. On the other hand, the IC_{50} value of XR9576 for $P_{\mathrm{app,BA}}$ of paclitaxel was only 15.6-fold lower than that of mitoxantrone. Pick et al. have reported that the IC_{50} value of XR9576 for P-gp-mediated Hoechst 33342 transport is approximately 20.1-fold lower than that for BCRP-mediated Hoechst 33342 transport [48]. These observations are in accordance with our present results. To summarize these findings, XR9576 and LY335979, particularly LY335979, were found to be potent and selective P-gp inhibitors.

Then, we evaluated the effect of WK-X-34 and LY335979 as a dual inhibitor and P-gp-selective inhibitor, respectively, on the intestinal absorption of paclitaxel in vivo. So far, several P-gp inhibitors have been reported to be evaluated their effects on the intestinal absorption of paclitaxel in vivo [35,49,50]. However, most of those studies determined the pharmacokinetic parameters of paclitaxel from the plasma concentration in systemic circulation. On the other hand, here, we applied the P-S difference method to determine the pharmacokinetic parameters of paclitaxel because this method would be useful for obtaining the exact F_aF_g values.

We observed that WK-X-34 delayed the elimination of paclitaxel, suggesting that WK-X-34 inhibits not only efflux transporters, including P-gp and BCRP, but also metabolic enzymes. It has been reported that paclitaxel is mainly metabolized by CYP2C8 and CYP3A4 [51,52]. In addition, we also confirmed that the AUC_{pv} of paclitaxel after oral administration in WT mice pretreated with WK-X-34 was only 1.6-fold higher than that in non-treated *mdr1a/1b* KO mice, and the F_aF_g value in WT mice pretreated with WK-X-34 was only half as high as that in non-treated *mdr1a/1b* KO mice. This may be due to the incomplete inhibition of P-gp by 40 mg/kg of WK-X-34 and the shorter action of WK-X-34. This would be the first report evaluating the effect of WK-X-34 on intestinal drug absorption by its oral administration. For effective and safe use of WK-X-34, further studies are needed to evaluate its appropriate dose in view of the influence on the metabolic enzymes and toxicity on mice.

In contrast to WK-X-34, the AUC_{sys} value of paclitaxel after oral administration in WT mice pretreated with LY335979 was approximately 2.9-fold higher than that in non-treated WT mice and comparable to that in *mdr1a/1b* KO mice. Moreover, LY335979 hardly affected the elimination process of paclitaxel. Dantzig et al. has demonstrated that the affinity of LY335979 for CYP3A4 is approximately 60-fold lower than that for P-gp [53]. This observation supports our results. However, the F_aF_g value of paclitaxel after oral administration in WT mice pretreated with LY335979 was higher than that in non-treated *mdr1a/1b* KO mice, suggesting that LY335979 could inhibit CYP3A4 in small intestinal epithelial cells.

To further assess the effect of P-gp inhibitors on P-gp-mediated efflux of paclitaxel in mice without their influence on the metabolic process of paclitaxel, we carried out the measurement of plasma concentration of paclitaxel at the early phase after oral administration with a lower concentration of LY335979. The C_{sys} of paclitaxel at 10 min after oral administration in WT mice pretreated with P-gp inhibitors did not significantly differ from that in *mdr1a/1b* KO mice. These results indicate that the P-S difference method would achieve the evaluation of the effect of P-gp inhibitors on the intestinal absorption of paclitaxel with minimal influence on the metabolic process. In addition, we also observed that the C_{sys} and C_{pv} of topotecan at 30 min after oral administration in WT mice pretreated with LY335979 was almost as same as those in WT mice and *mdr1a/1b* KO mice. These results indicate that LY335979 hardly affects the BCRP-mediated intestinal drug absorption.

In conclusion, the present study has revealed that LY335979 would be the most valuable P-gp inhibitor for evaluating the sole contribution of P-gp to drug absorption. Using LY335979, we have also succeeded in the evaluation of the impact of P-gp on intestinal drug absorption without the influence on the metabolic process by using absorption rate. Since LY335979 inhibits P-gp function by allosterically interfering ATP hydrolysis [54], the present approach would be available for evaluating the contribution of P-gp to the intestinal absorption of various drugs, including BCS class IV drugs, without an increase in the dose of LY335979. On the other hand, multidrug resistance-associated protein 2 (MRP2) is expressed on the apical membrane of the intestinal epithelial cells as well as P-gp and BCRP, and therefore, further studies considering MRP2 are needed to demonstrate the selectivity of LY335979 for P-gp. Nevertheless, these findings make a valuable contribution toward evaluating the contribution of P-gp to drug absorption without using *mdr1a/1b* KO mice.

Supplementary Materials: The following are available online at https://www.mdpi.com/1999-4923/13/3/388/s1, Figure S1: Relative mRNA expression levels of MDR1, BCRP, MRP2, and CYP3A4 in human small intestine, colon and Caco-2 cells. Relative mRNA expression levels were determined by real-time RT-PCR. GAPDH was selected as an endogenous RNA control to normalize for difference in amount of total RNA. Figure S2: Bidirectional transport of paclitaxel across Caco-2 cell monolayers. The apical-to-basal (A) and basal-to-apical (B) transport of paclitaxel (5 μM) in the presence or absence of various concentrations of P-gp inhibitors. Data are represented as mean ± S.D. for 3 experiments using different well in a single passage of Caco-2 cells. Figure S3: Efflux ratio (*ER*) of paclitaxel and mitoxantrone in Caco-2 cells with P-gp inhibitors. The *ER* values were calculated using the mean values of $P_{app,AB}$ and $P_{app,BA}$ of paclitaxel and mitoxantrone in Caco-2 cells in the presence or absence of various concentrations of P-gp inhibitors. Figure S4: Bidirectional transport of mitoxantrone across Caco-2 cell monolayers. The apical-to-basal (A) and basal-to-apical (B) transport of mitoxantrone (5 μM) in the presence or absence of various concentrations of P-gp inhibitors. Data are represented as mean ± S.D. for 3 experiments using different well in a single passage of Caco-2 cells.

Author Contributions: Conceptualization, A.Y. and T.F.; methodology, T.F.; validation, T.F.; formal analysis, Y.K., I.K., K.S., H.M., and I.N.; investigation, Y.K., I.K., K.S., H.M., and I.N.; data curation, T.F.; writing—original draft preparation, Y.K.; writing—review and editing, Y.K., I.K., and T.F.; visualization, Y.K. and T.F.; supervision, A.Y. and T.F.; project administration, T.F. All authors have read and agreed to the published version of the manuscript.

Funding: This study was supported by a grant from the Strategic Research Foundation at Private Universities and Grant-in-Aids for Scientific Research (C) (17K08430) from the Ministry of Education, Culture, Sports, Science and Technology of Japan; the Ritsumeikan Global Innovation Research Organization (R-GIRO) Project at Ritsumeikan University.

Institutional Review Board Statement: The study was conducted according to the guidelines of the Declaration of Helsinki, and approved by the Ethics Committee of Kyoto Pharmaceutical University (2005-239 (April 2005)) and Ritsumeikan University (BKC2010-27 (April 2011) and BKC2017-048 (Apirl 2018)).

Informed Consent Statement: Not applicable.

Data Availability Statement: Data is contained within the article and its supplementary materials.

Acknowledgments: We would like to thank Satoyo Nishikawa (Kyoto Pharmaceutical University) for their technical assistance.

Conflicts of Interest: The authors declare no conflict of interest.

References

1. Shekhawat, P.B.; Pokharkar, V.B. Understanding Peroral Absorption: Regulatory Aspects and Contemporary Approaches to Tackling Solubility and Permeability Hurdles. *Acta Pharm. Sin. B* **2017**, *7*, 260–280. [CrossRef]
2. Matsuda, Y.; Konno, Y.; Hashimoto, T.; Nagai, M.; Taguchi, T.; Satsukawa, M.; Yamashita, S. In Vivo Assessment of the Impact of Efflux Transporter on Oral Drug Absorption Using Portal Vein–Cannulated Rats. *Drug Metab. Dispos.* **2013**, *41*, 1514–1521. [CrossRef]
3. Miyata, K.-I.; Nakagawa, Y.; Kimura, Y.; Ueda, K.; Akamatsu, M. Structure–Activity Relationships of Dibenzoylhydrazines for the Inhibition of P-Glycoprotein-Mediated Quinidine Transport. *Bioorganic Med. Chem.* **2016**, *24*, 3184–3191. [CrossRef]
4. Matheny, C.J.; Lamb, M.W.; Brouwer, K.L.R.; Pollack, G.M. Pharmacokinetic and Pharmacodynamic Implications of P-glycoprotein Modulation. *Pharmacother. J. Hum. Pharmacol. Drug Ther.* **2001**, *21*, 778–796. [CrossRef]
5. Terao, T.; Hisanaga, E.; Sai, Y.; Tamai, I.; Tsuji, A. Active Secretion of Drugs from the Small Intestinal Epithelium in Rats by P-Glycoprotein Functioning as an Absorption Barrier. *J. Pharm. Pharmacol.* **1996**, *48*, 1083–1089. [CrossRef]
6. Jones, C.R.; Hatley, O.J.D.; Ungell, A.-L.; Hilgendorf, C.; Peters, S.A.; Rostami-Hodjegan, A. Gut Wall Metabolism. Application of Pre-Clinical Models for the Prediction of Human Drug Absorption and First-Pass Elimination. *AAPS J.* **2016**, *18*, 589–604. [CrossRef]
7. Sambuy, Y.; De Angelis, I.; Ranaldi, G.; Scarino, M.L.; Stammati, A.; Zucco, F. The Caco-2 Cell Line as a Model of the Intestinal Barrier: Influence of Cell and Culture-Related Factors on Caco-2 Cell Functional Characteristics. *Cell Biol. Toxicol.* **2005**, *21*, 1–26. [CrossRef]
8. Van Breemen, R.B.; Li, Y. Caco-2 Cell Permeability Assays to Measure Drug Absorption. *Expert Opin. Drug Metab. Toxicol.* **2005**, *1*, 175–185. [CrossRef]
9. Volpe, D.A. Variability in Caco-2 and MDCK Cell-Based Intestinal Permeability Assays. *J. Pharm. Sci.* **2008**, *97*, 712–725. [CrossRef]
10. Oostendorp, R.L.; Buckle, T.; Beijnen, J.H.; Van Tellingen, O.; Schellens, J.H.M. The Effect of P-gp (Mdr1a/1b), BCRP (Bcrp1) and P-gp/BCRP Inhibitors on the in Vivo Absorption, Distribution, Metabolism and Excretion of Imatinib. *Investig. New Drugs* **2009**, *27*, 31–40. [CrossRef] [PubMed]
11. Holmstock, N.; Mols, R.; Annaert, P.; Augustijns, P. In Situ Intestinal Perfusion in Knockout Mice Demonstrates Inhibition of Intestinal P-Glycoprotein by Ritonavir Causing Increased Darunavir Absorption. *Drug Metab. Dispos.* **2010**, *38*, 1407–1410. [CrossRef]
12. Kawahara, I.; Nishikawa, S.; Yamamoto, A.; Kono, Y.; Fujita, T. Assessment of Contribution of BCRP to Intestinal Absorption of Various Drugs Using Portal-Systemic Blood Concentration Difference Model in Mice. *Pharmacol. Res. Perspect.* **2019**, *8*, 00544. [CrossRef] [PubMed]
13. Sababi, M.; Borgå, O.; Hultkvist-Bengtsson, U. The Role of P-Glycoprotein in Limiting Intestinal Regional Absorption of Digoxin in Rats. *Eur. J. Pharm. Sci.* **2001**, *14*, 21–27. [CrossRef]
14. Dey, S.; Gunda, S.; Mitra, A.K. Pharmacokinetics of Erythromycin in Rabbit Corneas after Single-Dose Infusion: Role of P-Glycoprotein as a Barrier to in Vivo Ocular Drug Absorption. *J. Pharmacol. Exp. Ther.* **2004**, *311*, 246–255. [CrossRef] [PubMed]
15. König, J.; Müller, F.; Fromm, M.F. Transporters and Drug-Drug Interactions: Important Determinants of Drug Disposition and Effects. *Pharmacol. Rev.* **2013**, *65*, 944–966. [CrossRef]
16. Wacher, V.J.; Wu, C.-Y.; Benet, L.Z. Overlapping Substrate Specificities and Tissue Distribution of Cytochrome P450 3A and P-Glycoprotein: Implications for Drug Delivery and Activity in Cancer Chemotherapy. *Mol. Carcinog.* **1995**, *13*, 129–134. [CrossRef] [PubMed]
17. Kim, R.B.; Wandel, C.; Leake, B.; Cvetkovic, M.; Fromm, M.F.; Dempsey, P.J.; Roden, M.M.; Belas, F.; Chaudhary, A.K.; Roden, D.M.; et al. Interrelationship Between Substrates and Inhibitors of Human CYP3A and P-Glycoprotein. *Pharm. Res.* **1999**, *16*, 408–414. [CrossRef]
18. Varma, M.V.; Ashokraj, Y.; Dey, C.S.; Panchagnula, R. P-Glycoprotein Inhibitors and Their Screening: A Perspective from Bioavailability Enhancement. *Pharmacol. Res.* **2003**, *48*, 347–359. [CrossRef]
19. Modok, S.; Mellor, H.; Callaghan, R. Modulation of Multidrug Resistance Efflux Pump Activity to Overcome Chemoresistance in Cancer. *Curr. Opin. Pharmacol.* **2006**, *6*, 350–354. [CrossRef]
20. Jekerle, V.; Klinkhammer, W.; Scollard, D.A.; Breitbach, K.; Reilly, R.M.; Piquette-Miller, M.; Wiese, M. In Vitro Andin Vivo Evaluation of WK-X-34, a Novel Inhibitor of P-Glycoprotein and BCRP, Using Radio Imaging Techniques. *Int. J. Cancer* **2006**, *119*, 414–422. [CrossRef]
21. Lin, J.H. Drug–Drug Interaction Mediated by Inhibition and Induction of P-Glycoprotein. *Adv. Drug Deliv. Rev.* **2003**, *55*, 53–81. [CrossRef]
22. Yahanda, A.M.; Alder, K.M.; Fisher, G.A.; Brophy, N.; Halsey, J.; Hardy, R.I.; Gosland, M.P.; Lum, B.L.; Sikic, B.I. Phase I Trial of Etoposide with Cyclosporine as a Modulator of Multidrug Resistance. *J. Clin. Oncol.* **1992**, *10*, 1624–1634. [CrossRef]
23. Guns, E.S.; Denyssevych, T.; Dixon, R.; Bally, M.B.; Mayer, L. Drug Interaction Studies between Paclitaxel (Taxol) and OC144-093—A New Modulator of MDR in Cancer Chemotherapy. *Eur. J. Drug Metab. Pharmacokinet.* **2002**, *27*, 119–126. [CrossRef]

24. Callies, S.; De Alwis, D.P.; Wright, J.G.; Sandler, A.; Burgess, M.; Aarons, L. A Population Pharmacokinetic Model for Doxorubicin and Doxorubicinol in the Presence of a Novel MDR Modulator, Zosuquidar Trihydrochloride (LY335979). *Cancer Chemother. Pharmacol.* **2003**, *51*, 107–118. [CrossRef] [PubMed]
25. Litman, T.; Brangi, M.; Hudson, E.; Fetsch, P.; Abati, A.; Ross, D.D.; Miyake, K.; Resau, J.H.; Bates, S.E. The Multidrug-Resistant Phenotype Associated with Overexpression of the New ABC Half-Transporter, MXR (ABCG2). *J. Cell Sci.* **2000**, *113*, 2011–2021.
26. Kodaira, H.; Kusuhara, H.; Ushiki, J.; Fuse, E.; Sugiyama, Y. Kinetic Analysis of the Cooperation of P-Glycoprotein (P-gp/Abcb1) and Breast Cancer Resistance Protein (Bcrp/Abcg2) in Limiting the Brain and Testis Penetration of Erlotinib, Flavopiridol, and Mitoxantrone. *J. Pharmacol. Exp. Ther.* **2010**, *333*, 788–796. [CrossRef]
27. De Vries, N.A.; Zhao, J.; Kroon, E.; Buckle, T.; Beijnen, J.H.; Van Tellingen, O. P-Glycoprotein and Breast Cancer Resistance Protein: Two Dominant Transporters Working Together in Limiting the Brain Penetration of Topotecan. *Clin. Cancer Res.* **2007**, *13*, 6440–6449. [CrossRef]
28. Newman, M.J.; Rodarte, J.C.; Bendatoul, K.D.; Romano, S.J.; Zhang, C.; Krane, S.; Moran, E.J.; Uyeda, R.T.; Dixon, R.; Guns, E.S.; et al. Discovery and Characterization of OC144-093, a Novel Inhibitor of P-Glycoprotein-Mediated Multidrug Resistance. *Cancer Res.* **2000**, *60*, 2964–2972.
29. Zhang, H.; Xu, H.; Ashby, C.R., Jr.; Assaraf, Y.G.; Chen, Z.-S.; Liu, H.-M. Chemical Molecular-Based Approach to Overcome Multidrug Resistance in Cancer by Targeting P-Glycoprotein (P-gp). *Med. Res. Rev.* **2021**, *41*, 525–555. [CrossRef]
30. Hamid, K.A.; Lin, Y.; Gao, Y.; Katsumi, H.; Sakane, T.; Yamamoto, A. The Effect of Wellsolve, a Novel Solubilizing Agent, on the Intestinal Barrier Function and Intestinal Absorption of Griseofulvin in Rats. *Biol. Pharm. Bull.* **2009**, *32*, 1898–1905. [CrossRef]
31. Kawahara, I.; Nishikawa, S.; Yamamoto, A.; Kono, Y.; Fujita, T. The Impact of Breast Cancer Resistance Protein (BCRP/ABCG2) on Drug Transport Across Caco-2 Cell Monolayers. *Drug Metab. Dispos.* **2020**, *48*, 491–498. [CrossRef] [PubMed]
32. Roger, E.; Lagarce, F.; Garcion, E.; Benoit, J.-P. Reciprocal Competition between Lipid Nanocapsules and P-GP for Paclitaxel Transport across Caco-2 Cells. *Eur. J. Pharm. Sci.* **2010**, *40*, 422–429. [CrossRef]
33. Sugihara, N.; Kuroda, N.; Watanabe, F.; Choshi, T.; Kamishikiryo, J.; Seo, M. Effects of Catechins and Their Related Compounds on Cellular Accumulation and Efflux Transport of Mitoxantrone in Caco-2 Cell Monolayers. *J. Food Sci.* **2017**, *82*, 1224–1230. [CrossRef]
34. Hoffman, D.J.; Seifert, T.; Borre, A.; Nellans, H.N. Method to Estimate the Rate and Extent of Intestinal Absorption in Conscious Rats Using an Absorption Probe and Portal Blood Sampling. *Pharm. Res.* **1995**, *12*, 889–894. [CrossRef]
35. Tabata, K.; Yamaoka, K.; Fukuyama, T.; Nakagawa, T. Evaluation of Intestinal Absorption into the Portal System in Enterohepatic Circulation by Measuring the Difference in Portal–Venous Blood Concentrations of Diclofenac. *Pharm. Res.* **1995**, *12*, 880–883. [CrossRef] [PubMed]
36. Chae, S.W.; Lee, J.; Park, J.H.; Kwon, Y.; Na, Y.; Lee, H.J. Intestinal P-Glycoprotein Inhibitors, Benzoxanthone Analogues. *J. Pharm. Pharmacol.* **2018**, *70*, 234–241. [CrossRef] [PubMed]
37. Fu, Q.; Sun, X.; Lustburg, M.B.; Sparreboom, A.; Hu, S. Predicting Paclitaxel Disposition in Humans With Whole-Body Physiologically-Based Pharmacokinetic Modeling. *CPT Pharmacomet. Syst. Pharmacol.* **2019**, *8*, 931–939. [CrossRef]
38. Zhang, S.; Wang, X.; Sagawa, K.; Morris, M.E. Flavonoids Chrysin and Benzoflavone, Potent Breast Cancer Resistance Protein Inhibitors, Have No Significant Effect on Topotecan Pharmacokinetics in Rats or MDR1A/1B (−/−) Mice. *Drug Metab. Dispos.* **2004**, *33*, 341–348. [CrossRef]
39. Davies, B.; Morris, T. Physiological Parameters in Laboratory Animals and Humans. *Pharm. Res.* **1993**, *10*, 1093–1095. [CrossRef] [PubMed]
40. Bardelmeijer, H.A.; Ouwehand, M.; Beijnen, J.H.; Schellens, J.H.M.; van Tellingen, O. Efficacy of Novel P-Glycoprotein Inhib-Itors to Increase the Oral Uptake of Paclitaxel in Mice. *Investig. New. Drugs.* **2004**, *22*, 219–229. [CrossRef]
41. Troutman, M.D.; Thakker, D.R. Efflux Ratio Cannot Assess P-Glycoprotein-Mediated Attenuation of Absorptive Transport: Asymmetric Effect of P-Glycoprotein on Absorptive and Secretory Transport across Caco-2 Cell Monolayers. *Pharm. Res.* **2003**, *20*, 1200–1209. [CrossRef]
42. Jonker, J.W.; Smit, J.W.; Brinkhuis, R.F.; Maliepaard, M.; Beijnen, J.H.; Schellens, J.H.M.; Schinkel, A.H. Role of Breast Cancer Resistance Protein in the Bioavailability and Fetal Penetration of Topotecan. *J. Natl. Cancer Inst.* **2000**, *92*, 1651–1656. [CrossRef]
43. Lagas, J.S.; Van Waterschoot, R.A.; Van Tilburg, V.A.; Hillebrand, M.J.; Lankheet, N.; Rosing, H.; Beijnen, J.H.; Schinkel, A.H. Brain Accumulation of Dasatinib Is Restricted by P-Glycoprotein (ABCB1) and Breast Cancer Resistance Protein (ABCG2) and Can Be Enhanced by Elacridar Treatment. *Clin. Cancer Res.* **2009**, *15*, 2344–2351. [CrossRef] [PubMed]
44. Tang, S.C.; Nguyen, L.N.; Sparidans, R.W.; Wagenaar, E.; Beijnen, J.H.; Schinkel, A.H. Increased Oral Availability and Brain Accumulation of the ALK Inhibitor Crizotinib by Coadministration of the P-Glycoprotein (ABCB1) and Breast Cancer Resistance Protein (ABCG2) Inhibitor Elacridar. *Int. J. Cancer* **2013**, *134*, 1484–1494. [CrossRef] [PubMed]
45. Wu, Y.; Pan, M.; Dai, Y.; Liu, B.; Cui, J.; Shi, W.; Qiu, Q.; Huang, W.; Qian, H. Design, Synthesis and Biological Evaluation of LBM-A5 Derivatives as Potent P-Glycoprotein-Mediated Multidrug Resistance Inhibitors. *Bioorganic Med. Chem.* **2016**, *24*, 2287–2297. [CrossRef] [PubMed]
46. Minderman, H.; O'Loughlin, K.L.; Pendyala, L.; Baer, M.R. VX-710 (Biricodar) Increases Drug Retention and Enhances Chemosensitivity in Resistant Cells Overexpressing P-Glycoprotein, Multidrug Resistance Protein, and Breast Cancer Resistance Protein. *Clin. Cancer Res.* **2004**, *10*, 1826–1834. [CrossRef]

47. Shepard, R.L.; Cao, J.; Starling, J.J.; Dantzig, A.H. Modulation of P-Glycoprotein but not MRP1-or BCRP-Mediated Drug Resistance by LY335979. *Int. J. Cancer* **2002**, *103*, 121–125. [CrossRef] [PubMed]
48. Pick, A.; Müller, H.; Wiese, M. Structure–Activity Relationships of New Inhibitors of Breast Cancer Resistance Protein (ABCG2). *Bioorg. Med. Chem.* **2008**, *16*, 8224–8236. [CrossRef] [PubMed]
49. Hendrikx, J.J.; Lagas, J.S.; Rosing, H.; Schellens, J.H.; Beijnen, J.H.; Schinkel, A.H. P-Glycoprotein and Cytochrome P450 3A Act Together in Restricting the Oral Bioavailability of Paclitaxel. *Int. J. Cancer* **2012**, *132*, 2439–2447. [CrossRef]
50. Lee, K.; Chae, S.W.; Xia, Y.; Kim, N.H.; Kim, H.J.; Rhie, S.; Lee, H.J. Effect of Coumarin Derivative-Mediated Inhibition of P-Glycoprotein on Oral Bioavailability and Therapeutic Efficacy of Paclitaxel. *Eur. J. Pharmacol.* **2014**, *723*, 381–388. [CrossRef] [PubMed]
51. Rahman, A.; Korzekwa, K.R.; Grogan, J.; Gonzalez, F.J.; Harris, J.W. Selective Biotransformation of Taxol to 6 α-Hydroxytaxol by Human Cytochrome P450 2C8. *Cancer Res.* **1994**, *54*, 5543–5546. [PubMed]
52. Sonnichsen, D.S.; Liu, Q.; Schuetz, E.G.; Schuetz, J.D.; Pappo, A.; Relling, M.V. Variability in Human Cytochrome P450 Paclitaxel Metabolism. *J. Pharmacol. Exp. Ther.* **1995**, *275*, 566–575. [PubMed]
53. Dantzig, A.H.; Shepard, R.L.; Law, K.L.; Tabas, L.; Pratt, S.; Gillespie, J.S.; Binkley, S.N.; Kuhfeld, M.T.; Starling, J.J.; Wrighton, S.A. Selectivity of the Multidrug Resistance Modulator, LY335979, for P-Glycoprotein and Effect on Cytochrome P-450 Activities. *J. Pharmacol. Exp. Ther.* **1999**, *290*, 854–862. [PubMed]
54. Dastvan, R.; Mishra, S.; Peskova, Y.B.; Nakamoto, R.K.; Mchaourab, H.S. Mechanism of Allosteric Modulation of P-Glycoprotein by Transport Substrates and Inhibitors. *Science* **2019**, *364*, 689–692. [CrossRef]

pharmaceutics MDPI

Article

Oleacein Intestinal Permeation and Metabolism in Rats Using an In Situ Perfusion Technique

Anallely López-Yerena [1], Maria Pérez [1,2], Anna Vallverdú-Queralt [1,3], Eleftherios Miliarakis [4], Rosa M. Lamuela-Raventós [1,3] and Elvira Escribano-Ferrer [3,5,6,*]

[1] Department of Nutrition, Food Science and Gastronomy XaRTA, Faculty of Pharmacy and Food Sciences, Institute of Nutrition and Food Safety (INSA-UB), University of Barcelona, 08028 Barcelona, Spain; naye.yerena@gmail.com (A.L.-Y.); mariaperez@ub.edu (M.P.); avallverdu@ub.edu (A.V.-Q.); lamuela@ub.edu (R.M.L.-R.)
[2] Laboratory of Organic Chemistry, Faculty of Pharmacy and Food Sciences, University of Barcelona, 08028 Barcelona, Spain
[3] CIBER Physiopathology of Obesity and Nutrition (CIBEROBN), Institute of Health Carlos III, 28029 Madrid, Spain
[4] Department of Chemistry, Voutes Campus, University of Crete, 70013 Heraklion, Greece; leytmil@gmail.com
[5] Biopharmaceutics and Pharmacokinetics Unit, Department of Pharmacy and Pharmaceutical Technology and Physical Chemistry, Faculty of Pharmacy and Food Sciences, Institute of Nanoscience and Nanotechnology (IN2UB), University of Barcelona, 08028 Barcelona, Spain
[6] Pharmaceutical Nanotechnology Group I+D+I Associated Unit to CSIC, University of Barcelona, 08028 Barcelona, Spain
* Correspondence: eescribano@ub.edu, Fax: +34-9340-35937

Citation: López-Yerena, A.; Pérez, M.; Vallverdú-Queralt, A.; Miliarakis, E.; Lamuela-Raventós, R.M.; Escribano-Ferrer, E. Oleacein Intestinal Permeation and Metabolism in Rats Using an In Situ Perfusion Technique. *Pharmaceutics* **2021**, *13*, 719. https://doi.org/10.3390/pharmaceutics13050719

Academic Editor: Im-Sook Song

Received: 27 April 2021
Accepted: 12 May 2021
Published: 14 May 2021

Abstract: Oleacein (OLEA) is one of the most important phenolic compounds in extra virgin olive oil in terms of concentration and health-promoting properties, yet there are insufficient data on its absorption and metabolism. Several non-human models have been developed to assess the intestinal permeability of drugs, among them, single-pass intestinal perfusion (SPIP), which is commonly used to investigate the trans-membrane transport of drugs in situ. In this study, the SPIP model and simultaneous luminal blood sampling were used to study the absorption and metabolism of OLEA in rats. Samples of intestinal fluid and mesenteric blood were taken at different times and the ileum segment was excised at the end of the experiment for analysis by LC–ESI–LTQ–Orbitrap–MS. OLEA was mostly metabolized by phase I reactions, undergoing hydrolysis and oxidation, and metabolite levels were much higher in the plasma than in the lumen. The large number of metabolites identified and their relatively high abundance indicates an important intestinal first-pass effect during absorption. According to the results, OLEA is well absorbed in the intestine, with an intestinal permeability similar to that of the highly permeable model compound naproxen. No significant differences were found in the percentage of absorbed OLEA and naproxen (48.98 ± 12.27% and 43.96 ± 7.58%, respectively).

Keywords: bioavailability; extra virgin olive oil; secoiridoids; metabolism; phenolic compounds; intestinal permeability

1. Introduction

The small intestine is the main site for drug absorption after oral administration [1,2], and the intestinal epithelial membrane is the principle physiological barrier that chemicals must cross to enter the bloodstream and become bioavailable [3]. Many in silico, in vitro, in situ, and in vivo models have been developed to investigate the transport mechanisms, intestinal permeability, and plasma pharmacokinetic profile of chemicals [4]. The in vivo models are the most clinically relevant because they include all the physiological factors that can affect absorption and bioavailability [1,4], but they are less useful for mechanistic studies. The in situ models, such as single-pass intestinal perfusion (SPIP), are commonly used to investigate trans-membrane chemical transport. SPIP allows for intestinal effective permeability to be determined on the basis of the disappearance of the compound from the intestinal segment or its appearance in plasma after a venous sampling procedure [5–9], with the latter being especially suitable for poorly permeating substances [8]. Moreover, SPIP is the most similar alternative to an in vivo model in that it includes a mucus layer, blood irrigation, and innervation [4,6,7].

Intestinal permeability depends on the physicochemical properties and molecular structure and size of the drug or other xenobiotic molecules [2]. Lipophilicity, solubility, and the acid–base character can also affect the rate and extent of absorption, distribution, and transport through biological membranes [3]. In addition, the absorption rate is affected by the expression of transporter proteins and enzymes [1,3,10,11] that are highly region-dependent [2] and other biological factors [2,12].

The benefits of dietary phenolics have been extensively reported [13,14], especially as a protection from cardiovascular diseases. In extra virgin olive oil (EVOO), secoiridoids such as oleacein (OLEA) represent by far the most abundant group of phenolic compounds (>90%) [15] and are thought to be responsible for the healthy properties of the oil, although mediated by other components. In the review by Naruszewicz et al. (2015), OLEA is described as a substance with high pharmacological potential [16]. As well as various antioxidant and anti-inflammatory properties [17,18], OLEA exhibits anti-proliferative and anti-metastatic effects in the SH-SY5Y human neuroblastoma cell line [19].

Numerous studies have explored the bioavailability of phenolic compounds after the ingestion of EVOO or a phenolic extract, both in humans [20–25] and rats [26–29]. However, among the secoiridoids, most attention has been focused on oleuropein and hydroxytyrosol and its derivatives [30,31], and little information is available on OLEA. Thus, further animal and human studies using purified OLEA are needed to clarify whether the biological effects attributed to it are due to OLEA itself or its metabolites. In addition, as explained above, in situ studies are required to obtain detailed information on the intestinal permeability of OLEA and to verify the potential sites of its metabolization after oral administration.

To the best of our knowledge, no studies have been previously performed on pure OLEA using SPIP in rats. With this model, OLEA and its metabolites were simultaneously monitored in the intestinal lumen and mesenteric blood plasma, with the aim of shedding light on its intestinal permeability and metabolism. The resulting information will be useful for a better understanding of the biological effects attributed to OLEA. The highly permeable naproxen was included in the study as a reference drug.

2. Materials and Methods

2.1. Reagents and Materials

OLEA ($\geq$90% purity) was purchased from Toronto Research Chemicals (North York, ON, Canada). Naproxen and phenol red were purchased from Sigma-Aldrich (Madrid, Spain). Heparin sodium salt from porcine intestinal mucosa, Hanks' balanced salt solution (HBBS), and HEPES 1M solution were also obtained from Sigma-Aldrich (Madrid, Spain). Pentobarbital sodium 200 mg/mL (Dolethal) was supplied by Vetoquinol (Madrid, Spain) and isoflurane by Laboratorios Esteve (Barcelona, Spain). The solvents acetonitrile and methanol, and the chemical formic acid were acquired from PanReac AppliChem (Panreac Quimica SLU, Barcelona, Spain). Finally, a Milli-Q purification system was used to obtain ultrapure water (Millipore, Bedford, MA, USA).

2.2. Work Solutions

The transport medium (TM; pH 7, 9.7 g/L HBSS buffered with HEPES 10 mM) was used to infuse the compounds via the intestine. The secoiridoid OLEA (Figure 1) was assayed at 0.15 mg/mL (468.3 μM), a concentration chosen after taking into account both the OLEA concentration in EVOO (around 300 mg/kg) and the daily ingestion of EVOO recommended by the European Food Safety Authority (EFSA) (at least 5 mg of hydroxytyrosol and its derivatives per 20 g of olive oil) [32]. In accordance with its high dose strength, naproxen was assayed at 2.2 mg/mL in 250 mL of TM, as recommended [33]. Red phenol was assayed at 0.1 mg/mL. The stability of these test compounds, sampled at different times, was monitored in the perfusion solution at 37 °C for 60 min.

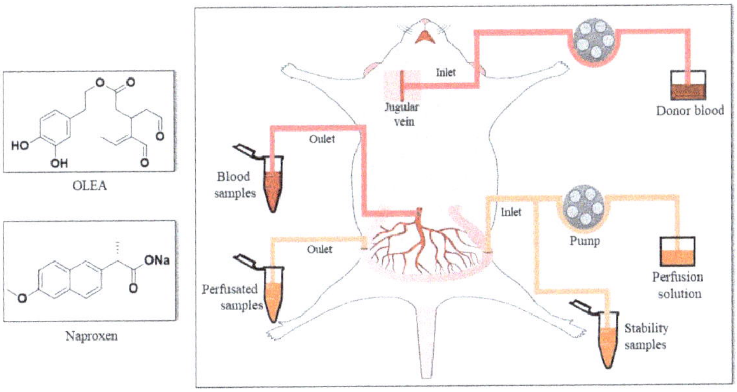

Figure 1. Chemical structure of the perfused compounds (OLEA and naproxen) and surgical procedure.

2.3. *Animals*

The Animal Experimentation Ethics Committee of the University of Barcelona, Spain (trial no. CEEA 124/16), and Generalitat de Catalunya (no. 6435, 27 June 2019) approved the study protocol. For each compound, four male Sprague-Dawley rats (Envigo RMS Spain SL, Sant Feliu de Codines, Barcelona, Spain) were used per intestinal perfusion experiment and four as blood donors (body weight 285 ± 6 g and 300–400 g, respectively). The animals arrived at the animal facility 10 days before the experiment and were kept with water and food ad libitum, with a 12 h light and dark cycle, at 21 °C and humidity-controlled (55 ± 10%).

2.4. *Single-Pass Intestinal Perfusion Studies*

The SPIP studies were performed in anesthetized rats according to the method described by López-Yerena and coworkers [6]; the donor blood and surgical procedure (Figure 1) were as described in that study. Regarding the procedure of donor blood, the rats were anesthetized by isoflurane inhalation (2.5%), and the whole blood was collected via cardiac puncture. The blood was diluted with heparin (50 u/mL TM) to 80% blood and kept in a 20 mL syringe for the in situ SPIP experiment. In the case of the rats that underwent surgery, the rats received intraperitoneal administration of pentobarbital sodium (Dolethal) at a dose of 60 mg/kg, and a maintenance dose of isoflurane (1.5%) was given 50 min after the induction dose. Body temperature was maintained at 37 ± 0.5 °C throughout the experiment by means of a homeothermic blanket. An ileal segment of approximately 7–10 cm was cannulated. The intestinal perfusion was started by delivering the perfusion solution containing OLEA or naproxen (in separate experiments) and phenol red at a flow rate of 0.2 mL/min to the cannulated intestinal segment, and the blood was supplied though the jugular vein at a rate of 0.3 mL/min. The phenol red included in the perfusion solution was used as non-absorbable marker for measuring water transport. To avoid the oxidation of OLEA, we carried out the SPIP experiments in a laboratory room with infrared light. Samples of both the intestinal lumen and mesenteric blood were collected simultaneously at 5 min intervals for 60 min. The outflow perfusate samples were collected in 2 mL amber vials and the blood was collected in pre-weighed lithium-heparinized tubes (BD Vacutainer). Next, the perfusate samples were centrifuged (7516× *g* for 10 min at 4 °C), and the tubes with blood samples were weighed and centrifuged (3000× *g* for 10 min at 4 °C). The supernatants were collected and immediately stored at −80 °C awaiting analysis by LC–ESI–LTQ–Orbitrap–MS.

2.5. Biological Sample Treatment

Plasma: The extraction of OLEA and its metabolites was carried out with protein precipitation. Initially, the samples were thawed and centrifuged (11,000× *g*, 10 min at 4 °C). To precipitate proteins, we blended 100 µL of plasma with cold acetonitrile containing 2% of formic acid (1:5 *v*/*v*). Samples were vortex-mixed for 1 min and kept at −20 °C for 20 min. The samples were then centrifuged (11,000× *g*, 4 °C, 10 min), and finally 100 µL of the supernatant was transferred to vials for analysis.

With regard to naproxen, the plasma samples were deproteinized following the methodology proposed by Elsinghorst and colleagues [34], with some modifications. Rat plasma samples (100 µL) were deproteinized by the addition of 200 µL of acetonitrile. After thorough vortex-mixing, the samples were centrifuged (2733× *g*, 4 °C, 10 min), and the supernatant was mixed with 0.02 M ammonium acetate buffer (pH 4.0) (1:1 *v*/*v*). Again, they were vortex-mixed and after centrifugation, and 100 µL of the supernatant was transferred to vials for analysis by LC–MS/MS.

Stability study and lumen samples: The stability and perfusate OLEA samples were defrosted and centrifuged (11,000× *g*, 4 °C, 10 min), and 100 µL of the upper phase was transferred to vials for analysis. The equivalent naproxen samples were thawed and centrifuged (11,000× *g*, 4 °C, 10 min), and the upper phase was diluted with TM in a ratio of 5:95 (stability samples) and 1:9 (*v*/*v*) (perfusate samples) and transferred to vials.

Ileum tissue: The intestinal segment perfunded with OLEA in the SPIP experiments was also analyzed to quantify the OLEA and its metabolites retained in the tissue. First, the intestinal segment was rinsed by several perfusions with TM and then cut into small sections and homogenized after the addition of water/acetonitrile (1:1 (*v*/*v*) with 0.1% ascorbic acid) with a small tissue disruptor (T10 basic ULTRA-TURRAX®, IKA laboratory technology, Staufen, Germany). The samples were sonicated in an ice bath (5 min), shaken for 1 min, and centrifuged (11,000× *g*, 4 °C, 10 min). To precipitate proteins, we blended 100 µL of the upper layer with cold acetonitrile containing 2% of formic acid (1:3 *v*/*v*) [35]. Samples were vortex-mixed for 1 min, kept at −20 °C for 20 min, and centrifuged again (11,000× *g*, 4 °C, 10 min) before analyzing the supernatant.

2.6. Analytical Technique

2.6.1. OLEA Analysis

The quantification of OLEA and red phenol in the samples and the profiling and structural characterization of OLEA metabolites was carried out using LC–ESI–LTQ–Orbitrap–MS. LC separation was performed using an Accela chromatograph (Thermo Scientific, Hemel Hempstead, UK) equipped with a quaternary pump, a photodiode array detector, and a thermostated autosampler. A 5-µL sample aliquot was injected onto an Acquity™ UPLC® BEH C_{18} Column (2.1 × 100 mm, i.d., 1.7 µm particle size) coupled to an Acquity™ UPLC® BEH C_{18} Pre-Column (2.1 × 5 mm, i.d., 1.7 µm particle size) (Waters Corporation®, Wexford, Ireland) with the column temperature set at 50 °C. Eluent A was 0.05% (*v*/*v*) formic acid in water, and eluent B was 0.05% formic acid in methanol. The total run time was 11 min. The elution gradient (0.6 mL/min) started at 0% B and was increased via a linear gradient to 53.6% B after 6 min. The gradient was then increased for 2 min to 100% B and held for 1 min before returning to 0% B for 1.9 min to re-equilibrate the column.

The mass spectrometer used for the analysis was an LTQ Orbitrap Velos (Thermo Scientific, Hemel Hempstead, UK) equipped with an electrospray (ESI) source. The ESI source was operated in negative mode [M–H] with the following conditions: source voltage, 4 kV; capillary temperature, 275 °C (FT Automatic gain control (AGC) target 5·105 for MS mode and 5·104 for MS^n mode); sheath gas (ultra-pure nitrogen, >99.9%); flow rate 20; auxiliary gas flow rate 10; and sweep gas flow rate 2. In the case of the last 3 parameters, the arbitrary units were initially used, Fourier transform mass spectrometry (FTMS) mode was then used to analyze at a resolving power of 30,000 at *m*/*z* 600, and the data-dependent MS/MS events were acquired at a resolving power of 15,000 at *m*/*z* 600. The most intense ions detected in FTMS mode triggered data-dependent scanning. Ions that were not intense enough for a data-dependent scan were analyzed in MS^n mode with the same orbitrap resolution (15,000 at m/z 600). Precursors were fragmented by collision-induced dissociation (CID) using a C-trap with normalized collision energy (35 V) and an activation time of 10 ms. The mass range in FTMS mode was from 100 to 600 (m/z). The system was controlled by Xcalibur 3.0 software (ThermoFisher Scientific, Hemel Hempstead, UK).

Accurate masses and the isotopic pattern (through the Formula Finder feature in Xcalibur 3.0 software (ThermoFisher Scientific, Hemel Hempstead, UK) were used to select the elemental composition of each OLEA derivative. In addition, metabolites were confirmed by comparison with those reported in the literature [21,22] and with a similar compound [6,36,37]. MS^n measurements were performed to obtain information about fragment ions generated in the linear ion trap within the same analysis.

The OLEA and phenol red calibration curves were prepared in TM (10–150 μg/mL). The OLEA calibration curves were also prepared in rat plasma (0.1–3 μg/mL) and ileum tissue (0.1–3 μg/mL). All calibration curves had an $R^2 > 0.97$. In the absence of a reference standard, OLEA derivatives were evaluated by considering the ratio between peak area metabolite and parent compound dosed (OLEA) [6].

2.6.2. Naproxen Analysis

All luminal, plasma, and stability samples were analyzed by ultra-high-performance liquid chromatography/ESI tandem mass spectrometry (UHPLC–ESI–MS/MS) following the procedure proposed by Elsinghorst et al. with some modifications [34]. The liquid chromatography system consisted of an Acquity™ UPLC (Waters; Milford, MA, USA). Chromatographic separations were performed on an XBridge™ C_{18} (4.6 × 50 mm, 5μm particle size) column (Waters Corporation®, Wexford, Ireland). The mobile phase consisted of 0.02 M ammonium acetate buffer (pH 4.0) and acetonitrile (30/70, v/v) and was delivered at a flow rate of 1.0 mL/min (column temperature at 30 °C). A total of 10 μL of sample was injected.

The detection and quantification of naproxen and red phenol were performed using an AB SCIEX API 3000™ triple quadrupole mass spectrometer with a turbo ion spray source. Ionization was performed by ESI in the negative mode [M–H] in the multiple monitoring mode (MRM). Arbitrary units were used for the nebulizer (10), curtain (12), and drying gas (450 °C) using N_2; the capillary voltage was −3500 V. To detect naproxen and red phenol with the highest signal, we optimized the collision energy and the declustering, focusing, and entrance potential by direct infusion. The system was operated by Analyst version 1.4.2 software supplied by ABSciex (ABSciex, Framingham, MA, USA).

The calibration curves with naproxen and phenol red were prepared in TM (10–150 μg/mL) and in rat plasma (0.5–20 μg/mL). The samples were adequately diluted to be interpolated in the calibration curves. All calibration curves had an $R^2 > 0.98$.

2.7. Data Analysis

The equations used to determine the effective permeability coefficient, the correction of outlet concentrations, and the apparent permeability coefficient through the ileum are as follows:

$$P_{\text{eff}} = \frac{-O_{in}}{2 * \pi * R * L} * Ln \frac{C_{out.cor}}{C_{in}} \tag{1}$$

$$C_{out.cor} = C_{out} * \frac{CPR_{in}}{CPR_{out}} \tag{2}$$

$$P_{\text{app}} = \frac{dQ}{dt} * \frac{1}{A\ x\ C_0} \tag{3}$$

where O_{in} is the perfusion solution flow (0.2 mL/min), C_{in} and $C_{out.cor}$ are the respective inlet and corrected outlet steady-state concentrations of the tested product, R is the radius of the intestinal segment (set to 0.2 cm), and L is the length of intestinal segment determined after completion of the perfusion experiment.

The outlet concentrations were corrected for water transport by measuring the phenol red (*PR*) marker according to Equation (2), where C_{out} is the concentration of OLEA or naproxen in the perfusate at the specified time interval, and CPR_{in} and CPR_{out} are the phenol red concentrations in the inlet and outlet solutions at the specific time intervals, respectively.

The P_{app} was calculated using Equation (3), where Q is the cumulative number of tested compounds (OLEA or naproxen) appearing in the mesenteric blood as a function of time t in steady state conditions, A is the surface area of the exposed intestinal segment, and C_0 is the tested compounds initial concentration in the perfusate.

All in situ perfusion experiments were replicated in four rats. Data are presented as the arithmetic mean $\pm$ the standard deviation (SD). Statistical analysis was performed using Statgraphics Centurion XVI software (Statpoint Technologies Inc., Warrenton, VA, USA). The concentrations estimated at a range of times (stability samples) and the concentration of metabolites and OLEA at different times were compared using a parametric statistical assay (ANOVA test). Statistical differences in the concentration of metabolites between plasma and perfusion samples were analyzed using were evaluated using an ANOVA test, followed by the LSD post hoc test. The P_{eff} and P_{app} of OLEA and naproxen were compared using a Mann–Whitney U test. Differences were considered significant at $p < 0.05$.

3. Results and Discussion

3.1. Stability of OLEA

The stability of OLEA and the reference standard naproxen was evaluated prior to carrying out the intestinal permeability study, and both remained stable in the perfusion solution at 37 °C ($p > 0.05$) for the length of the experiments, i.e., over 60 min (Figure S1). The absence of degradation products such as M2 and elenolic acid was also verified, although traces of a hydrated form of OLEA (M5) were detected, probably due to interaction of the aldehyde groups with the aqueous TM during the analysis.

3.2. Qualitative and Quantitative Characterization of OLEA and Its Metabolites

The lumen, plasma, and ileum samples were analyzed by HPLC–ESI–LTQ–Orbitrap–MS to identify OLEA and its metabolites. The FTMS scan and MS^n experiments allowed for the identification of OLEA (M1), four phase I metabolites (M2, M3, M4, and M5), and six phase II metabolites (M6, M7, M8, M9, M10, and M11). These metabolites and their precursor ions (measured), tentative formula, mass error, retention times, and major fragments are presented in Table 1. An example of a chromatogram for each metabolite and the parent compound is shown in the supporting information (Figure S2), and the structure for the detected fragments is also proposed in Figure S3.

Table 1. Identification of OLEA and its metabolites in lumen, plasma, and ileum tissue samples by LTQ–Orbitrap–MS.

	Compound	Precursor Ion Measured m/z $[M-H]^-$	Tentative Formula $[M-H]^-$	Mass Error (ppm)	RT (min)	MS/MS
M1	OLEA	319.1184	$C_{17}H_{19}O_6$	0.785	6.81	153/183
Phase	I					
M2	OH-TY	153.0554	$C_8H_9O_3$	0.779	3.67	123
M3	OLEA + H_2	321.1337	$C_{17}H_{21}O_6$	0.435	7.05	185/199/143
M4	OLEA + OH	335.1128	$C_{17}H_{19}O_7$	0.271	6.82	131/199
M5	OLEA + H_2O	337.1282	$C_{17}H_{21}O_7$	0.021	6.69	201/133
Phase	II					
M6	OLEA + CH_3	333.1348	$C_{18}H_{21}O_6$	0.835	8.51	167
M7	OLEA + OH + CH_3	349.1277	$C_{18}H_{21}O_7$	−0.479	7.38	167/199
M8	OLEA + H_2O + CH_3	351.1445	$C_{18}H_{23}O_7$	1.771	7.20	215/167
M9	OLEA + H_2 + Glucu	497.1665	$C_{23}H_{29}O_{12}$	1.247	6.53	199/329
M10	OLEA + H_2O + Glucu	513.1621	$C_{23}H_{29}O_{13}$	1.833	6.43	329/215
M11	OLEA + H_2O + CH_3 + Glucu	527.1743	$C_{24}H_{31}O_{13}$	0.963	6.50	343/201

RT: retention time; Glucu: glucuronic acid; OH-TY: hydroxytyrosol.

OLEA metabolites have been studied previously, but their structures have not been reported [21,22]. As mentioned above, on the basis of the fragmentation pattern of each detected metabolite and in comparison with related phenolic compounds [6,36], we proposed tentative structures for the OLEA derivatives (Figure 2).

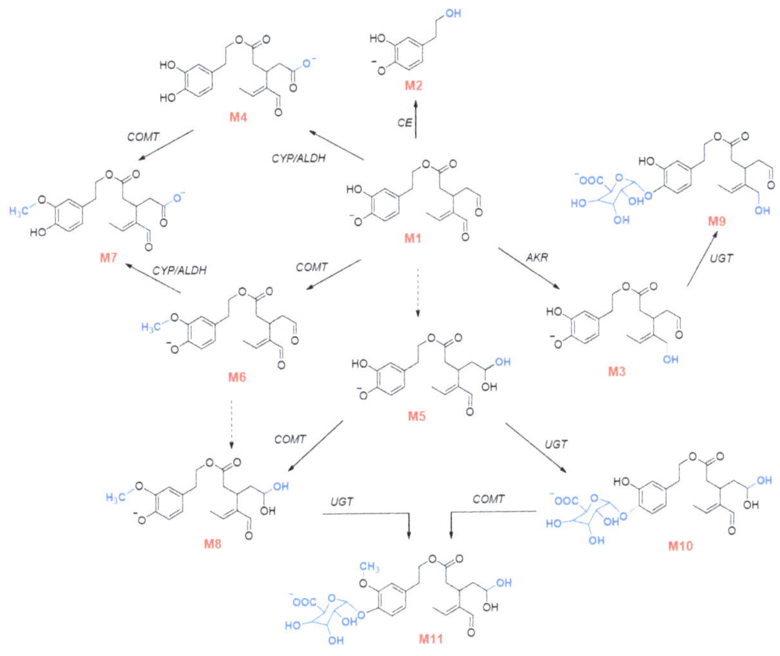

Figure 2. Proposed metabolic pathway of OLEA (M1) with phase I and phase II reactions. The chemical structures of M1 to M11 were identified in the plasma, lumen, and/or ileum samples after the SPIP study. CE: carboxylesterases; AKR: aldo-keto reductases; CYP3A: subfamily of cytochrome P450 enzymes; UGTs: glucuronosyltransferases; COMT: catechol-O-methyltransferase; ALDH: aldehyde dehydrogenase.

3.3. Phase I Metabolism

OLEA metabolites arising from phase I reactions both in lumen and plasma samples are shown in Figure 3. For the first time, the metabolic profile of OLEA in the ileum of rats after an SPIP assay has been evaluated. It is worth noting that the metabolite levels were much higher in plasma than the lumen, e.g., levels of M2 and M4 were 27- and 29-fold higher at 60 min, respectively. In the ileum tissue samples, the main metabolite was M2 ($p < 0.05$). The main phase I metabolites detected in plasma and lumen samples were M2 and M4, and its concentration was favored in time reaching the higher concentration at 55 and 60 min, respectively ($p < 0.05$). The large number of metabolites identified and their relatively high abundance (peak area metabolite/parent ratio up to 15 in plasma) indicates an important intestinal first-pass effect during the absorption of OLEA and that the metabolites formed are mainly transferred to the systemic circulation.

Hydrolysis is known to be a common process in phase I drug metabolism. Carboxylesterases (CEs) catalyze the hydrolysis of esters, thioesters, amides, and carbamates, with carboxylic acids and alcohols as the hydrolysis products [38,39]. Among the enzymes of this family, CES2 is present in the small intestine in both humans and rats [40]. The hydrolysis of OLEA can lead to the formation of hydroxytyrosol (M2) and elenolic acid [27]. In our study, M2 was found in lumen, plasma, and ileum tissue, but elenolic acid was not detected in any sample. Similar results were obtained in the study of Pinto et al. (2011), where the M2 metabolite was detected in Caco-2 cells and in the in vitro study of isolated intestine (in the serosal fluid of the jejunum and ileum), but not elenolic acid [41]. Similarly, only the conjugated forms of M2 were detected in the stomach, intestinal and caecum content, and feces of rats fed for 21 days with a diet supplemented with an extract composed mainly of OLEA [27], although elenolic acid was found in plasma and urine. The absence of elenolic acid in our samples could be explained by its rapid absorption from the hydrolyzed OLEA fraction. In the study of Kano et al. (2016), M2 was also the main metabolite found in the plasma of portal blood after oral administration of OLEA to rats [29]. In addition, M2 was not detected in human urine after EVOO intake [21,22].

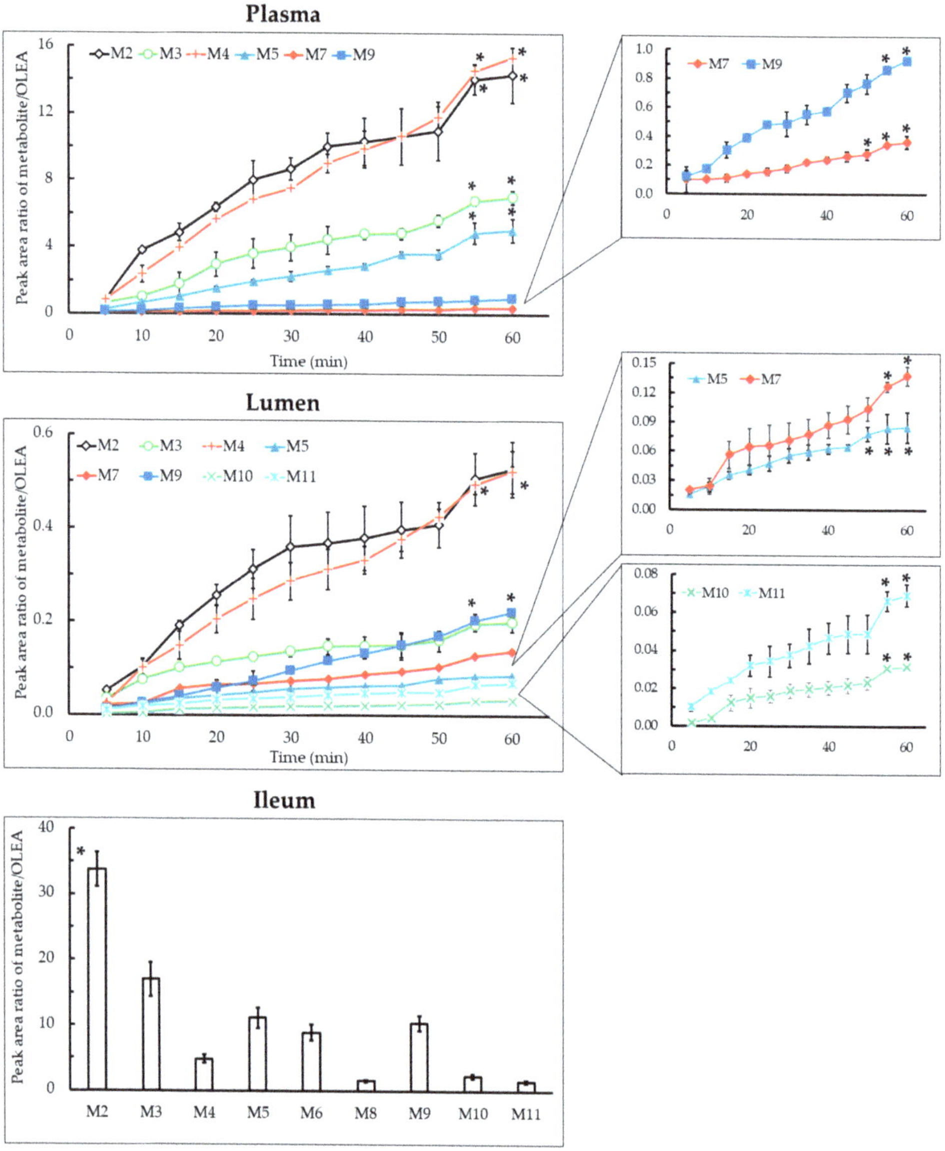

Figure 3. Peak area ratio of metabolite/OLEA as a function of time in plasma, lumen, and ileum tissue samples. Results are expressed as the mean ± standard deviation. * $p < 0.05$, one-way ANOVA.

Hydrogenated (M3), oxidated (M4), and hydrated (M5) forms of OLEA were detected in lumen, plasma, and ileum tissue (Figure 3). Major phase I enzymes include oxidases (especially monooxygenases), reductases, and hydrolases [10]. The hydrogenation of OLEA (M3) can arise from a reduction reaction catalyzed by NADPH-dependent aldo-keto reductases located in the small intestine epithelium. The reduction of aldehydes to primary alcohols can occur in OLEA because it contains the dialdehydic form of the linked elenolic acid [42]. In addition, the intestinal redox potential provides a reducing environment due to low oxygen tension, whereas oxidation is favored in tissues such as the liver [43]. Pinto et al. [41] proposed a structure for M3 but they were unable to confirm which of the carbonyl functional groups had undergone reduction, as the reaction at either site yielded similar fragmentation patterns. In our study, on the basis of the fragment detected (mass 143), we proposed a hydrogenation of the unsaturated aldehyde, although this cannot be confirmed without an NMR spectrum or the fragmentation analysis of a previously synthesized structure (Figure S3).

Cytochrome P450 enzymes (CYP), monooxygenases found in the epithelium of the small intestine [44], are responsible for the oxidative biotransformation of xenobiotics and other compounds [38,45]. In our work, the OLEA derivatives M4 and M5 could have been produced by the microbiome, as many bacterial CYP are soluble [46], or by the CYP expressed in the enterocytes, as shown in our luminal and tissue samples (Figure 3). However, non-CYP-mediated oxidative reactions can play an important role in the metabolism of xenobiotics [47]. Regarding carboxylic acids, as they are products of aldehyde oxidation, they could also be generated by aldehyde dehydrogenase enzyme catalysis. While only traces of M5 were detected in the TM (stability study), the high amount in both lumen and plasma samples indicates a metabolic reaction during its transport across the intestinal membrane. In 2010, Garcia-Villalba and co-workers found the same OLEA derivatives (M3, M4, and M5) in human urine after olive oil intake [21]. Although these derivatives were not found in plasma and urine samples of healthy volunteers in the study of Silva and co-workers [22], a hydrated OLEA metabolite was observed (OLE + CH_3 + H_2O + glucuronide). In fact, the metabolic profile of phenolic compounds from EVOO has been previously studied [23,26,41], but OLEA derivatives have not yet been reported.

3.4. *Phase II Metabolism*

Phase II biotransformation reactions, also known as conjugation reactions, generally serve as a detoxifying step in xenobiotic metabolism, increasing hydrophilicity and therefore excretion, as well as the metabolic inactivation of pharmacologically active compounds [48,49]. Phase II derivatives detected in plasma (M7 and M9), lumen (M7 and M9-M11), and ileum tissue samples (M6, M8, M9, and M11) are presented in Figure 3. The main product of phase II biotransformation reactions in all the samples was M9, with the highest relative abundance in plasma at 45–60 min, and in lumen samples at 55–60 min ($p < 0.05$).

It is well known that the enzyme that catalyzes *O*-methylation is catechol-*O*-methyl transferase, which mediates the transfer of a methyl moiety from the *S*-adenosyl-L-methionine cofactor to a hydroxyl group on the xenobiotic [50]. In rats and humans [51], catechol-*O*-methyltransferase is most active in the liver, kidney, intestine, and brain [52]. In agreement with the computational study carried out by Cuyàs et al. (2019), which concluded that meta-methylation at the O5 position of the catechol residue of OLEA occurs preferentially, we proposed the methylated derivative M6 (Figure 2) [50]. Among the three methylated metabolites, M6 and M8 were found in ileum tissue samples but not in the plasma and lumen (Figure 3), whereas M7 (OLEA + OH + CH_3) was detected in plasma and, after being secreted by an efflux membrane protein, in lumen samples. Previously reported results for these methylated forms are contradictory, being detected in human urine samples by Garcia-Villalba et al. [21] but not in other studies in rats [26,29,41]. Differences in experimental procedures may explain these discrepancies.

The glucuronidation reaction consists of transferring a glucuronyl moiety from the co-substrate UDP-glucuronic acid to one or more electrophilic groups of a hydrophobic molecules. The family of uridine diphosphate (UDP) glucuronosyltransferases are the enzymes that catalyze this reaction [53]. Glucuronidation often occurs as a secondary step after the production of primary metabolites in phase I reactions such as hydrolysis, hydroxylation, and dealkylation [54], as can be observed in M9 and M10, in which a glucuronic acid is attached to the hydrated and hydrogenated OLEA. Similarly, M11 arises from the addition of a methyl group and a glucuronic acid in a previously hydrated molecule of OLEA. M11 was detected in lumen and ileum tissue samples but not in plasma. The glucuronidation of hydrogenated OLEA has been previously reported in perfused segments of jejunum and ileum in rats [41]. Two different studies in humans obtained similar results: García-Villalba et al. [21] detected all glycoconjugates (M9, M10, and M11), while Silva et al. [22] only found M9 and M11. The bioavailability of phenolic compounds in EVOO depends not only on their concentration but also other dietary components and the individual genomic profile, which can affect enzymatic activity involved in the digestion and metabolism processes [22]. Polymorphism of conjugation enzymes or individual variations in digestive enzymes or bile salts could underlie the variations observed [1,2,17]. The aforementioned studies on humans reported three additional glycoconjugates (OLEA + glucuronide, OLEA + CH_3 + glucuronide, and OLEA + CH_3 + OH + glucuronide) not identified in our work, which may have been due to differences in the species and model used to evaluate the intestinal metabolism (in vivo vs. in situ models) [1]. The presence of these metabolites in humans can also be explained by the hepatic metabolism that OLEA or its derivatives may undergo after absorption.

In the present work, the observed phase I (M2-M5) and phase II (M7 and M9) OLEA derivatives in both lumen and plasma samples can be attributed to the presence of specific membrane transporters expressed in the apical (MDR1, BCRP, MRP2) or basal membrane (MRP1) of the enterocytes [55]. The OLEA derivatives recognized by these efflux transporters would thus be secreted to the intestinal lumen. On the basis of the results obtained, Figure 4 depicts the metabolic fate of OLEA in the small intestine, showing possible interactions with metabolic enzymes and carriers during transport across the enterocyte.

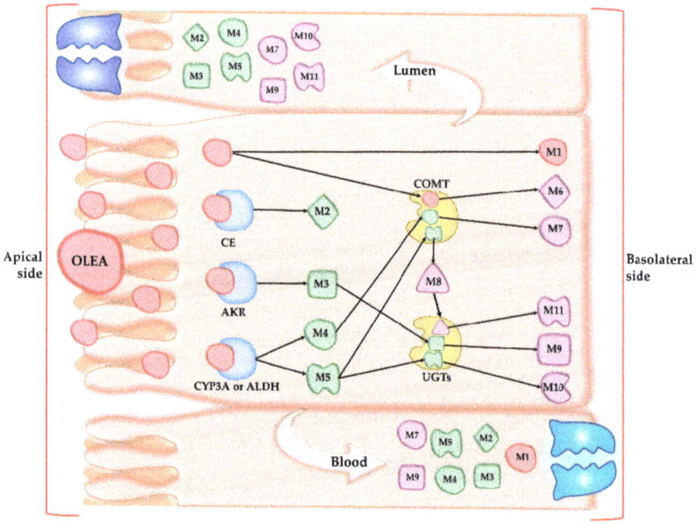

Figure 4. Tentative interactions of oleacein (OLEA) with metabolic enzymes and transporters. CE: carboxylesterases; AKR: aldo-keto reductases; CYP3A: subfamily of cytochrome P450 enzymes; UGTs: glucuronosyltransferases; COMT: catechol-*O*-methyltransferase; ALDH: aldehyde dehydrogenase.

3.5. Absorption Study

To investigate the intestinal permeability of OLEA, we carried out a comparative study with the anti-inflammatory drug naproxen. A highly permeable standard [55], naproxen has an oral bioavailability close to 100% [33] and was tested with the same in situ perfusion technique and conditions as OLEA.

The SPIP model is used in general screening for the intestinal membrane permeability of orally administered drugs and xenobiotics and to predict the effective permeability coefficient (P_{eff}). In this study, the ileum permeability of the tested compounds was based on luminal disappearance as well as appearance in mesenteric blood plasma, a suitable option for substances with low membrane permeability, as the differences in perfusate concentrations may be too small to determine accurately [8]. To obtain information about the intestinal metabolism of OLEA (see Sections 3.3 and 3.4), we analyzed perfusate and plasma samples for potential derivatives. The results of the absorption study are presented in Table 2, together with previously reported data for comparison. As can be observed, the P_{eff} values we obtained for naproxen agreed with those in the literature, indicating the validity of the methodology employed. However, as the variability between laboratories is relatively high, the data from individual studies should be interpreted separately [56].

Table 2. Intestinal effective permeability coefficient (P_{eff}), apparent permeability coefficient (P_{app}), and percentage of absorption after SPIP (mean ± SD, n = 4) for OLEA and the reference standard naproxen. Reported data are also included.

Compound	Segment	$P_{eff} \times 10^{-4}$ (cm/s) ± SD	$P_{app} \times 10^{-4}$ (cm/s) ± SD	Absorption (%)	Study
OLEA	Ileum	1.83 ± 0.18	0.607 * ± 0.202	48.98 ± 12.27	Current study
Naproxen	Ileum	1.47 ± 0.44	0.19 ± 0.018	43.96 ± 7.58	Current study
		1.17 ± 0.23			[57]
		1.78 ± 0.52			[56]
	Jejunum	1.17 ± 0.23			[58]
		1.19 ± 0.12			[33]
		1.47 ± 0.25			[56]
		2.10 ± 0.41			[59]
	Colon	2.06 ± 1.04			[56]

* $p < 0.05$ differences OLEA vs. naproxen (Mann–Whitney U test).

Despite the broad range of promising biological effects of secoiridoids from EVOO [17], the P_{eff} value of OLEA has not been previously reported. The mean permeability ratio (P_{eff}) of OLEA/naproxen was 1.24, without significant differences between them ($p > 0.05$), which indicates that the intestinal permeability of OLEA is comparable with that of the highly permeable standard. No significant differences were found for the percentage of drug absorbed (48.98 ± 12.27% and 43.96 ± 7.58% for OLEA and naproxen, respectively). These results are coherent with the lipophilicity (expressed as log P (octanol/water)) and molecular weight of OLEA (1.53 [60]; 1.02 [16], and 320.3 g/mol, respectively), which favor intestinal membrane transport by passive mechanisms [61].

In the mesenteric blood plasma, in our experimental conditions, the P_{app} of naproxen was significantly lower than that of OLEA (Figure 5B). As naproxen has a complete oral bioavailability, this result could be explained by a higher retention in or interaction with the lipid membranes (apical and basolateral), attributable to its high lipophilicity (log P = 3.18 [62]) and molecular structure, rather than a presystemic intestinal metabolism. Other authors have described an affinity of naproxen and other nonsteroidal anti-inflammatory drugs (NSAIDs) for the phosphatidylcholine of biological membranes [63,64]. It would therefore have been interesting to extend the study time from 60 min to, for example, 90 min.

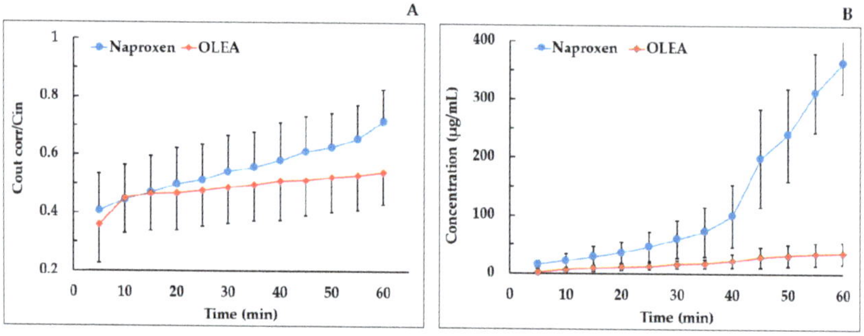

Figure 5. (**A**) Plot of the mean concentration ratio of the corrected outlet and inlet concentrations vs. time for naproxen and OLEA in SPIP in rats; (**B**) mean mesenteric plasma concentration of naproxen and OLEA vs. time. Error bars represent S.D.

To the best of our knowledge, this is the first study to report the intestinal and apparent permeability coefficients of OLEA in rats. Pinto et al. (2011), who investigated the metabolism of OLEA in an in vitro intestinal preparation from rats, also described its transport through the small intestine, observing OLEA in the receptor medium in an in vitro assay with Caco-2 cells [41]. Kano et al. (2016), who studied the absorption, metabolism, and excretion of OLEA after oral administration (300 mg/kg) in rats, did not observe OLEA in the portal plasma, possibly because its detection was hindered by binding to plasma components such as serum albumin, serum lipoprotein, and glycoprotein [29]; phenolic compounds and their metabolites are known to form complexes with plasma proteins [65]. Although further investigation is required, the amount of OLEA metabolites found in the perfusate and plasma in our study suggests that the bioavailability of this phenolic compound is incomplete. In conclusion, the important role of the small intestine in the bioavailability of OLEA has been demonstrated in terms of absorption and membrane transport as well as metabolic reactions that contribute to its elimination.

4. Conclusions

This is the first in situ study to simultaneously assess the absorption and intestinal metabolism of OLEA in rats. The SPIP model was used to determine the intestinal effective permeability of OLEA on the basis of its disappearance from the intestinal segment and its appearance in mesenteric blood. The range and abundance of metabolites found in the perfusate and plasma suggest that the oral bioavailability of OLEA in rats is incomplete. The results indicate that the small intestine plays an important role in the bioavailability of OLEA, considering its high intestinal permeability and the metabolic reactions that contribute to its elimination. The metabolites arising from hydrolysis (M2) and hydroxylation (M4) were the main circulating metabolites of OLEA detected in plasma and the lumen. The higher metabolite levels in plasma suggests that the intestinal metabolism of OLEA occurs mainly during the transport of the compound across the intestinal membrane.

Supplementary Materials: The following are available online at https://www.mdpi.com/article/10.3390/pharmaceutics13050719/s1, Figure S1. Concentration of NAP (right Y-axis scale) and OLEA (left Y-axis scale) in the TM and 37 °C as a function of time in the stability study. Figure S2. Chromatogram and retention time of OLEA and its metabolites. Figure S3. Molecular structure of OLEA and derivatives and proposed fragments with their masses through LQT–Orbitrap–MS analysis.

Author Contributions: Conceptualization, A.L.-Y., E.E.-F., and R.M.L.-R.; methodology, A.L.-Y., E.E.-F., E.M., and A.V.-Q.; software, A.L.-Y., E.E.-F., and A.V.-Q.; validation, A.L.-Y., E.E.-F., and R.M.L.-R.; formal analysis, A.L.-Y. and E.E.-F.; investigation, A.L.-Y. and E.E.-F.; resources, R.M.L.-R.; data curation, A.L.-Y., E.E.-F., M.P., and A.V.-Q.; writing—original draft preparation, A.L.-Y. and E.E.-F.; writing—review and editing, A.L.-Y., E.M., and E.E.-F.; visualization, A.L.-Y., M.P., and E.E.-F.; supervision, E.E.-F. and R.M.L.-R.; project administration, E.E.-F. and R.M.L.-R.. All authors have read and agreed to the published version of the manuscript.

Funding: This research was funded by CICYT [AGL2016-75329-R], CIBEROBN from the Instituto de Salud Carlos III, ISCIII from the Ministerio de Ciencia, Innovación y Universidades, (AEI/FEDER, UE), and Generalitat de Catalunya (GC) [2017SGR 196]. A.L.-Y. wishes to thank the Consejo Nacional de Ciencia y Tecnología (CONACYT) of Mexico for the doctoral scholarship. M.-P. thanks the Ministry of Science Innovation (MICIU/FEDER) for the project (RTI2018-093974-B-I00). A.V.-Q. thanks the Ministry of Science Innovation and Universities for the Ramon y Cajal contract (RYC-2016-19355). E.M. thanks the technical university of CRETA (TUC) and from Athens University of Economics and Business (AUEB) for the Erasmus scholarship.

Institutional Review Board Statement: The Animal Experimentation Ethics Committee of the University of Barcelona, Spain (trial no. CEEA 124/16), and Generalitat de Catalunya (no. 6435) approved the study protocol.

Informed Consent Statement: Not applicable.

Data Availability Statement: Data is contained within the article or supplementary material. The data presented in this study are available in Figures 1–5. In addition, the information is also presented in Tables 1 and 2.

Acknowledgments: The authors wish to thank the CCiT-UB for the mass spectrometry equipment.

Conflicts of Interest: R.M.L.-R. reports receiving lecture fees from Cerveceros de España and receiving lecture fees and travel support from Adventia. The other authors declare no conflict of interest. The funders had no role in the design of the study; in the collection, analyses, or interpretation of data; in the writing of the manuscript; or in the decision to publish the results.

References

1. Billat, P.-A.; Roger, E.; Faure, S.; Lagarce, F. Models for Drug Absorption from the Small Intestine: Where Are We and Where Are We Going? *Drug Discov. Today* **2017**, *22*, 761–775. [CrossRef] [PubMed]
2. Zhu, L.; Lu, L.; Wang, S.; Wu, J.; Shi, J.; Yan, T.; Xie, C.; Li, Q.; Hu, M.; Liu, Z. Oral Absorption Basics: Pathways and Physicochemical and Biological Factors Affecting Absorption. In *Developing Solid Oral Dosage Forms*; Academic Press: Cambridge, MA, USA, 2017; pp. 297–329. ISBN 978-0-12-802447-8.
3. Chmiel, T.; Mieszkowska, A.; Kempińska-Kupczyk, D.; Kot-Wasik, A.; Namieśnik, J.; Mazerska, Z. The Impact of Lipophilicity on Environmental Processes, Drug Delivery and Bioavailability of Food Components. *Microchem. J.* **2019**, *146*, 393–406. [CrossRef]
4. Dahlgren, D.; Lennernäs, H. Intestinal Permeability and Drug Absorption: Predictive Experimental, Computational and In Vivo Approaches. *Pharmaceutics* **2019**, *11*, 411. [CrossRef] [PubMed]
5. Mudra, D.R.; Borchardt, R.T. Absorption Barriers in the Rat Intestinal Mucosa: 1. Application of an in Situ Perfusion Model to Simultaneously Assess Drug Permeation and Metabolism. *J. Pharm. Sci.* **2010**, *99*, 982–998. [CrossRef]
6. López-Yerena; Vallverdú-Queralt; Mols; Augustijns; Lamuela-Raventós; Escribano-Ferrer Absorption and Intestinal Metabolic Profile of Oleocanthal in Rats. *Pharmaceutics* **2020**, *12*, 134. [CrossRef]
7. Griffin, B.; O'Driscoll, C. Models of the small intestine. In *Drug Absorption Studies*; Springer: Boston, MA, USA, 2008; pp. 34–76.
8. Dahlgren, D.; Roos, C.; Peters, K.; Lundqvist, A.; Tannergren, C.; Sjögren, E.; Sjöblom, M.; Lennernäs, H. Evaluation of Drug Permeability Calculation Based on Luminal Disappearance and Plasma Appearance in the Rat Single-Pass Intestinal Perfusion Model. *Eur. J. Pharm. Biopharm.* **2019**, *142*, 31–37. [CrossRef]
9. Brouwers, J.; Mols, R.; Annaert, P.; Augustijns, P. Validation of a Differential in Situ Perfusion Method with Mesenteric Blood Sampling in Rats for Intestinal Drug Interaction Profiling. *Biopharm. Drug Dispos.* **2010**. [CrossRef] [PubMed]
10. Mao, Q.; Lai, Y.; Wang, J. Drug Transporters in Xenobiotic Disposition and Pharmacokinetic Prediction. *Drug Metab. Dispos.* **2018**, *46*, 561–566. [CrossRef]
11. Barthea, L.; Woodleya, J.; Houin, G. Gastrointestinal Absorption of Drugs: Methods and Studies. *Fundam. Clin. Pharmacol.* **1999**, *13*, 154–168. [CrossRef]
12. Lennernäs, H. Intestinal Permeability and Its Relevance for Absorption and Elimination. *Xenobiotica* **2007**, *37*, 1015–1051. [CrossRef]
13. Tresserra-Rimbau, A.; Rimm, E.B.; Medina-Remón, A.; Martínez-González, M.A.; De la Torre, R.; Corella, D.; Salas-Salvadó, J.; Gómez-Gracia, E.; Lapetra, J.; Arós, F. Inverse Association between Habitual Polyphenol Intake and Incidence of Cardiovascular Events in the PREDIMED Study. *Nutr. Metab. Cardiovasc. Dis.* **2014**, *24*, 639–647. [CrossRef] [PubMed]

14. Tresserra-Rimbau, A.; Rimm, E.B.; Medina-Remón, A.; Martínez-González, M.A.; López-Sabater, M.C.; Covas, M.I.; Corella, D.; Salas-Salvadó, J.; Gómez-Gracia, E.; Lapetra, J. Polyphenol Intake and Mortality Risk: A Re-Analysis of the PREDIMED Trial. *BMC Med.* **2014**, *12*, 1–11. [CrossRef] [PubMed]
15. López-Yerena, A.; Ninot, A.; Lozano-Castellón, J.; Escribano-Ferrer, E.; Romero-Aroca, A.J.; Belaj, A.; Vallverdú-Queralt, A.; Lamuela-Raventós, R.M. Conservation of Native Wild Ivory-White Olives from the MEDES Islands Natural Reserve to Maintain Virgin Olive Oil Diversity. *Antioxidants* **2020**, *13*, 1009. [CrossRef] [PubMed]
16. Naruszewicz, M.; Czerwinska, M.; Kiss, A. Oleacein. Translation from Mediterranean Diet to Potential Antiatherosclerotic Drug. *Curr. Pharm. Des.* **2015**, *21*, 1205–1212. [CrossRef] [PubMed]
17. Lozano-Castellón, J.; López-Yerena, A.; Rinaldi de Alvarenga, J.F.; Romero del Castillo-Alba, J.; Vallverdú-Queralt, A.; Escribano-Ferrer, E.; Lamuela-Raventós, R.M. Health-Promoting Properties of Oleocanthal and Oleacein: Two Secoiridoids from Extra-Virgin Olive Oil. *Crit. Rev. Food Sci. Nutr.* **2020**, *60*, 2532–2548. [CrossRef]
18. Filipek, A.; Czerwińska, M.E.; Kiss, A.K.; Wrzosek, M.; Naruszewicz, M. Oleacein Enhances Anti-Inflammatory Activity of Human Macrophages by Increasing CD163 Receptor Expression. *Phytomedicine* **2015**, *22*, 1255–1261. [CrossRef]
19. Cirmi, S.; Celano, M.; Lombardo, G.E.; Maggisano, V.; Procopio, A.; Russo, D.; Navarra, M. Oleacein Inhibits STAT3, Activates the Apoptotic Machinery, and Exerts Anti-Metastatic Effects in the SH-SY5Y Human Neuroblastoma Cells. *Food Funct.* **2020**, *11*, 3271–3279. [CrossRef]
20. De Bock, M.; Thorstensen, E.B.; Derraik, J.G.B.; Henderson, H.V.; Hofman, P.L.; Cutfield, W.S. Human Absorption and Metabolism of Oleuropein and Hydroxytyrosol Ingested as Olive (*Olea europaea* L.) Leaf Extract. *Mol. Nutr. Food Res.* **2013**, *57*, 2079–2085. [CrossRef]
21. García-Villalba, R.; Carrasco-Pancorbo, A.; Nevedomskaya, E.; Mayboroda, O.A.; Deelder, A.M.; Segura-Carretero, A.; Fernández-Gutiérrez, A. Exploratory Analysis of Human Urine by LC–ESI-TOF MS after High Intake of Olive Oil: Understanding the Metabolism of Polyphenols. *Anal. Bioanal. Chem.* **2010**, *398*, 463–475. [CrossRef]
22. Silva, S.; Garcia-Aloy, M.; Figueira, M.E.; Combet, E.; Mullen, W.; Bronze, M.R. High Resolution Mass Spectrometric Analysis of Secoiridoids and Metabolites as Biomarkers of Acute Olive Oil Intake-An Approach to Study Interindividual Variability in Humans. *Mol. Nutr. Food Res.* **2018**, *62*, 1700065. [CrossRef]
23. Rubió, L.; Farràs, M.; de La Torre, R.; Macià, A.; Romero, M.-P.; Valls, R.M.; Solà, R.; Farré, M.; Fitó, M.; Motilva, M.-J. Metabolite Profiling of Olive Oil and Thyme Phenols after a Sustained Intake of Two Phenol-Enriched Olive Oils by Humans: Identification of Compliance Markers. *Food Res. Int.* **2014**, *65*, 59–68. [CrossRef]
24. Khymenets, O.; Farré, M.; Pujadas, M.; Ortiz, E.; Joglar, J.; Covas, M.I.; de la Torre, R. Direct Analysis of Glucuronidated Metabolites of Main Olive Oil Phenols in Human Urine after Dietary Consumption of Virgin Olive Oil. *Food Chem.* **2011**, *126*, 306–314. [CrossRef]
25. Suárez, M.; Valls, R.M.; Romero, M.-P.; Macià, A.; Fernández, S.; Giralt, M.; Solà, R.; Motilva, M.-J. Bioavailability of Phenols from a Phenol-Enriched Olive Oil. *Br. J. Nutr.* **2011**, *106*, 1691–1701. [CrossRef]
26. Serra, A.; Rubió, L.; Borràs, X.; Macià, A.; Romero, M.-P.; Motilva, M.-J. Distribution of Olive Oil Phenolic Compounds in Rat Tissues after Administration of a Phenolic Extract from Olive Cake. *Mol. Nutr. Food Res.* **2012**, *56*, 486–496. [CrossRef] [PubMed]
27. López de las Hazas, M.-C.; Piñol, C.; Macià, A.; Romero, M.-P.; Pedret, A.; Solà, R.; Rubió, L.; Motilva, M.-J. Differential Absorption and Metabolism of Hydroxytyrosol and Its Precursors Oleuropein and Secoiridoids. *J. Funct. Foods* **2016**, *22*, 52–63. [CrossRef]
28. Domínguez-Perles, R.; Auñón, D.; Ferreres, F.; Gil-Izquierdo, A. Gender Differences in Plasma and Urine Metabolites from Sprague–Dawley Rats after Oral Administration of Normal and High Doses of Hydroxytyrosol, Hydroxytyrosol Acetate, and DOPAC. *Eur. J. Nutr.* **2017**, *56*, 215–224. [CrossRef]
29. Kano, S.; Komada, H.; Yonekura, L.; Sato, A.; Nishiwaki, H.; Tamura, H. Absorption, Metabolism, and Excretion by Freely Moving Rats of 3,4-DHPEA-EDA and Related Polyphenols from Olive Fruits (*Olea europaea*). *J. Nutr. Metab.* **2016**, *2016*, 9104208. [CrossRef]
30. Radić, K.; Jurišić Dukovski, B.; Vitali Čepo, D. Influence of Pomace Matrix and Cyclodextrin Encapsulation on Olive Pomace Polyphenols' Bioaccessibility and Intestinal Permeability. *Nutrients* **2020**, *12*, 669. [CrossRef] [PubMed]
31. Edgecombe, S.C.; Stretch, G.L.; Hayball, P.J. Oleuropein, an Antioxidant Polyphenol from Olive Oil, Is Poorly Absorbed from Isolated Perfused Rat Intestine. *J. Nutr.* **2000**, *130*, 2996–3002. [CrossRef]
32. EFSA Scientific Opinion on the Substantiation of Health Claims Related to Polyphenols in Olive and Protection of LDL Particles from Oxidative Damage (ID **1333**, *1638*, 1639, 1696, 2865), Maintenance of Normal Blood HDL Cholesterol Concentrations (ID 1639), Mainte. *EFSA J.* **2011**, *9*, 2033–2058. [CrossRef]
33. Kim, J.-S.; Mitchell, S.; Kijek, P.; Tsume, Y.; Hilfinger, J.; Amidon, G.L. The Suitability of an in Situ Perfusion Model for Permeability Determinations: Utility for BCS Class I Biowaiver Requests. *Mol. Pharm.* **2006**, *3*, 686–694. [CrossRef]
34. Elsinghorst, P.W.; Kinzig, M.; Rodamer, M.; Holzgrabe, U.; Sörgel, F. An LC–MS/MS Procedure for the Quantification of Naproxen in Human Plasma: Development, Validation, Comparison with Other Methods, and Application to a Pharmacokinetic Study. *J. Chromatogr. B* **2011**, *879*, 1686–1696. [CrossRef] [PubMed]
35. Polson, C.; Sarkar, P.; Incledon, B.; Raguvaran, V.; Grant, R. Optimization of Protein Precipitation Based upon Effectiveness of Protein Removal and Ionization Effect in Liquid Chromatography-Tandem Mass Spectrometry. *J. Chromatogr. B Analyt. Technol. Biomed. Life Sci.* **2003**, *785*, 263–275. [CrossRef]

36. López-Yerena, A.; Vallverdú-Queralt, A.; Mols, R.; Augustijns, P.; Lamuela-Raventós, R.M.; Escribano-Ferrer, E. Reply to "Comment on López-Yerena et al. 'Absorption and Intestinal Metabolic Profile of Oleocanthal in Rats' Pharmaceutics **2020**, *12*, 134.". *Pharmaceutics* **2020**, *12*, 1221. [CrossRef]
37. López-Yerena, A.; Vallverdú-Queralt, A.; Jáuregui, O.; Garcia-Sala, X.; Lamuela-Raventós, R.M.; Escribano-Ferrer, E. Tissue Distribution of Oleocanthal and Its Metabolites after Oral Ingestion in Rats. *Antioxidants* **2021**, *10*, 688. [CrossRef] [PubMed]
38. Chen, G. Xenobiotic metabolism and disposition. In *An Introduction to Interdisciplinary Toxicology*; Academic Press: Cambridge, MA, USA, 2020; pp. 31–42.
39. Wang, D.; Zou, L.; Jin, Q.; Hou, J.; Ge, G.; Yang, L. Human Carboxylesterases: A Comprehensive Review. *Acta Pharm. Sin. B* **2018**, *8*, 699–712. [CrossRef]
40. Taketani, M.; Shii, M.; Ohura, K.; Ninomiya, S.; Imai, T. Carboxylesterase in the Liver and Small Intestine of Experimental Animals and Human. *Life Sci.* **2007**, *81*, 924–932. [CrossRef]
41. Pinto, J.; Paiva-Martins, F.; Corona, G.; Debnam, E.S.; Jose Oruna-Concha, M.; Vauzour, D.; Gordon, M.H.; Spencer, J.P.E. Absorption and Metabolism of Olive Oil Secoiridoids in the Small Intestine. *Br. J. Nutr.* **2011**, *105*, 1607–1618. [CrossRef] [PubMed]
42. Penning, T.M. The Aldo-Keto Reductases (AKRs): Overview. Chem. *Biol. Interact.* **2015**, *234*, 236–246. [CrossRef]
43. Kang, M.J.; Kim, H.G.; Kim, J.S.; Oh, D.G.; Um, Y.J.; Seo, C.S.; Han, J.W.; Cho, H.J.; Kim, G.H.; Jeong, T.C.; et al. The Effect of Gut Microbiota on Drug Metabolism. *Expert Opin. Drug Metab. Toxicol.* **2013**, *9*, 1295–1308. [CrossRef]
44. Dressman, J.B.; Thelen, K. Cytochrome P450-Mediated Metabolism in the Human Gut Wall. *J. Pharm. Pharmacol.* **2009**, *61*, 541–558. [CrossRef] [PubMed]
45. Spanogiannopoulos, P.; Bess, E.N.; Carmody, R.N.; Turnbaugh, P.J. The Microbial Pharmacists within Us: A Metagenomic View of Xenobiotic Metabolism. *Nat. Publ. Group* **2016**, *14*, 273–287. [CrossRef] [PubMed]
46. Clarke, G.; Sandhu, K.V.; Griffin, B.T.; Dinan, T.G.; Cryan, J.F.; Hyland, N.P. Gut Reactions: Breaking Down Xenobiotic—Microbiome Interactions. *Pharmacol. Rev.* **2019**, 198–224. [CrossRef] [PubMed]
47. Strolin Benedetti, M.; Whomsley, R.; Baltes, E. Involvement of Enzymes Other than CYPs in the Oxidative Metabolism of Xenobiotics. *Expert Opin. Drug Metab. Toxicol.* **2006**, *2*, 895–921. [CrossRef]
48. Jancova, P.; Anzenbacher, P.; Anzenbacherova, E. Phase II Drug Metabolizing Enzymes. *Biomed. Pap.* **2010**, *154*, 103–116. [CrossRef]
49. Xu, C.; Li, C.Y.-T.; Kong, A.-N.T. Induction of Phase I, II and III Drug Metabolism/Transport by Xenobiotics. *Arch. Pharm. Res.* **2005**, *28*, 249–268. [CrossRef]
50. Cuyàs, E.; Verdura, S.; Lozano-Sánchez, J.; Viciano, I.; Llorach-Parés, L.; Nonell-Canals, A.; Bosch-Barrera, J.; Brunet, J.; Segura-Carretero, A.; Sanchez-Martinez, M.; et al. The Extra Virgin Olive Oil Phenolic Oleacein Is a Dual Substrate-Inhibitor of Catechol-O-Methyltransferase. *Food Chem. Toxicol.* **2019**, *128*, 35–45. [CrossRef]
51. Nissinen, E.; Tuominen, R.; Perhoniemi, V.; Kaakkola, S. Catechol-O-Methyltransferase Activity in Human and Rat Small Intestine. *Life Sci.* **1988**, *42*, 2609–2614. [CrossRef]
52. Taskinen, J.; Ethell, B.T.; Pihlavisto, P.; Hood, A.M.; Burchell, B.; Coughtrie, M.W.H. Conjugation of Catechols by Recombinant Human Sulfotransferases, UDP-Glucuronosyltransferases, and Soluble Catechol O-Methyltransferase: Structure-Conjugation Relationships and Predictive Models. *Drug Metab. Dispos.* **2003**, *31*, 1187–1197. [CrossRef]
53. Shipkova, M.; Wieland, E. Glucuronidation in Therapeutic Drug Monitoring. *Clin. Chim. Acta* **2005**, *358*, 2–23. [CrossRef]
54. Yang, G.; Ge, S.; Singh, R.; Basu, S.; Shatzer, K.; Zen, M.; Liu, J.; Tu, Y.; Zhang, C.; Wei, J.; et al. Glucuronidation: Driving Factors and Their Impact on Glucuronide Disposition. *Drug Metab. Rev.* **2017**, *49*, 105–138. [CrossRef] [PubMed]
55. FDA. *Waiver of In Vivo Bioavailability and Bioequivalence Studies for Immediate-Release Solid Oral Dosage Forms Based on a Biopharmaceutics Classification System*; US Department of Health and Human Services Food andDrug Administration: Rockville, MD, USA, 2017.
56. Dubbelboer, I.R.; Dahlgren, D.; Sjögren, E.; Lennernäs, H. Rat Intestinal Drug Permeability: A Status Report and Summary of Repeated Determinations. *Eur. J. Pharm. Biopharm.* **2019**, *142*, 364–376. [CrossRef] [PubMed]
57. Fagerholm, U.; Lindahl, A.; Lennernäs, H. Regional Intestinal Permeability in Rats of Compounds with Different Physicochemical Properties and Transport Mechanisms. *J. Pharm. Pharmacol.* **1997**, *49*, 687–690. [CrossRef] [PubMed]
58. Zakeri-Milani, P.; Barzegar-Jalali, M.; Tajerzadeh, H.; Azarmi, Y.; Valizadeh, H. Simultaneous Determination of Naproxen, Ketoprofen and Phenol Red in Samples from Rat Intestinal Permeability Studies: HPLC Method Development and Validation. *J. Pharm. Biomed. Anal.* **2005**, *39*, 624–630. [CrossRef] [PubMed]
59. Lennernaäs, H. Human Intestinal Permeability. *J. Pharm. Sci.* **1998**, *87*, 403–410. [CrossRef] [PubMed]
60. ChemAxon. Available online: https://foodb.ca/compounds/FBD016341 (accessed on 24 February 2021).
61. Avdeef, A. Physicochemical Profiling (Solubility, Permeability and Charge State). *Curr. Top. Med. Chem.* **2001**, *1*, 277–351. [CrossRef]
62. Hansch, C.; Leo, A.; Hoekman, D.; Livingstone, D. *Exploring QSAR: Hydrophobic, Electronic, and Steric Constants*; American Chemical Society: Washington, DC, USA, 1995; Volume 48.
63. Lichtenberger, L.M.; Zhou, Y.; Jayaraman, V.; Doyen, J.R.; O'Neil, R.G.; Dial, E.J.; Volk, D.E.; Gorenstein, D.G.; Boggara, M.B.; Krishnamoorti, R. Insight into NSAID-Induced Membrane Alterations, Pathogenesis and Therapeutics: Characterization of Interaction of NSAIDs with Phosphatidylcholine. Biochim. Biophys. *Acta BBA-Mol. Cell Biol. Lipids* **2012**, *1821*, 994–1002. [CrossRef]
64. Pereira-Leite, C.; Figueiredo, M.; Burdach, K.; Nunes, C.; Reis, S. Unraveling the Role of Drug-Lipid Interactions in NSAIDs-Induced Cardiotoxicity. *Membranes* **2021**, *11*, 24. [CrossRef]
65. López-Yerena, A.; Perez, M.; Vallverdú-Queralt, A.; Escribano-Ferrer, E. Insights into the Binding of Dietary Phenolic Compounds to Human Serum Albumin and Food-Drug Interactions. *Pharmaceutics* **2020**, *12*, 1123. [CrossRef]

pharmaceutics MDPI

Article

Assessment of Metabolic Interaction between Repaglinide and Quercetin via Mixed Inhibition in the Liver: In Vitro and In Vivo

Ji-Min Kim †, Seong-Wook Seo †, Dong-Gyun Han, Hwayoung Yun * and In-Soo Yoon *

Department of Manufacturing Pharmacy, College of Pharmacy, Pusan National University, Busan 46241, Korea; jiminkim@pusan.ac.kr (J.-M.K.); sswook@pusan.ac.kr (S.-W.S.); hann9607@pusan.ac.kr (D.-G.H.)
* Correspondence: hyun@pusan.ac.kr (H.Y.); insoo.yoon@pusan.ac.kr (I.-S.Y.); Tel.: +82-51-510-2810 (H.Y.); +82-51-510-2806 (I.-S.Y.)
† These authors contributed equally to this work.

Abstract: Repaglinide (RPG), a rapid-acting meglitinide analog, is an oral hypoglycemic agent for patients with type 2 diabetes mellitus. Quercetin (QCT) is a well-known antioxidant and antidiabetic flavonoid that has been used as an important ingredient in many functional foods and complementary medicines. This study aimed to comprehensively investigate the effects of QCT on the metabolism of RPG and its underlying mechanisms. The mean (range) IC_{50} of QCT on the microsomal metabolism of RPG was estimated to be 16.7 (13.0–18.6) μM in the rat liver microsome (RLM) and 3.0 (1.53–5.44) μM in the human liver microsome (HLM). The type of inhibition exhibited by QCT on RPG metabolism was determined to be a mixed inhibition with a K_i of 72.0 μM in RLM and 24.2 μM in HLM as obtained through relevant graphical and enzyme inhibition model-based analyses. Furthermore, the area under the plasma concentration versus time curve (AUC) and peak plasma concentration (C_{max}) of RPG administered intravenously and orally in rats were significantly increased by 1.83- and 1.88-fold, respectively, after concurrent administration with QCT. As the protein binding and blood distribution of RPG were observed to be unaltered by QCT, it is plausible that the hepatic first-pass and systemic metabolism of RPG could have been inhibited by QCT, resulting in the increased systemic exposure (AUC and C_{max}) of RPG. These results suggest that there is a possibility that clinically significant pharmacokinetic interactions between QCT and RPG could occur, depending on the extent and duration of QCT intake from foods and dietary supplements.

Keywords: drug-phytochemical interaction; hepatic metabolism; mixed inhibition; quercetin; repaglinide

Citation: Kim, J.-M.; Seo, S.-W.; Han, D.-G.; Yun, H.; Yoon, I.-S. Assessment of Metabolic Interaction between Repaglinide and Quercetin via Mixed Inhibition in the Liver: In Vitro and In Vivo. *Pharmaceutics* **2021**, *13*, 782. https://doi.org/10.3390/pharmaceutics13060782

Academic Editor: Im-Sook Song

Received: 17 March 2021
Accepted: 20 May 2021
Published: 23 May 2021

1. Introduction

Repaglinide (RPG; Figure 1), a rapid-acting meglitinide analogue, is an oral hypoglycemic agent for patients with type 2 diabetes mellitus [1]. It lowers postprandial blood glucose levels by promoting insulin secretion from pancreatic β-cells [2]. RPG reduces the risk of hypoglycemia by stimulating insulin secretion only when blood glucose levels are higher than normal, whereas sulfonylureas induce insulin secretion even at low blood glucose levels [3,4]. Additionally, treatment with RPG has been shown to improve oxidative stress indices in type 2 diabetic patients, potentially reducing the risk of diabetes-associated vascular disease [5]. The oral absorption of RPG is rapid and complete but its bioavailability is low because of considerable first-pass metabolism [6]. RPG is primarily eliminated via cytochrome P450 (CYP)-mediated oxidative metabolism in the liver; in particular, both CYP2C8 and CYP3A4 are the principal CYP isoforms responsible for the biotransformation of RPG [7,8].

Over the past decades, bioactive flavonoids from various medicinal herbs and dietary supplements have gained increasing interest because of their important roles in complementary and alternative medicines [9,10]. A previous literature review of 18 studies over

9 countries indicated that the prevalence of complementary and alternative medicine use among people with diabetes ranges from 17% to 72.8% [11]. Quercetin (QCT; Figure 1), one of the most extensively explored flavonoids, is commonly found in many fruits, vegetables, and grains [12,13]. QCT is a widely recognized nutraceutical commercially available in capsule and tablet forms, consumed at a daily dose of 1 g or more [14]. It is a potent antioxidant and anti-inflammatory phytochemical that exerts a wide range of protective and therapeutic activities against arthritis, cancer, cardiovascular disease, diabetes, neurodegenerative disease, and obesity [15]. In particular, the mechanisms of the antidiabetic action of QCT include the inhibition of intestinal glucose absorption, stimulation of insulin secretion, and enhancement of peripheral glucose utilization, which contribute to improving whole-body glucose homeostasis [16]. Thus, there is a possibility that QCT can be used as a complementary medicine concurrently with RPG for the prevention and treatment of type 2 diabetes.

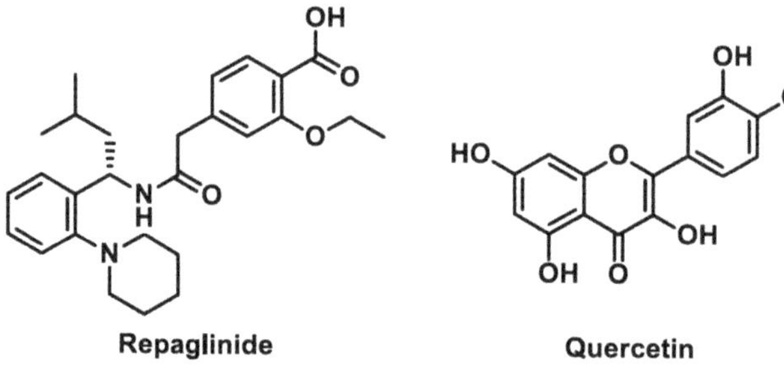

Figure 1. Chemical structures of repaglinide and quercetin.

QCT is eliminated mainly through phase II metabolism, such as glucuronidation, sulfation, and methylation in the liver [17]. QCT has been used as a selective CYP2C8 inhibitor in CYP phenotyping studies [18–20]; however, some reports have shown the inhibitory effects of QCT on other CYP isozymes [21,22]. In particular, a previous study revealed that QCT profoundly inhibited the activity of several CYPs including CYP2C8 and CYP3A4 [23], while another more recent study reported that QCT significantly inhibited CYP3A4 activity with a K_i of 15.4 μM [24]. Furthermore, it is important to note that several studies have reported significant drug interactions of RPG with CYP2C8 and CYP3A4 inhibitors. Systemic exposure to orally administered RPG was significantly increased by CYP2C8 inhibitors such as trimethoprim (1.6–2-fold) and clopidogrel (3.1–5.1-fold) [25,26] and by CYP3A4 inhibitors such as telithromycin (1.8-fold) and itraconazole (1.4-fold) [27,28]. Indeed, a previous study reported that QCT (25 μM) inhibited the in vitro metabolism of RPG (0.2 μM) by 58% in human liver microsome (HLM) [8], and another study reported the K_i of 0.61 μM for the inhibitory effect of QCT on in vitro metabolism of RPG in HLM [29]. Thus, there is a possibility of in vivo herb–drug interactions between QCT and RPG, but relevant information is currently lacking. This strongly suggests an immediate need for further investigation on this issue to avoid adverse reactions and optimize drug therapy.

Therefore, the present study aimed to comprehensively investigate the effects of QCT on the metabolism and pharmacokinetics of RPG. The inhibitory effect of QCT on the metabolism of RPG and its mechanisms were studied in HLM and rat liver microsomes (RLM). Next, the in vivo pharmacokinetic interactions between QCT and RPG were evaluated in a rat model. The protein binding and blood distribution of RPG were also examined.

2. Materials and Methods

2.1. Materials

RPG (purity > 98%), QCT (purity ≥ 95%), and ketoconazole (used as an internal standard; purity ≥ 98%) were purchased from Tokyo Chemical Industry Co. (Tokyo, Japan) Ethanol, dimethyl sulfoxide, polyethylene glycol 400 (PEG 400), carboxymethyl cellulose

(CMC), potassium phosphate monobasic/dibasic, β-Nicotinamide adenine dinucleotide phosphate (NADPH), and phosphate-buffered saline (PBS) were purchased from Sigma-Aldrich (St. Louis, MO, USA). Pooled male Sprague-Dawley rat plasma and pooled male human plasma were purchased from Innovative Research, Inc. (Novi, MI, USA) Pooled HLM and RLM were purchased from BD-Genetech (Woburn, MA, USA).

2.2. Protein Binding and Blood Distribution Studies

The unbound fractions of RPG and QCT in plasma (f_{uP}) and hepatic microsomes (f_{uMIC}) were measured through an equilibrium dialysis method using a rapid equilibrium dialysis (RED) device (Thermo Fisher Scientific, Inc., Waltham, MA, USA) as described previously [30–33]. The microsomes and 20-fold diluted plasma were spiked with either RPG alone or in combination with QCT yielding final concentrations of 5 μM for both compounds. A 200 μL spiked samples and 400 μL PBS were placed into the "sample" and "buffer" chambers of the RED device, respectively. After 4-h incubation to equilibrate between the buffer and plasma compartments, the RED plate was sampled from both compartments. The samples were matrix-matched for analysis by addition of either diluted plasma or buffer; (a) blank diluted plasma added to the buffer samples and (b) blank buffer added to the diluted plasma sample, at a ratio of 50:50 *v*/*v*. The unbound fractions in microsomes and diluted plasma were determined by dividing the analyte/IS peak area ratios of the (a) sample by those of the (b) sample. The unbound fraction in diluted plasma ($f_{u,d}$) was converted to the unbound fraction in undiluted plasma (f_u) using a Kalvass equation as below (DF: dilution factor) [33].

$$f_u = \frac{1/DF}{[(1/f_{u,d}) - 1] + 1/DF} \tag{1}$$

The blood-to-plasma concentration ratio (R_B) of RPG was determined as described previously [34]. Briefly, 1 mL of fresh blood was spiked with either RPG alone or in combination with QCT, yielding a final concentration of 5 μM for both compounds, and then incubated at 37 °C for 60 min. A plasma sample was obtained by centrifugation of the blood sample at 2000× *g* for 5 min. The concentrations of RPG in 50 μL of the plasma samples were determined using a validated high-performance liquid chromatography (HPLC) method.

2.3. In Vitro Microsomal Metabolism Study

The concentration-dependent disappearance of RPG in the RLM and HLM was evaluated to investigate the kinetics of the hepatic CYP-mediated metabolism of RPG. A microsomal reaction mixture consisting of microsomes (0.3 mg/mL), 1 mM NADPH, 50 mM phosphate buffer, and 1–500 μM RPG in distilled water (DW) was prepared, at a total volume of 200 μL. At 0, 30, and 60 min after starting the metabolic reaction, a 50 μL aliquot of the incubation mixture was sampled and transferred to a clean 1.5-mL microcentrifuge tube containing 150 μL of ice-cold acetonitrile to terminate the metabolic reaction. Following centrifugation at 15,000× *g* for 10 min, 150 μL of the resultant supernatant was obtained and the concentration of RPG in the sample was determined using the HPLC method.

2.4. In Vitro Metabolic Inhibition Study

To construct dose–response curves to determine the inhibitory effect of QCT on the hepatic metabolism of RPG, a microsomal incubation mixture consisting of RLM or HLM (0.5 mg/mL microsomal protein), 1 mM NADPH, 50 mM potassium phosphate buffer, 3 μM RPG, and nine different concentrations of QCT (0, 0.1, 0.5, 1, 5, 10, 50, 100, and 200 μM) were prepared, at a total volume of 200 μL. To construct Dixon plots for the inhibitory effects of QCT on the hepatic metabolism of RPG, five different concentrations of RPG (1, 3, 10, 30, and 100 μM), and five different concentrations of QCT (0, 1, 30, 100, and 200 μM) were used. Microsomal incubation and sample preparation were performed as described in the Section 2.3.

2.5. Animals

Sprague-Dawley rats (approximately 250 g) were purchased from Samtako Bio Korea Co. (Gyeonggi-do, South Korea) Rats were housed in ventilated rat cages (Tecniplast USA, West Chester, PA, USA) with access to standard rat chow (Agribrands Purina Canada Inc., Levis, Canada) and water ad libitum, and were allowed to acclimatize for one week prior to the experiments. Protocols for the animal studies were reviewed and approved in accordance with the guidelines of the Institutional Animal Care and Use Committee of Pusan National University (Busan, South Korea; date of approval: 4 May 2020; approval number: PNU-2020-2602).

2.6. In Vivo Pharmacokinetic Study in Rats

Rats were anesthetized via intramuscular injection of 10 mg/kg zoletil [35]. The femoral vein and artery of the rats were cannulated using a polyethylene tube (BD Medical, Franklin Lakes, NJ, USA). After recovery from anesthesia, a single intravenous or oral dose (0.4 mg/kg) of RPG with or without a single simultaneous intravenous dose (25 mg/kg) or oral dose (100 mg/kg) of QCT was administered to the rats. The vehicle solutions for the intravenous and oral doses were composed of PEG 400 and aqueous 0.3% CMC solution (50:50 *v*/*v*). Approximately 300 μL of blood was collected via the femoral artery at 0, 1, 5, 15, 30, 60, 90, 120, 180, and 240 min after intravenous injection and at 10, 20, 30, 45, 60, 90, 120, 180, and 240 min after oral administration. After centrifugation of the blood sample at 2000× *g* at 4 °C for 5 min, 120 μL of the resulting supernatant (plasma) was obtained and the concentration of RPG in the sample was determined using the HPLC method.

2.7. HPLC Analysis

The concentrations of RPG and QCT in the buffer, microsomes, and (diluted) plasma samples were determined as reported previously [36,37], with slight modifications. For RPG, 50 μL of the sample (or 120 μL of the plasma sample obtained from the in vivo pharmacokinetic study) was deproteinized with 300 μL of acetonitrile that contain ketoconazole (internal standard; 100 ng/mL). For QCT, 200 μL of the microsome sample or diluted plasma was deproteinized with 400 μL of acetonitrile that contained lapatinib (internal standard; 2000 ng/mL). After vortex mixing and centrifugation at 15,000× *g* for 10 min, the resulting supernatant was transferred to a clean 1.5-mL microcentrifuge tube and dried under nitrogen gas at room temperature. The residue was reconstituted with 50 μL of a mobile phase. After vortex mixing and centrifugation at 15,000× *g* for 10 min, 40 μL of the resulting supernatant was injected into the HPLC column (length 250 mm, inner diameter 4.6 mm, particle size 5 μm, pore size 100 Å; Phenomenex, Torrance, CA, USA). For RPG, isocratic elution of a mobile phase consisting of 10 mM phosphate buffer (pH 6.0) and acetonitrile (46.4:53.6, *v*/*v*) was performed at a flow rate of 1 mL/min; the column effluent was monitored by a fluorescence detector (RF-20A; Shimadzu Co., Kyoto, Japan) at 240 nm (λ_{ex})/380 nm (λ_{em}) at room temperature. For QCT, gradient elution of a mobile phase consisting of 0.1% TFA in water (solvent A) and acetonitrile (solvent B) was performed at a flow rate of 1 mL/min, and the procedure was as follows (solvent A: solvent B, *v*/*v*): started at 75:25 at 0 min, ramped from 75:25 to 60:40 for 13 min, back to 75:25 for 0.1 min, and maintained for 6.9 min (total run time: 20 min); the column effluent was monitored by an ultraviolet detector (SPD-20A; Shimadzu Co., Kyoto, Japan) at 254 nm at 40 °C. The lower limit of quantitation limit (LLOQ) of the HPLC methods were 10 ng/mL (buffer and plasma samples) and 50 ng/mL (microsome samples) for RPG and 100 ng/mL for QCT. The validation parameters for the HPLC methods were listed in Tables S1 and S2.

2.8. Data Analysis

A single-site Michaelis–Menten Equation was simultaneously fitted to the substrate (RPG) concentration ([S]; μM) as follows versus initial metabolic rate (V; pmol/min/mg protein):

$$V = \frac{V_{max} \times [S]}{K_m + [S]} \tag{2}$$

where V_{max} and K_m are the maximal metabolic rate and Michaelis–Menten constant, respectively. The intrinsic metabolic clearance (CL_{int}) was calculated as V_{max}/K_m. The half maximal inhibitory concentration (IC_{50}) of QCT for the hepatic metabolism of RPG was determined via nonlinear regression using GraphPad Prism software (version 5.01; GraphPad Software, San Diego, CA, USA) according to the four-parameter logistic equation:

$$Y = Min + \frac{Max - Min}{1 + (\frac{X}{IC_{50}})^{-P}} \tag{3}$$

where X and Y are the inhibitor concentrations and response, respectively. Max and Min are the initial and final Y values, respectively, and the power P represents the Hill coefficient. The type of inhibition of QCT on the hepatic metabolism of RPG was determined graphically using a Dixon plot. The inhibition constant K_i of QCT on the hepatic metabolism of RPG was determined via nonlinear regression using a GraphPad Prism, according to the mixed-model enzyme inhibition equation:

$$Y = \frac{V_{max} \times X}{K_m \times (1 + \frac{I}{K_i}) + X \times (1 + \frac{I}{\alpha \times K_i})} \tag{4}$$

where X, Y, and I are the substrate concentration, enzyme activity, and inhibitor concentration, respectively. V_{max} and K_m are the same as those defined in Equation (2). The parameter α is indicative of the inhibition type. The mixed model is a general equation that includes competitive, uncompetitive, and noncompetitive inhibition as special cases. When $\alpha = 1$, the mixed model is identical to a noncompetitive inhibition. When α is very large ($\alpha \to \infty$) or very small ($\alpha \to 0$), the mixed model becomes identical to competitive inhibition or uncompetitive inhibition, respectively. In the other cases ($\alpha \neq 1$), the mixed model describes mixed inhibition.

Non-compartmental analysis (WinNonlin, version 3.1, NCA200 and 201; Certara, Inc., Princeton, NJ, USA) was conducted to estimate the following pharmacokinetic parameters: total area under the plasma concentration–time curve from time zero to time infinity (AUC); total body clearance (CL, calculated as dose/AUC); terminal half-life ($t_{1/2}$); and apparent volume of distribution at steady state (V_{ss}). For comparison, the extent of absolute oral bioavailability (F; expressed as percent of dose administered) was calculated by dividing the dose-normalized AUC after oral administration by the dose-normalized AUC after intravenous injection. The peak plasma concentration (C_{max}) and time to reach C_{max} (T_{max}) were obtained directly from the measured experimental data.

2.9. Statistical Analysis

p-values < 0.05 were considered statistically significant. They were calculated using the unpaired *t*-test for comparison between two means or one-way analysis of variance (ANOVA) with post-hoc Tukey's honestly significant difference test for comparison among three means. Unless indicated otherwise, all data are expressed as the mean ± standard deviation, except for T_{max}, which is expressed as median (range), rounded to three significant figures.

3. Results

3.1. Effects of QCT on the Protein Binding and Blood Distribution of RPG

The f_{uP}, f_{uMIC}, and R_B of RPG in the absence and presence of QCT are shown in Figure 2. The f_{uP} of RPG was 0.0533 ± 0.0060 and 0.0761 ± 0.0094 in human and rat plasma, respectively, indicating extensive plasma protein binding. The f_{uMIC} of RPG was 0.620 ± 0.152 and 0.671 ± 0.009 in HLM and RLM, respectively, indicating low to moderate microsomal protein binding. The f_{uP} and f_{uMIC} of RPG were not significantly altered by the presence of QCT ($p \geq 0.0609$). The rat and human R_B of RPG observed in the present study were 0.869 ± 0.043 and 0.847 ± 0.021, respectively, and they were not significantly altered by the presence of QCT ($p \geq 0.054$). These results indicated minimal effects of QCT on the protein binding and blood distribution of RPG.

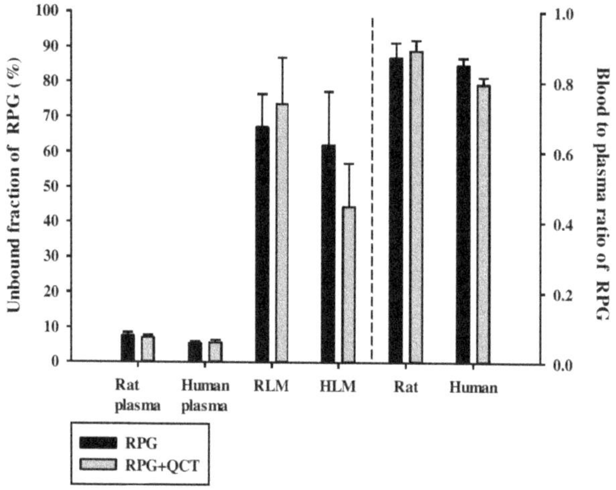

Figure 2. Unbound fractions of RPG in plasma (f_{uP}) and liver microsomes (f_{uMIC}) in the absence or presence of QCT, and the blood-to-plasma concentration ratios (R_B) of RPG in rat and human whole blood in the absence or presence of QCT. The rectangular bars and their error bars represent the means and standard deviations, respectively (n = 5).

3.2. *Hepatic Microsomal Metabolism of RPG*

The concentration dependence of RPG metabolism in the RLM and HLM was also investigated. As shown in Figure 3, saturable and concentration-dependent metabolic profiles were observed and well-described via Michaelis–Menten kinetics in both RLM and HLM, assuming the presence of one saturable component (r^2 = 0.982–0.996). The V_{max}, K_m, and CL_{int} of RPG in the RLM were estimated to be 1990–4560 pmol/min/mg protein, 16.0–92.2 μM, and 49.5–124 μL/min/mg protein, respectively. The V_{max}, K_m, and CL_{int} of RPG in the HLM were estimated to be 2380–3240 pmol/min/mg protein, 27.0–69.4 μM, and 46.6–89.2 μL/min/mg protein, respectively. There were no significant differences in the metabolic parameters of RPG between RLM and HLM (p = 0.656 for V_{max}, 0.972 for K_m, and 0.394 for CL_{int}), indicating negligible species differences.

3.3. *Effects of QCT on the Hepatic Microsomal Metabolism of RPG*

The inhibitory effects of QCT at various concentrations up to 200 μM on the metabolism of QCT in RLM and HLM were assessed by constructing dose–response curves (Figure 4). They were readily described using the sigmoidal logistic equation (Equation (3); r^2 = 0.990–0.999). The mean (range) of the IC_{50} of QCT on the microsomal metabolism of RPG was estimated to be 16.7 (13.0–18.6) μM in RLM and 3.03 (1.53–5.44) μM in HLM (Table 1). The IC_{50} values were significantly lower in the HLM than in the RLM (p = 0.000133). The inhibition mechanism of QCT on RPG metabolism was assessed through the construction of Dixon plots. In both RLM (Figure 5A) and HLM (Figure 5B), the plot lines intersected at a point near the x-axis in the upper-left quadrant of the plot, indicating mixed inhibition [38]. The K_i of QCT on the microsomal metabolism of RPG was estimated by fitting the data to the mixed inhibition model equation (Equation (4)), as listed in Table 1.

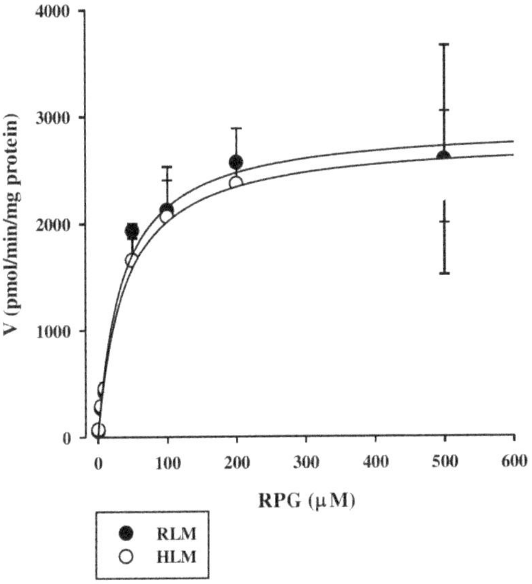

Figure 3. Concentration dependence of the disappearance of RPG in RLM and HLM. The closed circles and their error bars represent the means and standard deviations, respectively ($n = 4$). The solid lines represent the fitted nonlinear regression curves.

3.4. *In Vivo Intravenous and Oral Pharmacokinetic Studies in Rats*

The plasma concentration versus time profiles of intravenous RPG with or without the concurrent administration of intravenous QCT in rats are shown in Figure 6, and the relevant pharmacokinetic parameters are listed in Table 2. The AUC and $t_{1/2}$ of RPG were significantly higher by 83.4% ($p < 0.0001$) and 40.8% ($p = 0.0022$), respectively, whereas its CL was significantly lower by 44.9% ($p < 0.0001$) in rats with concurrent administration of QCT than in control rats. There were no significant differences in the V_{ss} of RPG between the two groups ($p = 0.061$). The plasma concentration versus time profiles of oral RPG with or without the concurrent administration of oral QCT in rats are shown in Figure 7, and the relevant pharmacokinetic parameters are listed in Table 3. The AUC and C_{max} of RPG were significantly higher by 87.6% and 84.2%, respectively, in rats that received a concurrent administration of QCT than in control rats ($p = 0.000263$ and 0.00479, respectively).

Table 1. Enzyme kinetic parameters for the metabolism of RPG and its inhibition by QCT in RLM and HLM.

Parameter	RLM	HLM
	Metabolism of RPG	
V_{max} (pmol/min/mg protein)	3070 ± 960	2850 ± 417
K_m (μM)	43.3 ± 29.7	42.8 ± 16.7
CL_{int} (μL/min/mg protein)	85.5 ± 29.2	71.8 ± 17.7
	Inhibition of RPG metabolism by QCT	
IC_{50} (μM)	16.7 ± 2.6	3.03 ± 1.84 *
K_i (μM)	72.0	24.2
α	2.88	14.4
Type	Mixed	Mixed

* Significantly different from the 'RLM' group ($p < 0.05$).

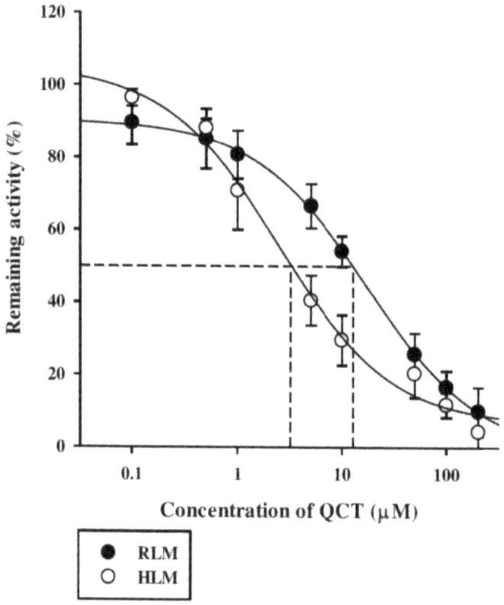

Figure 4. Dose versus response curves for the inhibitory effect of QCT on the disappearance of RPG of 3 μM (well below its K_m of 43 μM) in RLM and HLM. The closed circles and their error bars represent the means and standard deviations, respectively (n = 4). The solid lines represent the fitted nonlinear regression curves.

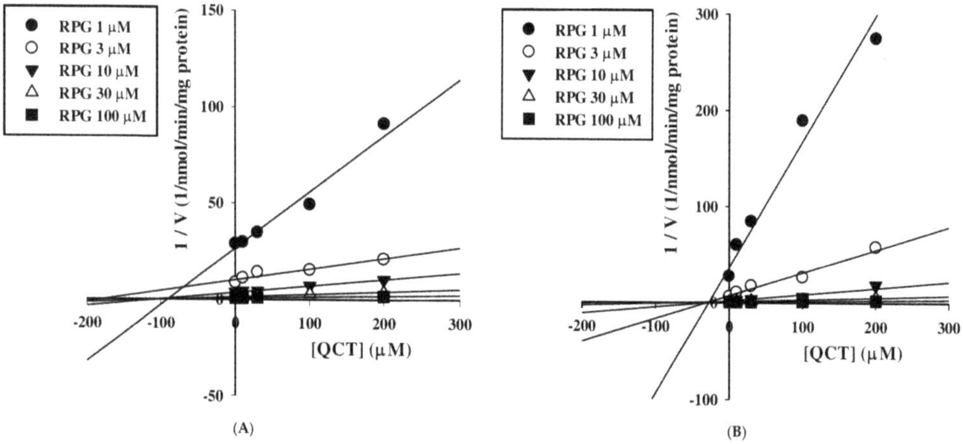

Figure 5. Dixon plots for the inhibitory effects of QCT on the metabolism of RPG in RLM (**A**) and HLM (**B**).

Table 2. Pharmacokinetic parameters of RPG following its intravenous administration at 0.4 mg/kg without or with simultaneous intravenous administration of QCT at 25 mg/kg in rats (n = 7).

Parameter	RPG alone	RPG with QCT
AUC (μg·min/mL)	50.7 ± 3.0	92.9 ± 11.8 *
$t_{1/2}$ (min)	40.8 ± 4.2	57.4 ± 10.6 *
CL (mL/min/kg)	7.92 ± 0.47	4.36 ± 0.54 *
Ae_U (% of dose)	1.60 ± 0.77	1.32 ± 0.88
Ae_{GI} (% of dose)	ND	ND
V_{ss} (mL/kg)	293 ± 18	269 ± 25

* Significantly different from the control (RPG alone) group ($p < 0.05$).

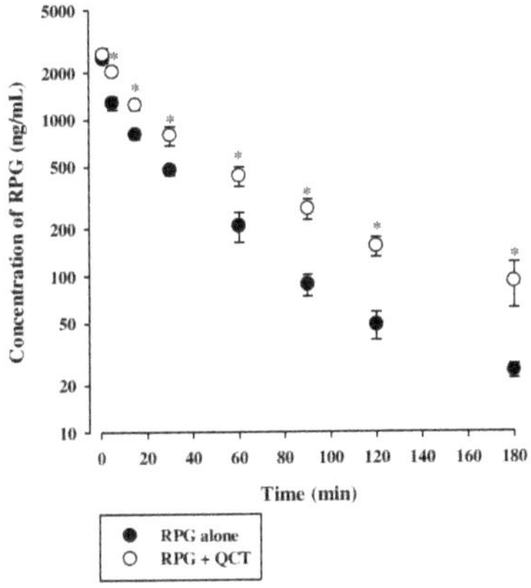

Figure 6. Plasma concentration versus time profiles of RPG following its intravenous administration at 0.4 mg/kg without or with intravenous QCT at 25 mg/kg in rats. The circles and their error bars represent the means and standard deviations, respectively ($n = 7$). The asterisks indicate statistical significance when compared to the control (RPG alone) group ($p < 0.05$).

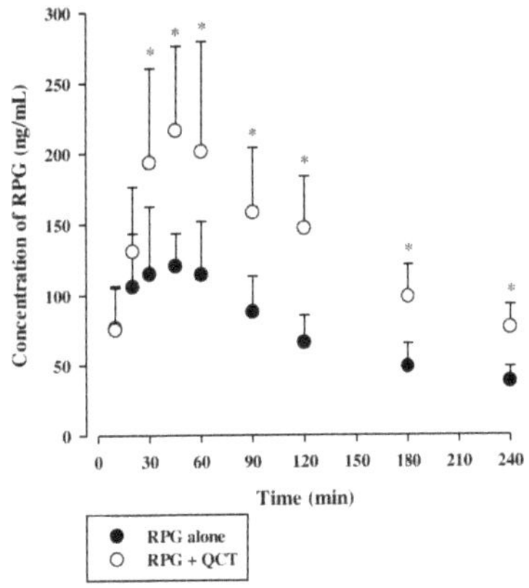

Figure 7. Plasma concentration versus time profiles of RPG following its oral administration at 0.4 mg/kg without or with oral QCT at 100 mg/kg in rats. The circles and their error bars represent the means and standard deviations, respectively ($n = 7$). The asterisks indicate statistical significance when compared to the control (RPG alone) group ($p < 0.05$).

Table 3. Pharmacokinetic parameters of RPG following its oral administration at 0.4 mg/kg without or with simultaneous oral administration of QCT at 100 mg/kg in rats ($n = 7$).

Parameter	RPG Alone	RPG with QCT
AUC (μg·min/mL)	25.7 ± 6.6	48.2 ± 9.6 *
$t_{1/2}$ (min)	139 ± 66	148 ± 49
C_{max} (ng/mL)	129 ± 33	238 ± 76 *
T_{max} (min)	45 (30–45)	45 (30–60)
Ae_U (% of dose)	0.458 ± 0.441	0.371 ± 0.336
Ae_{GI} (% of dose)	3.41 ± 1.65	2.90 ± 2.50
F (%)	50.7	95.1

* Significantly different from the control (RPG alone) group ($p < 0.05$).

4. Discussion

This study aimed to systematically investigate the potential metabolic drug–phytochemical interactions between RPG and QCT. A previous study reported that the metabolism of RPG (at 0.2 and 2 μM) in HLM was significantly inhibited by the presence of 25 μM QCT [8]. To our knowledge, however, the present study is the first systematic investigation of the kinetic mechanisms of the inhibitory actions of QCT on the metabolism of RPG and their possible species differences. Since CYP2C8- and CYP3A4-mediated metabolism are principally responsible for the elimination of RPG in humans [7,8], the results of the present in vitro microsomal metabolic interaction studies can be interpreted and discussed based on the principles and guidelines of CYP-mediated drug–drug interactions. The apparent K_i values represent the dissociation constant for the interaction between the inhibitor and the enzyme [39]. As the concentration of the inhibitor (QCT) increased from 0 μM to 200 μM in the present K_i estimation study, the V_{max} of RPG metabolism tended to decrease (RLM: 2016 to 928 pmol/min/mg protein; HLM: 1507 to 818 pmol/min/mg protein) and the K_m of RPG metabolism tended to increase (RLM: 53 to 81 μM; HLM: 23 to 111 μM). These results are typical diagnostic signatures of mixed inhibition [40], which are consistent with the graphical analysis of the constructed Dixon plots (Figure 5). A mixed inhibitor can bind to the enzyme–substrate complex as well as free enzymes, but it has a higher affinity for one state than the other [41]. In our present results, the α value (representing the extent to which the binding affinity between enzyme and substrate is changed by the inhibitor) was much greater than 1, implying that the inhibitor (QCT) may bind with a higher affinity to the free enzyme (CYP2C8/3A4) than the enzyme-substrate (RPG) complex [42]. Collectively, it is plausible that QCT can inhibit the hepatic metabolism of RPG in vitro via a mixed mechanism and the inhibition potency is weak in rats and moderate in humans.

To investigate the in vivo consequences of the aforementioned in vitro metabolic inhibition data, the pharmacokinetics of RPG with or without concurrent administration of QCT was assessed in rats. The in vivo intravenous and oral doses of RPG and QCT were selected based on previous rat pharmacokinetic studies [43–46]. In our present rat study, the urinary and fecal excretion of RPG administered intravenously was negligible (≤1.60% of the dose) [36], suggesting that RPG is primarily eliminated via metabolic routes. Assuming that RPG is metabolized exclusively by the liver, the hepatic clearance (CL_H) of RPG becomes equivalent to its blood clearance (calculated as CL/R_B = 9.11 mL/min/kg). Thus, the hepatic extraction ratio (E_H) of RPG can be estimated to be 0.114–0.182, by dividing the CL_H by the rat hepatic blood flow (Q_H, 50–80 mL/min/kg) [47]. The CL_H of a drug with a low E_H primarily depends on its unbound fraction in the blood (f_B) and CL_{int}, based on the well-stirred hepatic clearance model. Because the f_B (=f_P/R_B) of RPG was not significantly altered by the presence of QCT, the reduced CL of intravenous RPG by the co-administration of QCT (Table 1) could be attributed to a decrease in the CL_{int} of RPG, resulting from the observed inhibitory effects of QCT on RPG metabolism.

The F of RPG was known to be approximately 62.5% in humans [6], which coincides closely with that observed in the present rat study (Table 3). F can be determined by the fraction absorbed (F_{abs}), intestinal availability (F_G), and hepatic availability (F_H) as follows: $F = F_{abs} \times F_G \times F_H = F_{abs} \times (1 - E_G) \times (1 - E_H)$, where E_G is the GI extraction ratio. Consistent with intravenous RPG, the fecal excretion of oral RPG was observed to be minimal (2.21–5.78% of the dose administered). Thus, F_{abs} can be assumed to be 1, and the F_H of RPG in rats can be estimated to be 0.818–0.886 from our present rat data. The F_G of RPG can be calculated to be 0.572–0.620 in rats using the equation mentioned above, suggesting that considerable gut first-pass effects of RPG may occur, which warrants further investigation. Thus, in our present oral study using a combination of RPG and QCT, it is plausible that the gut and hepatic first-pass and hepatic systemic metabolism of RPG could have been inhibited by QCT, resulting in the increased systemic exposure (AUC and C_{max}) of RPG.

Notably, oral administration of QCT increased the AUC of orally administered RPG by 1.88-fold, indicating that QCT can be classified as an weak inhibitor of in vivo metabolism and systemic exposure of RPG in rats [48]. This suggests that a single oral QCT dose of 100 mg/kg achieved GI and hepatic QCT levels sufficient to significantly inhibit the first-pass and systemic metabolism of RPG in vivo. Previous clinical studies have reported controversial results regarding the pharmacokinetic interactions between QCT and therapeutic drugs. In healthy subjects, oral treatment with QCT at 500 mg/day for 21 days did not significantly change the pharmacokinetics of rosiglitazone [49], whereas the systemic exposure (AUC and/or C_{max}) of chlorzoxazone and caffeine were significantly increased by oral treatment with QCT at 1000 mg/day for 10 days and 500 mg/day for 14 days, respectively [14,50]. Based on the FDA guidelines [51], the magnitude of in vivo clinical herb–drug interactions between RPG and QCT was predicted from the in vitro protein binding and metabolism data. The ratio of the AUC of RPG in the presence and absence of QCT was predicted to be 1.03–1.54 by the basic (simple static) model (for a detailed calculation process, see Table S3 in the Supplementary Information). This suggests that QCT could act as a significant inhibitor for RPG metabolism in clinical settings, and there is a possibility that clinically significant pharmacokinetic interactions between QCT and RPG could occur, depending on the extent and duration of QCT intake from food products and dietary supplements.

5. Conclusions

This study clearly indicates that QCT can inhibit the hepatic metabolism of RPG in vitro via a mixed mechanism. Furthermore, the in vivo systemic exposure of RPG following intravenous and oral administration in rats was significantly increased by the concurrent administration of QCT. Based on the FDA guidelines, the magnitude of in vivo clinical herb–drug interactions between RPG and QCT was predicted to be a 1.03–1.54-fold increase in the AUC of RPG. These results suggest that clinically significant pharmacokinetic interactions between QCT and RPG could occur, which warrant further systematic clinical investigation.

Supplementary Materials: The following are available online at https://www.mdpi.com/article/10.3390/pharmaceutics13060782/s1, Figure S1: Cornish-Bowden plots for the inhibitory effects of QCT on the metabolism of RPG in RLM and HLM, Table S1: Within-run and between-run precision and accuracy of the present bioanalytical method for the quantification of RPG in biological matrices, Table S2: Within-run and between-run precision and accuracy of the present bioanalytical method for the quantification of QCT in biological matrices, Table S3: Parameters related to the estimation of R value. References [51,52] are cited in the supplementary materials.

Author Contributions: Conceptualization, J.-M.K., S.-W.S., H.Y. and I.-S.Y.; Data curation, J.-M.K. and S.-W.S.; Formal analysis, J.-M.K., S.-W.S. and D.-G.H.; Funding acquisition, H.Y. and I.-S.Y.; Investigation, J.-M.K., S.-W.S. and D.-G.H.; Methodology, J.-M.K. and S.-W.S.; Project administration, I.-S.Y.; Software, J.-M.K., S.-W.S. and H.Y.; Supervision, H.Y. and I.-S.Y.; Validation, J.-M.K. and S.-W.S.; Writing—original draft, J.-M.K.; Writing—review and editing, H.Y. and I.-S.Y. All authors have read and agreed to the published version of the manuscript.

Funding: This work was supported by the National Research Foundation of Korea (NRF) grants funded by the Ministry of Science and ICT (NRF-2020R1C1C1011061) and the Bio & Medical Technology Development Program of the National Research Foundation (NRF) funded by the Korea government (MSIT) (NRF-2017M3A9G7072568).

Institutional Review Board Statement: The study was approved by the Institutional Animal Care and Use Committee at Pusan National University (approval number: PNU-2019-2217, date of approval: 17 April 2019).

Informed Consent Statement: Not applicable.

Data Availability Statement: The data presented in this study are available in the paper.

Conflicts of Interest: The authors declare no conflict of interest.

References

1. Marbury, T.C.; Ruckle, J.L.; Hatorp, V.; Andersen, M.P.; Nielsen, K.K.; Huang, W.C.; Strange, P. Pharmacokinetics of repaglinide in subjects with renal impairment. *Clin. Pharmacol. Ther.* **2000**, *67*, 7–15. [CrossRef]
2. Sekhar, M.C.; Reddy, P.J. Influence of atorvastatin on the pharmacodynamic and pharmacokinetic activity of repaglinide in rats and rabbits. *Mol. Cell Biochem.* **2012**, *364*, 159–164. [CrossRef]
3. Riefflin, A.; Ayyagari, U.; Manley, S.E.; Holman, R.R.; Levy, J.C. The effect of glibenclamide on insulin secretion at normal glucose concentrations. *Diabetologia* **2015**, *58*, 43–49. [CrossRef]
4. Campbell, I.W. Nateglinide-current and future role in the treatment of patients with type 2 diabetes mellitus. *Int. J. Clin. Pract.* **2005**, *59*, 1218–1228. [CrossRef]
5. Tankova, T.; Koev, D.; Dakovska, L.; Kirilov, G. The effect of repaglinide on insulin secretion and oxidative stress in type 2 diabetic patients. *Diabetes Res. Clin. Pract.* **2003**, *59*, 43–49. [CrossRef]
6. Hatorp, V.; Oliver, S.; Su, C.A. Bioavailability of repaglinide, a novel antidiabetic agent, administered orally in tablet or solution form or intravenously in healthy male volunteers. *Int. J. Clin. Pharmacol. Ther.* **1998**, *36*, 636–641.
7. Bidstrup, T.B.; Bjornsdottir, I.; Sidelmann, U.G.; Thomsen, M.S.; Hansen, K.T. CYP2C8 and CYP3A4 are the principal enzymes involved in the human in vitro biotransformation of the insulin secretagogue repaglinide. *Br. J. Clin. Pharmacol.* **2003**, *56*, 305–314. [CrossRef]
8. Kajosaari, L.I.; Laitila, J.; Neuvonen, P.J.; Backman, J.T. Metabolism of repaglinide by CYP2C8 and CYP3A4 in vitro: Effect of fibrates and rifampicin. *Basic Clin. Pharmacol. Toxicol.* **2005**, *97*, 249–256. [CrossRef] [PubMed]
9. Egert, S.; Rimbach, G. Which sources of flavonoids: Complex diets or dietary supplements? *Adv. Nutr.* **2011**, *2*, 8–14. [CrossRef] [PubMed]
10. Han, D.-G.; Cho, S.-S.; Kwak, J.-H.; Yoon, I.-S. Medicinal plants and phytochemicals for diabetes mellitus: Pharmacokinetic characteristics and herb-drug interactions. *J. Pharm. Investig.* **2019**, *49*, 603–612. [CrossRef]
11. Chang, H.Y.; Wallis, M.; Tiralongo, E. Use of complementary and alternative medicine among people living with diabetes: Literature review. *J. Adv. Nurs.* **2007**, *58*, 307–319. [CrossRef]
12. Gruse, J.; Gors, S.; Tuchscherer, A.; Otten, W.; Weitzel, J.M.; Metges, C.C.; Wolffram, S.; Hammon, H.M. The effects of oral quercetin supplementation on splanchnic glucose metabolism in 1-week-old calves depend on diet after birth. *J. Nutr.* **2015**, *145*, 2486–2495. [CrossRef]
13. Hatahet, T.; Morille, M.; Hommoss, A.; Dorandeu, C.; Muller, R.H.; Begu, S. Dermal quercetin smartCrystals(R): Formulation development, antioxidant activity and cellular safety. *Eur. J. Pharm. Biopharm.* **2016**, *102*, 51–63. [CrossRef]
14. Bedada, S.K.; Neerati, P. The effect of quercetin on the pharmacokinetics of chlorzoxazone, a CYP2E1 substrate, in healthy subjects. *Eur. J. Clin. Pharmacol.* **2018**, *74*, 91–97. [CrossRef] [PubMed]
15. D'Andrea, G. Quercetin: A flavonol with multifaceted therapeutic applications? *Fitoterapia* **2015**, *106*, 256–271. [CrossRef] [PubMed]
16. Eid, H.M.; Haddad, P.S. The antidiabetic potential of quercetin: Underlying mechanisms. *Curr. Med. Chem.* **2017**, *24*, 355–364. [PubMed]
17. Almeida, A.F.; Borge, G.I.A.; Piskula, M.; Tudose, A.; Tudoreanu, L.; Valentová, K.; Williamson, G.; Santos, C.N. Bioavailability of quercetin in humans with a focus on interindividual variation. *Compr. Rev. Food Sci. Food Saf.* **2018**, *17*, 714–731. [CrossRef]
18. Komatsu, T.; Yamazaki, H.; Shimada, N.; Nakajima, M.; Yokoi, T. Roles of cytochromes P450 1A2, 2A6, and 2C8 in 5-fluorouracil formation from tegafur, an anticancer prodrug, in human liver microsomes. *Drug Metab. Dispos.* **2000**, *28*, 1457–1463.
19. Marill, J.; Capron, C.C.; Idres, N.; Chabot, G.G. Human cytochrome P450s involved in the metabolism of 9-cis- and 13-cis-retinoic acids. *Biochem. Pharmacol.* **2002**, *63*, 933–943. [CrossRef]
20. Projean, D.; Baune, B.; Farinotti, R.; Flinois, J.P.; Beaune, P.; Taburet, A.M.; Ducharme, J. In vitro metabolism of chloroquine: Identification of CYP2C8, CYP3A4, and CYP2D6 as the main isoforms catalyzing N-desethylchloroquine formation. *Drug Metab. Dispos.* **2003**, *31*, 748–754. [CrossRef]
21. Obach, R.S. Inhibition of human cytochrome P450 enzymes by constituents of St. John's Wort, an herbal preparation used in the treatment of depression. *J. Pharmacol. Exp. Ther.* **2000**, *294*, 88–95.
22. Zou, L.; Harkey, M.R.; Henderson, G.L. Effects of herbal components on cDNA-expressed cytochrome P450 enzyme catalytic activity. *Life Sci.* **2002**, *71*, 1579–1589. [CrossRef]
23. Walsky, R.L.; Obach, R.S.; Gaman, E.A.; Gleeson, J.P.; Proctor, W.R. Selective inhibition of human cytochrome P4502C8 by montelukast. *Drug Metab. Dispos.* **2005**, *33*, 413–418. [CrossRef]
24. Ostlund, J.; Zlabek, V.; Zamaratskaia, G. In vitro inhibition of human CYP2E1 and CYP3A by quercetin and myricetin in hepatic microsomes is not gender dependent. *Toxicology* **2017**, *381*, 10–18. [CrossRef]
25. Niemi, M.; Kajosaari, L.I.; Neuvonen, M.; Backman, J.T.; Neuvonen, P.J. The CYP2C8 inhibitor trimethoprim increases the plasma concentrations of repaglinide in healthy subjects. *Br. J. Clin. Pharmacol.* **2004**, *57*, 441–447. [CrossRef]
26. Tornio, A.; Filppula, A.M.; Kailari, O.; Neuvonen, M.; Nyronen, T.H.; Tapaninen, T.; Neuvonen, P.J.; Niemi, M.; Backman, J.T. Glucuronidation converts clopidogrel to a strong time-dependent inhibitor of CYP2C8: A phase II metabolite as a perpetrator of drug-drug interactions. *Clin. Pharmacol. Ther.* **2014**, *96*, 498–507. [CrossRef]
27. Niemi, M.; Backman, J.T.; Neuvonen, M.; Neuvonen, P.J. Effects of gemfibrozil, itraconazole, and their combination on the pharmacokinetics and pharmacodynamics of repaglinide: Potentially hazardous interaction between gemfibrozil and repaglinide. *Diabetologia* **2003**, *46*, 347–351. [CrossRef] [PubMed]

28. Kajosaari, L.I.; Niemi, M.; Backman, J.T.; Neuvonen, P.J. Telithromycin, but not montelukast, increases the plasma concentrations and effects of the cytochrome P450 3A4 and 2C8 substrate repaglinide. *Clin. Pharmacol. Ther.* **2006**, *79*, 231–242. [CrossRef] [PubMed]
29. VandenBrink, B.M.; Foti, R.S.; Rock, D.A.; Wienkers, L.C.; Wahlstrom, J.L. Evaluation of CYP2C8 inhibition in vitro: Utility of montelukast as a selective CYP2C8 probe substrate. *Drug Metab. Dispos.* **2011**, *39*, 1546–1554. [CrossRef] [PubMed]
30. Kim, S.B.; Lee, T.; Lee, H.S.; Song, C.K.; Cho, H.J.; Kim, D.D.; Maeng, H.J.; Yoon, I.S. Development and validation of a highly sensitive LC-MS/MS method for the determination of acacetin in human plasma and its application to a protein binding study. *Arch. Pharm. Res.* **2016**, *39*, 213–220. [CrossRef] [PubMed]
31. Isbell, J.; Yuan, D.; Torrao, L.; Gatlik, E.; Hoffmann, L.; Wipfli, P. Plasma Protein Binding of Highly Bound Drugs Determined With Equilibrium Gel Filtration of Nonradiolabeled Compounds and LC-MS/MS Detection. *J. Pharm. Sci.* **2019**, *108*, 1053–1060. [CrossRef] [PubMed]
32. Riccardi, K.; Cawley, S.; Yates, P.D.; Chang, C.; Funk, C.; Niosi, M.; Lin, J.; Di, L. Plasma Protein Binding of Challenging Compounds. *J. Pharm. Sci.* **2015**, *104*, 2627–2636. [CrossRef] [PubMed]
33. Kalvass, J.C.; Maurer, T.S. Influence of nonspecific brain and plasma binding on CNS exposure: Implications for rational drug discovery. *Biopharm. Drug Dispos.* **2002**, *23*, 327–338. [CrossRef]
34. Yoon, I.; Han, S.; Choi, Y.H.; Kang, H.E.; Cho, H.J.; Kim, J.S.; Shim, C.K.; Chung, S.J.; Chong, S.; Kim, D.D. Saturable sinusoidal uptake is rate-determining process in hepatic elimination of docetaxel in rats. *Xenobiotica* **2012**, *42*, 1110–1119. [CrossRef]
35. Kim, J.E.; Cho, H.J.; Kim, J.S.; Shim, C.K.; Chung, S.J.; Oak, M.H.; Yoon, I.S.; Kim, D.D. The limited intestinal absorption via paracellular pathway is responsible for the low oral bioavailability of doxorubicin. *Xenobiotica* **2013**, *43*, 579–591. [CrossRef] [PubMed]
36. Han, D.G.; Kwak, J.; Seo, S.W.; Kim, J.M.; Yoo, J.W.; Jung, Y.; Lee, Y.H.; Kim, M.S.; Jung, Y.S.; Yun, H.; et al. Pharmacokinetic Evaluation of Metabolic Drug Interactions between Repaglinide and Celecoxib by a Bioanalytical HPLC Method for Their Simultaneous Determination with Fluorescence Detection. *Pharmaceutics* **2019**, *11*, 382. [CrossRef]
37. Biasutto, L.; Marotta, E.; Garbisa, S.; Zoratti, M.; Paradisi, C. Determination of quercetin and resveratrol in whole blood–implications for bioavailability studies. *Molecules* **2010**, *15*, 6570–6579. [CrossRef]
38. Zhang, D.; Zhu, M.; Humphreys, W.G. *Drug Metabolism in Drug Design and Development: Basic Concepts and Practice*; John Wiley & Sons, Inc.: Hoboken, NJ, USA, 2007.
39. Kim, S.B.; Kim, K.S.; Kim, D.D.; Yoon, I.S. Metabolic interactions of rosmarinic acid with human cytochrome P450 monooxygenases and uridine diphosphate glucuronosyltransferases. *Biomed. Pharmacother.* **2019**, *110*, 111–117. [CrossRef] [PubMed]
40. Santos, J.A.; Kondo, M.Y.; Freitas, R.F.; dos Santos, M.H.; Ramalho, T.C.; Assis, D.M.; Juliano, L.; Juliano, M.A.; Puzer, L. The natural flavone fukugetin as a mixed-type inhibitor for human tissue kallikreins. *Bioorg. Med. Chem. Lett.* **2016**, *26*, 1485–1489. [CrossRef]
41. Copeland, R.A.; Horiuchi, K.Y. Kinetic effects due to nonspecific substrate-inhibitor interactions in enzymatic reactions. *Biochem. Pharmacol.* **1998**, *55*, 1785–1790. [CrossRef]
42. Kim, S.B.; Cho, H.J.; Kim, Y.S.; Kim, D.D.; Yoon, I.S. Modulation of Cytochrome P450 Activity by 18beta-Glycyrrhetic Acid and its Consequence on Buspirone Pharmacokinetics in Rats. *Phytother. Res.* **2015**, *29*, 1188–1194. [CrossRef]
43. Xu, Y.; Zhou, D.; Wang, Y.; Li, J.; Wang, M.; Lu, J.; Zhang, H. CYP2C8-mediated interaction between repaglinide and steviol acyl glucuronide: In vitro investigations using rat and human matrices and in vivo pharmacokinetic evaluation in rats. *Food Chem. Toxicol.* **2016**, *94*, 138–147. [CrossRef] [PubMed]
44. Choi, J.S.; Choi, I.; Choi, D.H. Effects of nifedipine on the pharmacokinetics of repaglinide in rats: Possible role of CYP3A4 and P-glycoprotein inhibition by nifedipine. *Pharmacol. Rep.* **2013**, *65*, 1422–1430. [CrossRef]
45. Yang, L.L.; Xiao, N.; Li, X.W.; Fan, Y.; Alolga, R.N.; Sun, X.Y.; Wang, S.L.; Li, P.; Qi, L.W. Pharmacokinetic comparison between quercetin and quercetin 3-O-beta-glucuronide in rats by UHPLC-MS/MS. *Sci. Rep.* **2016**, *6*, 35460. [CrossRef]
46. Liu, Y.; Luo, X.; Yang, C.; Yang, T.; Zhou, J.; Shi, S. Impact of quercetininduced changes in drugmetabolizing enzyme and transporter expression on the pharmacokinetics of cyclosporine in rats. *Mol. Med. Rep.* **2016**, *14*, 3073–3085. [CrossRef] [PubMed]
47. Seo, S.W.; Park, J.W.; Han, D.G.; Kim, J.M.; Kim, S.; Park, T.; Kang, K.H.; Yang, M.H.; Yoon, I.S. In Vitro and In Vivo Assessment of Metabolic Drug Interaction Potential of Dutasteride with Ketoconazole. *Pharmaceutics* **2019**, *11*, 673. [CrossRef] [PubMed]
48. Center for Drug Evaluation and Research. Clinical Interaction Studies: Cytochrome P450 Enzyme- and Transporter-Mediated Drug Interactions. *USA Food Drug Adm. Guid. Ind.* **2020**, 16–21. Available online: https://www.fda.gov/media/134581/download (accessed on 1 May 2021).
49. Kim, K.A.; Park, P.W.; Kim, H.K.; Ha, J.M.; Park, J.Y. Effect of quercetin on the pharmacokinetics of rosiglitazone, a CYP2C8 substrate, in healthy subjects. *J. Clin. Pharmacol.* **2005**, *45*, 941–946. [CrossRef] [PubMed]
50. Xiao, J.; Huang, W.H.; Peng, J.B.; Tan, Z.R.; Ou-Yang, D.S.; Hu, D.L.; Zhang, W.; Chen, Y. Quercetin significantly inhibits the metabolism of caffeine, a substrate of cytochrome P450 1A2 unrelated to CYP1A2*1C (-2964G>A) and *1F (734C>A) gene polymorphisms. *Biomed Res. Int.* **2014**, *2014*, 405071. [CrossRef]
51. Center for Drug Evaluation and Research. In Vitro Drug Interaction Studies: Cytochrome P450 Enzyme- and Transporter-Mediated Drug Interactions. *USA Food Drug Adm. Guid. Ind.* **2020**, 2–5. Available online: https://www.fda.gov/media/134582/download (accessed on 1 May 2021).
52. Ganio, M.S.; Armstrong, L.E.; Johnson, E.C.; Klau, J.F.; Ballard, K.D.; Michniak-Kohn, B.; Kaushik, D.; Maresh, C.M. Effect of quercetin supplementation on maximal oxygen uptake in men and women. *J. Sports Sci.* **2010**, *28*, 201–208. [CrossRef] [PubMed]

pharmaceutics

Article

Developing pH-Modulated Spray Dried Amorphous Solid Dispersion of Candesartan Cilexetil with Enhanced In Vitro and In Vivo Performance

Surendra Poudel and Dong Wuk Kim *

Vessel-Organ Interaction Research Center (VOICE, MRC), BK21 FOUR Community-Based Intelligent Novel Drug Discovery Education Unit, Research Institute of Pharmaceutical Sciences, College of Pharmacy, Kyungpook National University, Daegu 41566, Korea; surendrapoudel1016@gmail.com
* Correspondence: dkim17@knu.ac.kr; Tel.: +82-53-950-8579; Fax: +82-53-950-8557

Abstract: Candesartan cilexetil (CC), a prodrug and highly effective antihypertensive agent, is a poorly soluble (BCS Class II) drug with limited bioavailability. Here, we attempted to improve CC's bioavailability by formulating several CC-loaded amorphous solid dispersions with a hydrophilic carrier (PVPK30) and pH modifier (sodium carbonate) using the spray drying technique. Solubility, in vitro dissolution, and moisture content tests were used for screening the optimized formulation. We identified an optimized formulation of CC/PVPK30/SC, which at the ratio of 1:0.5:1 (*w*/*w*/*w*) exhibited a 30,000-fold increase in solubility and a more than 9-fold enhancement in dissolution compared to pure CC. Solid-state characterization revealed that in pH-modulated CC amorphous solid dispersion ($CCSD_{pM}$), CC's crystallinity was altered to an amorphous state with the absence of undesirable interactions. Stability studies also showed that the optimized formulation was stable with good drug content and drug release under accelerated conditions of up to 4 weeks and real-time stability conditions of up to 12 weeks. Furthermore, pharmacokinetic parameters, such as *AUC* and C_{max} of candesartan, had a 4.45-fold and 7.42-fold improvement, respectively, in $CCSD_{pM}$-treated rats compared to those in the CC-treated rats. Thus, these results suggest that $CCSD_{pM}$ is highly effective for increasing oral absorption. The application of these techniques can be a viable strategy to improve a drug's bioavailability.

Keywords: amorphous solid dispersion; candesartan Cilexetil; PVPK30; pH-modulation; spray drying; bioavailability

Citation: Poudel, S.; Kim, D.W. Developing pH-Modulated Spray Dried Amorphous Solid Dispersion of Candesartan Cilexetil with Enhanced In Vitro and In Vivo Performance. *Pharmaceutics* **2021**, *13*, 497. https://doi.org/10.3390/pharmaceutics13040497

Academic Editor: Im-Sook Song

Received: 4 March 2021
Accepted: 4 April 2021
Published: 6 April 2021

1. Introduction

Gradual shifts of drug therapeutics strategy toward targeting protein, ion channels, and synthesis/or regulation pathways have led to development of many lipophilic molecules or higher molecular weights molecules, or molecules with both properties. These lipophilic entities demonstrate low aqueous solubility, leading to erratic and limited oral bioavailability and poor therapeutic inefficacy [1–3]. As a result, formulation scientists face the significant challenges of improving the solubility and dissolution of lipophilic drugs in the gastrointestinal (GI) fluid. A promising way to increase a drug's dissolution rate in GI fluids is to alter the solubility or the surface area of the dissolving drugs, or both [4]. Different drug formulation strategies, such as micro or nanoparticle formation [5,6], solid dispersions (SD) [7–10], lipids-based formulation [11], inclusion complexation [12] and prodrugs [13,14] have been used to increase the rate of drug absorption in GI tract.

SD is a promising and widely accepted technique to increase the aqueous solubility of hydrophobic drugs [15,16]. Amorphous solid dispersion (ASD), a subset of SD, deals with molecular dispersion of drug molecules in an amorphous nontoxic hydrophilic carrier or matrix. The rationale behind ASD is to transform the crystalline form of drug into an amorphous form, a high-energy state, thus reducing the energy required to break crystal lattice and enhancing dissolution [17]. Technologies such as spray drying, KinetiSol® dispersing, and hot-melt extrusion give polymeric stabilized amorphous formulations. Spray drying is a popular solvent evaporation technique that atomizes a suspended or dissolved drug in a polymer solution or suspension with high pressure in a chamber with hot air to produce dried particles [18]. Commonly used polymers such as polyvinylpyrrolidone (PVP), sodium carboxymethyl cellulose (Na CMC), hydroxypropyl cellulose (HPC), and hydroxypropyl methylcellulose (HPMC) are highly water-soluble and help to increase the uptake of water in ASD. Spray drying techniques reduce particle size, whereas the hydrophilic polymer matrix provides an antiplasticization effect, stabilizing the amorphous form of a drug through its viscous properties, reducing the chemical potential of the drug and maintaining the drug's supersaturation in the GI lumen thus, improving the solubility and dissolution of drug candidate [18–20].

Polymer's physicochemical properties, such as melting point, glass transition temperature (T_g), solubility, molecular weight, viscosity, and miscibility with a drug molecule play an essential role in an ASD [21]. Usually drugs with higher melting temperature (T_m) have high lattice energy and drug with low glass transition temperature (Tg) have higher mobility. Both have high chances of crystallization and by forming ASD with polymer, the phenomena of recrystallization can be altered. The miscibility of polymer with drug decreases the T_m of drug while the Tg of ASD is increased [22,23]. Generally, the use of polymers with a higher glass transition temperature (Tg) in ASD increases the Tg of the dispersion system, enhancing the physiochemical stability of ASDs [24]. For example, Kollidon® 30 (polyvinylpyrrolidone K30, or PVPK30; Figure 1B) is a synthetic, almost white water-soluble polymer with a T_g at 163 °C. It is nontoxic and used for film-forming, solubilization, stabilizing, taste masking and supersaturation maintenance/precipitation inhibitor agent [25].

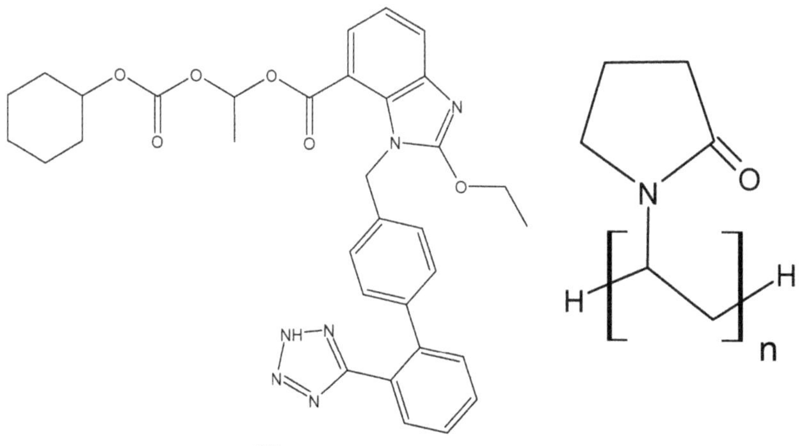

(A) (B)

Figure 1. *Cont.*

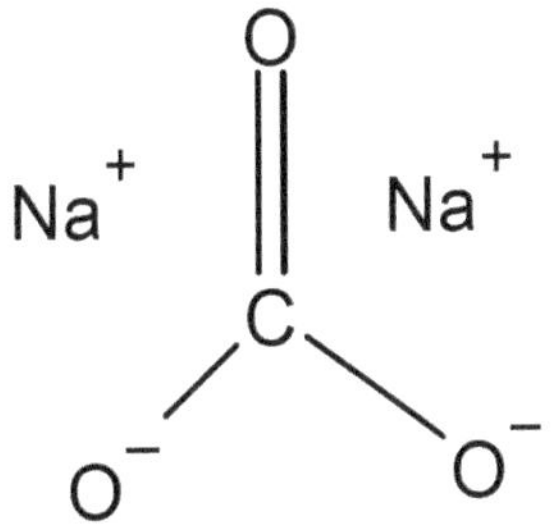

(C)

Figure 1. The chemical structure of candesartan cilexetil (CC) (**A**), Kollidon 30 (PVPK30) (**B**), and sodium carbonate (SC) (**C**).

Although ASD enhances the dissolution rate of hydrophobic drugs, inadequate drug solubility of polymers might result into limited enhancement. One of the commonly used strategies to maximize the aqueous solubility of weakly acidic or basic drugs is to use pH modifiers (pH_M) with a polymer. The intraluminal pH of GI tract is diversified from highly acidic in stomach to alkaline at the intestinal regions. Such variation largely affects the weakly acidic or basic drugs as the environmental pH plays crucial role in solubility and dissolution [26]. The pH_M used in formulation gets dissolved in the adjacent diffusion layer and alters the microenvironment pH which induces higher saturation solubility at diffusion layer. These phenomenon leads to increased drug dissolution with supersaturation at the bulk solution. Since the supersaturation at micro-level involves the risk of rapid precipitation and/or recrystallization of drug, use of polymer helps to stabilize and maintain the supersaturation state for longer period of time which directly affects the rate of absorption [27].

Candesartan cilexetil (CC) (Figure 1A) is an ester prodrug that is generally prescribed for management of hypertension and heart failure by itself or with ACE inhibitors, beta-blockers, and diuretics. CC is biotransformed into the active metabolite, candesartan, after ester hydrolysis in the GI tract. Candesartan is a potent angiotensin II receptor blocker that restricts the activity of vasoconstrictors and produces antihypertensive effects [28]. Despite its potent therapeutic effects, CC is a BCS Class II drug with low aqueous solubility (at less than 8×10^{-8} M, pKa 6.0) across various physiological pH environments, contributing to its incomplete absorption in the GI tract [29,30]. CC was selected as a drug candidate because of its erratic and low bioavailability (15% to 40%) after oral administration and high first-pass metabolism. Therefore, approaches enhancing drug solubility can be handy to enhance absorption and oral bioavailability of CC. Moreover, several studies have reported enhanced candesartan bioavailability using SD [31], nano-based system [6,32,33] but increasing solubility with pH modulation in ASD is an area of interest. However, the inclusion of pH modifier comes with challenges related to production and stability due to hygroscopicity of pH modifier so, formulation with less hydroscopic pH modifier and smaller amount of pH modifier were more desired to maintain integrity of ASD.

This study aimed to design and fabricate a novel optimized CC-loaded ASD with a pH modifier to improve candesartan oral bioavailability. The $CCSD_{pM}$ was prepared by the solvent evaporation technique with selected polymer and alkalizer in a spray dryer. The optimized formulation was characterized using solid-state characterization tools, such as scanning electron microscopy (SEM), Fourier transform infrared (FTIR) spectroscopy, differential scanning calorimetry (DSC), and X-ray diffraction (XRD). The in vitro dissolution of $CCSD_{pM}$ was assessed in various media. Finally, the bioavailability of $CCSD_{pM}$ was compared with pure drug CC in Sprague–Dawley rats.

2. Material and Methods

2.1. Materials

CC (Hanmi Fine Chemical Co. Ltd., Siheung, Korea), candesartan (purity > 99%; ALADDIN Biochemical Technology Co. Ltd., Shanghai, China), and Kollidon 30 (PVPK30; BASF Chemical Co., Ludwigshafen, Germany) were obtained. Sodium carbonate, sodium hydroxide, potassium hydroxide, and sodium bicarbonate were purchased from Duksan Chemicals Co. (Ansan, Korea). All other components and chemical agents were of analytical or HPLC grade; they were used without additional purification.

2.2. Saturation Solubility Studies of CC

The saturation solubility of candesartan cilexetil (CC) was examined in different pH (1.2, 4.0, 6.8, and 10) and deionized water. An excess amount of CC was added to an Eppendorf tube containing 1 mL of the test solution. The mixture was thoroughly vortexed and placed in an isothermal shaking water bath at 25 ± 0.5 °C at 100 rpm for five days. Then, the samples were centrifuged at 10,000× *g* for 5 min followed with filtration using a 0.45-μm membrane filter. Next, the filtrate was diluted with the deionized water to determine the drug concentration using UV spectroscopy.

2.3. Screening of Polymer Carrier and Alkalizers

Various polymers and alkalizers were screened with the saturation solubility method to select a suitable carrier and alkalizing agent. In short, an excess amount of CC was added to a tube containing 1% (*w*/*v*) of a polymer or an alkalizer followed by vortexing. All the samples were then incubated in a shaking water bath at 25 ± 0.5 °C and 100 rpm. After five days, the samples were centrifuged at 10,000× *g* for 5 min and filtered using a 0.45 μm membrane filter. Then, the filtrates were analyzed with a UV spectrophotometer at 254 nm.

2.4. Supersaturation Stabilization Assessment

Polymers are commonly known to stabilize or inhibit precipitation of supersaturated drugs [20,34,35]. A polymer's ability to stabilize supersaturation is studied using the solvent shift method [36]. A dissolution apparatus (ERWEKA; DT 620, Heusenstamm, Germany) was the ideal instrument to maintain the temperature and rpm of the test solution. For each test solution, a selected polymer was dissolved at the concentration of 0.05% and maintained at 37 °C and 50 rpm [37]. Here,1 mL of 25 mg/mL CC in DMSO was added into a 900 mL of the test solution; 2 mL of the mixture was withdrawn with subsequent equal replacement, filtered through a 0.22 mm Millipore filter at predetermined time intervals within 240 min, and analyzed using a UV spectrophotometer (see Section 2.6).

2.5. Preparation of ASD

The selected polymer and alkalizing agents were used to formulate different pH-modulated ASDs to identify the optimal formulation. A lab-scale spray dryer (ADL311S; Yamato Scientific, Tokyo, Japan) was used to prepare ternary SDs of the drug, polymer, and alkalizer. At 1 g of CC in 100 mL of methanol, the methanolic solution of CC was dispersed into 200 mL of deionized water containing different amounts of carrier and alkalizer (fixed at 1 g) with stirring to produce a clear homogenous solution (Table 1). The clear solutions were then transferred at a rate of 3.5 mL/min with a peristaltic pump through a nozzle with a 0.4-mm diameter. The air was heated to 120 °C in the drying chamber and the air escaping from the spray dryer was at 65–70 °C. The atomizing was maintained at 0.15 MPa. The average flow rate of drying air was adjusted at 0.13 m^3/min by setting the blower knob at 5.5. In total, five SDs were prepared for further evaluation to select the optimized ternary solid dispersion.

Table 1. Compositions of the pH-modulated amorphous solid dispersion (ASDs) with different polymer ratios.

Formulation	CC (g)	PVPK30 (g)	Na_2CO_3 (g)
F1	1	0.5	1
F2	1	1	1
F3	1	2	1
F4	1	4	1
F5	1	8	1

2.6. *UV-VIS Spectroscopy*

The quantitative measurement of CC was conducted with a UV-VIS spectrophotometer (UV-1800; Shimadzu, Kyoto, Japan). The standard calibration curve was drawn from known CC concentrations between 0.625 and 25 μg mL^{-1} in methanol measured at 254 nm using Beer–Lambert plots. A standard curve with linearity (R^2 = 0.9991) was used for the quantification of CC.

2.7. *Optimization of $CCSD_{pM}$*

2.7.1. Aqueous Saturated Solubility and In Vitro Dissolution Study

The solubility of the five $CCSD_{pM}$ formulations was examined to select the formulation with maximal solubility. An excess amount of an $CCSD_{pM}$ was added to a vial containing 1 mL of deionized water. The resultant suspension was maintained at 25 ± 0.5 °C and 100 rpm in an isothermal shaking water bath for five days. Next, the $CCSD_{pM}$ suspension was centrifuged at 10,000× *g* for 5 min and filtered to obtain a clear supernatant solution. The drug's concentration in the supernatant was determined with a UV spectrophotometer at 254 nm.

The in vitro dissolution behavior is one of the crucial criteria in determining ASD technique viability. The dissolution test of $CCSD_{pM}$ equivalent to 8 mg of CC and 8 mg of pure CC was performed using a USP Type II dissolution apparatus (ERWEKA; DT 620, Heusenstamm, Germany). The $CCSD_{pM}$ or the pure CC powder was placed in a capsule (size "0"), and a sinker was used to sink the capsule to the bottom of vessels filled with 900 mL of distilled water maintained at 37 ± 0.5 °C with continuous stirring at 50 rpm. Two mL of the medium was sampled at predetermined time intervals at 5, 10, 15, 30, 45, and 60 min; after each sampling, 2 mL of fresh medium was added to replenish the volume loss. The sampled medium was filtered through 0.45 μm PTFE syringe filter, and the drug released into the medium was analyzed using a UV spectrophotometer, as mentioned above.

2.7.2. Moisture Content Measurement

The moisture content of the formulations F1–F5 was analyzed by a moisture analyzer (OHAUS, MB 120). The instrument records the difference in the sample's weight before and, after heating up to 100 °C for 10 min. Finally, the difference in weight was displayed as percentage of moisture content (MC), an indicator of water content in the sample.

2.8. *Characterization of $CCSD_{pM}$*

2.8.1. Drug Content Assay

The estimation of drug loading is crucial to exclude drug loss by the spray drying process. For drug loading assay, 100 μg/mL of CC in methanol was prepared with the equivalent amount of $CCSD_{pM}$, filtered, and analyzed using UV spectroscopy (Section 2.6). The mathematical relation, drug content (%) = estimated drug content/theoretical drug content × 100, was used to determine drug content.

2.8.2. External Morphology

The surface morphology of pure drug, polymer, alkalizer, physical mixture (PM), and optimized $CCSD_{pM}$ was assessed using a scanning electron microscope (SEM) (SU8220; Hitachi; Tokyo, Japan). The physical mixture was composed of CC, Kollidon 30, and Na_2CO_3 in the weight ratio of 1:0.5:1. The samples were fixed on the brass post with two-sided adhesive tapes and sputter-coated for 4 min at 5.0 kV and 15 mA using a Sputter Coater (EMI Tech, K575 K; West Sussex, UK).

2.8.3. Differential Scanning Calorimetry (DSC)

The change in the physical properties of CC, Kollidon 30, Na2CO3, PM, and $CCSD_{pM}$, F1, along with temperature against time, was measured using a thermal analysis instrument (DSC Q20; Newcastle, DE, USA). Approximately 5 mg of a sample was placed in a non-hermetically enclosed aluminum pan and heated with dry nitrogen purge at 50 mL/min. The instrument was operated at a scan rate of 10 °C/min in a heating range of 30–220 °C.

2.8.4. X-ray Diffraction (XRD)

The X-ray diffraction (XRD) analysis of the pure drug, polymer, alkalizer, PM, and $CCSD_{pM}$ was performed using a D/MAX-2500 XR instrument (Rigaku, Japan) equipped with a Cu anode. The X-ray beam was operated at a voltage of 40 kV and a current of 40 mA. The scanning range was between 5°–35° (2θ) with a scanning speed of 0.05°/s. The diffractograms was plotted using the SIGMA PLOT 12.0 software.

2.8.5. Fourier Transform Infrared Spectroscopy (FTIR)

The percentage transmittance of the pure drug, polymer, alkalizer, PM, and F1 was analyzed with an FTIR spectrophotometer (Frontier; PerkinElmer, Norwalk, CT, USA). The samples were placed with a KBr disk and scanned from 4000 to 400 cm^{-1} at a 2 cm^{-1} resolution. The KBr pellets were a mixture of 1 g of sample and 200 mg of KBr.

2.9. Stability Assessment

The optimized pH-modulated ASD (F1) was investigated for the changes in its attributes over time under environmental conditions such as temperature and humidity. As per ICH guidelines, the samples were introduced into a stability chamber maintained at real-time (RT) at 25 ± 2°C, 60 ± 5% relative humidity (RH) and the accelerated stability conditions (ACC) of 40 ± 2 °C and 75 ± 5% RH [38]. At predetermined intervals, 1, 4, 8, and 12 weeks for RT and 1 and 4 weeks for ACC, the samples were analyzed for drug content and in vitro dissolution by UV spectroscopy.

2.10. Pharmacokinetic Study

2.10.1. Animal Handling and Blood Sampling

Sprague Dawley rats aged 7–9 weeks and weighing 280–343 g, were used for the in vivo experiments. The rats were adapted to the controlled conditions of 25 ± 2 °C, 55 ± 5% RH, and 12-h light/dark cycles for at least 3 days. The rats were abstained from food and had free access to water for at least 12 h ahead of the oral administration of the drugs. All the procedures were as per established codes at Kyungpook National University (Institutional Animal Care and Use Committee, License Number: 2019-0054, Authorization date: 1 March 2019).

Twelve rats are divided into two groups, with 6 per group (n = 6). Each rat was given 10 mg/kg CC aqueous suspension or F1 (the optimized $CCSD_{pM}$) at a single dose with oral gavage. The CC aqueous suspension was developed by dispersing the pure CC powder in 0.5% *w*/*v* in Na CMC. Subsequently, approximately 0.3 mL of the blood sample was collected in a heparinized tube at predetermined intervals of 0.083, 0.25, 0.5, 1, 2, 4, 8, 12, and 24 hr. Juglar vein was selected for blood sampling after the rats were anesthetized with diethyl ether. The collected blood samples were immediately centrifuged at 13,000× *g* for 10 min at 4 °C and stored at −20 °C.

2.10.2. Plasma Sample Analysis

A 90 µL plasma sample was vortexed with 40 µL of irbesartan (IS), internal standard, and 270 µL of ACN, a precipitating agent, for a few minutes, and centrifuged at 1000× *g* for 20 min. The final concentration of IS was maintained at 1 µg/mL. The clear supernatant liquid was transferred into an HPLC vial, and 20 µL of it was injected into a column (Capcell Pak C18, 4.6 × 250 mm) equilibrated at 25 °C with a mobile phase of ACN: MeOH: Potassium dihydrogen phosphate at pH 3.0 at a ratio of 30:30:40 (*v*:*v*:*v*). The samples were injected at a flow rate of 1.0 mL/min, and the quantification was done at λ_{max} 254 nm. A standard plasma curve was projected in the range of 25–5000 ng/mL, showing good linearity (R^2 = 0.9998).

2.10.3. Statistical Evaluation

The pharmacokinetics parameters of candesartan, such as the area under the concentration-time curve (*AUC*), half-life ($T_{1/2}$), peak plasma concentration (C_{max}), time for C_{max} (T_{max}), and elimination-rate constant (K_{el}) of each rat, were determined by fitting to a noncompartmental analysis using WinNonlin^{TM} (Pharsight Corp.; Mountain View, CA, USA). The $AUC_{0\text{–}24h}$ was estimated using the trapezoidal rule. Unpaired Student's *t*-test was used to analyze the level of statistical significance ($p < 0.05$).

3. Results and Discussion

3.1. Saturation Solubility and Screening Studies

Understanding the solubility profile of a drug in various test solutions would help select the carriers and solubilizers that are optimal for the preparation of ASDs. Polymers and other excipients must have good compatibility and affinity with the drug to achieve the desired in vitro dissolution rate, which is correlated to a favorable in vivo drug profile [9]. CC behaves like a weakly acidic drug and gets deprotonated in solutions with a high pH (pH > pKa), resulting increased solubility profile [39].

Among the test solutions with different pH values, CC had remarkably high solubility, at 3148.29 ± 338.32 µg/mL, at pH 10.0, and very low solubility at pH 1.2, 4.0, 6.8, and water (Figure 2A). These data demonstrate that ASD with alkaline pH modifiers will enhance CC's solubility. In the solubility screening of the alkalizers as pH modifiers, the CC in 1% *w*/*v* sodium hydroxide solution had the highest solubility at 78,254.85 ± 2239.49 µg/mL; in contrast, the CC in sodium bicarbonate had the lowest solubility at 34.67 ± 2.03 µg/mL (Figure 2B). Though the highest solubility was demonstrated by hydroxides of sodium and potassium, sodium carbonate was chosen because the hydroxides were strong alkalizing agents with more hygroscopicity properties that would impact the stability of formulations.

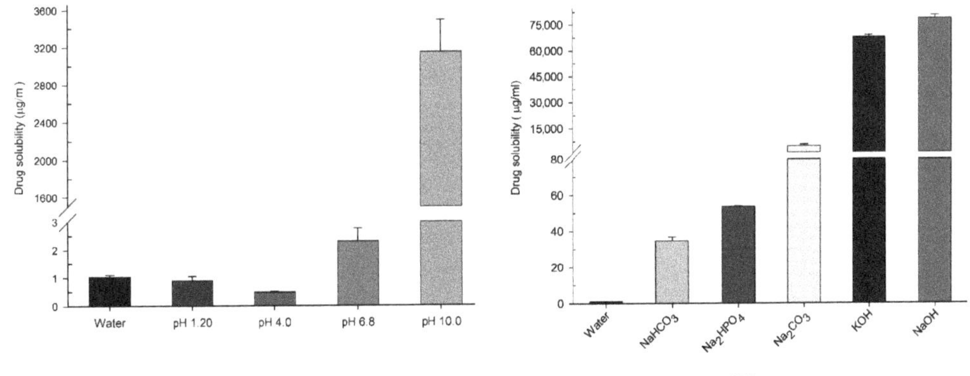

(A) (B)

Figure 2. Aqueous solubility of CC in (**A**) different pH conditions and (**B**) different alkalizers (1% *w*/*v*). Each value represents the mean of three experiments (n = 3), and the error bar represents the standard deviation.

Similarly, the solubility study (Figure 3A) of the polymeric carriers showed that Kollidon 30 (PVPK30) had the highest drug solubility at 31.60 ± 5.84 µg/mL whereas copovidone had the lowest drug solubility at 3.83 ± 0.67 µg/mL among the hydrophilic carriers. Kollidon 30 is a hydrophilic polymer with successful pharmaceutical applications. Its amorphous nature, higher T_g, and hydrophilicity indicate its suitability for the spray drying technique.

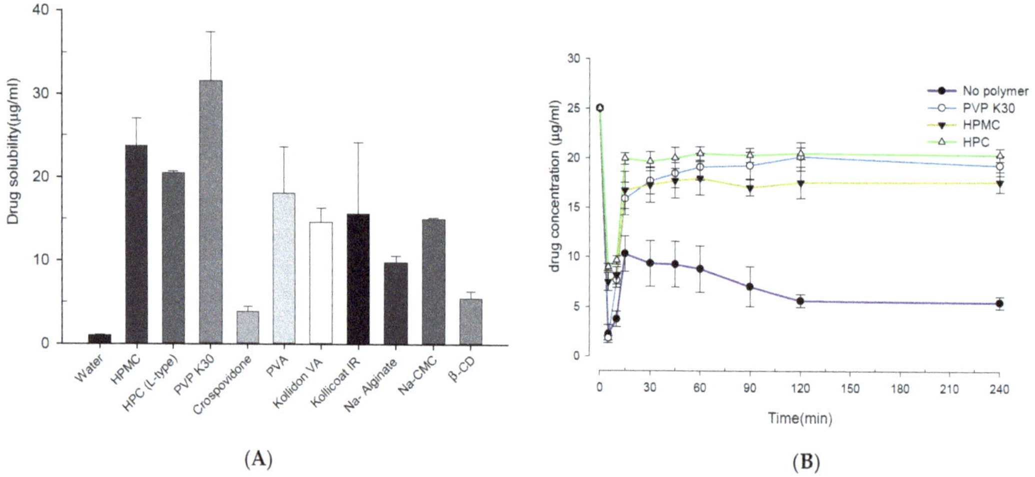

Figure 3. (**A**) The solubility of CC in different polymer solutions (1% *w*/*v*). (**B**) The concentration-time profile of CC in various test solutions. Each value represents the mean of three experiments (n = 3), and the error bar represents the standard deviation.

In addition to solubility screening, the supersaturation maintenance test was also conducted to analyze ability of polymer to stabilize or inhibit precipitate from saturated state of drug in a non-sink condition. Generally, ASD techniques generate drugs in an amorphous state that tends to precipitate rapidly in GI lumen; thus, polymeric stabilizers can extend and maintain a drug in a supersaturable state in GI lumen [40]. Here, PVPK30, HPMC, HPC, and distilled water were used as test solutions to study the supersaturation maintenance behavior for 4 h, which mimics intestinal transit. The supersaturation profile (concentration-time) of the individual polymers was examined (Figure 3B). In all the test solutions, a rapid decrease in CC concentration was observed immediately after the injection of concentrated CC; subsequently, CC concentration was maintained based on the polymer's supersaturation maintenance ability. HPC had highest ability to maintain CC concentration of 20.38 µg/mL for up to 240 min, whereas HPMC had least ability. In addition, PVPK30 could also maintain a CC concentration of approximately 19.3 µg/mL for up to 240 min. Similar behavior can be correlated with the saturation solubility study, as polymers can increase CC's solubility.

The stabilization of the supersaturation state is a complex phenomenon which can be regulated with increasing the solubility by reducing nucleation and crystal growths, increasing the viscosity by reducing molecular mobility, thus decreasing nucleation and crystal growth and altering the solvation level at the crystal/liquid interface [41]. A slight increase in supersaturation maintenance of CC by HPC could be related to the viscosity phenomenon by cellulose-based polymers, which in turn limits molecular mobility [42]. Considering the results from the solubility enhancement and supersaturation stabilization studies, PVPK30 was chosen for developing pH-modulated ASDs using the spray drying method.

3.2. Optimization of $CCSD_{pM}$ Formulations

Sprayed dried $CCSD_{pM}$ formulations (F1–F5) were prepared using a spray dryer (ADL311S; Yatamo Scientific) with PVPK30 as a hydrophilic carrier and SC as an alkalizer. The effect of varying weight ratios of PVPK30 on the solubility of a $CCSD_{pM}$ formulation was studied by assessing the solubility profiles of all the formulations (Figure 4A). The incorporation of SC and PVPK30 demonstrated a phenomenal enhancement of CC solubility, in $CCSD_{pM}$'s compared to the CC powder, at more than 15,000-fold, irrespective of the polymer ratios. Additionally, increasing PVPK30 did not consistently improve CC's solubility as F1 with the lowest PVPK30 showed maximum solubility.

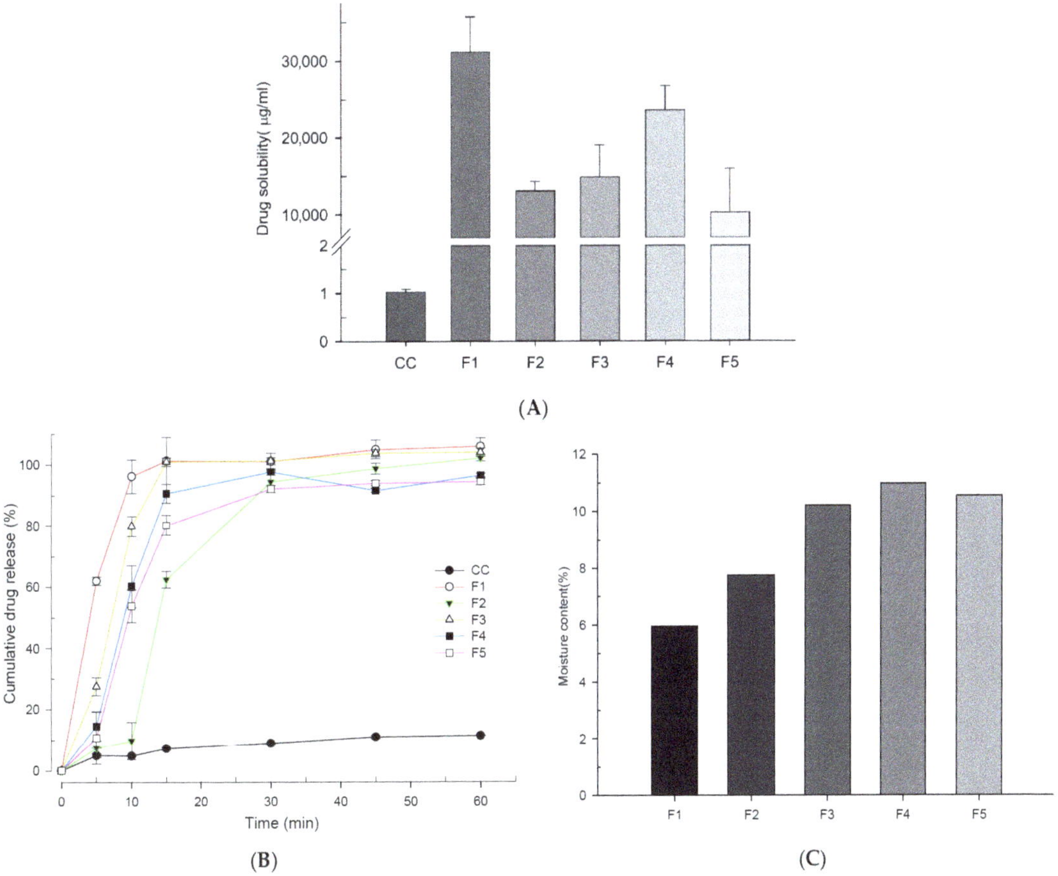

Figure 4. (**A**) The drug solubility of the $CCSD_{pM}$ formulations (F1–F5). (**B**) The in vitro release profiles of the pure drug from the capsules compared to that of the different $CCSD_{pM}$ formulations in distilled water. (**C**) The moisture content of the $CCSD_{pM}$ formulations.

The degree of pH modulation with SC in varying drug: polymer ratio is an important aspect for such differences in solubility of five formulations. The maximum enhancement in F1 could be due to adequate microenvironmental pH modulation with SC in given lower amount of PVPK30. Additionally, drug particles might have extensive size reduction achieving increased surface area with molecular dispersion into given amount of PVPK30 matrix [9]. Surprisingly, F2–F4 have increasing trends in solubility and F5 shows slight reduction in solubility enhancement. The uptrend of F2–F5 suggest that, SC doesn't have major effect as in F1 but the increasing amount of PVPK30 in presence of SC increased the solubility. However, in F5, there was not significant cumulative effect of PVPK30 and SC as amount of PVPK30 was highest. Although, there was slight reduction in solubility of F5, it still had more than 15,000-fold improvement in comparison with pure CC.

While the conventional SD system increases the solubility and dissolution profile of hydrophobic drugs, using large amount of polymer with exclusive or heavy use of organic solvent in the formulation had been a major issue. Organic solvents are not ideal from health, environmental and industrial-scale perspectives. Thus, the difference in solubility of polymers and drugs in an organic solvent and incomplete removal of organic solvents are significant limitations associate with conventional SD techniques [14,43]. We attempted to reduce the toxicity of an organic solvent by dissolving the drug in a relatively small volume of organic solvent followed with dispersion in the aqueous phase. In addition, a relatively small amount of polymer was used for solubilization in the presence of an alkalizer.

The dissolution study of the $CCSD_{pM}$ formulations in deionized water revealed that the incorporation of SC as an alkalizer and PVPK30 as a hydrophilic carrier greatly enhances their drug release rate compared to the CC powder. The CC powder's release rate was only about 11% at 60 min, while all the $CCSD_{pM}$ formulations released more than 90% of their drugs at 30 min. F2 had a slower release rate than others before 30 min, while other formulations had a similar release rate (Figure 4B). The difference in the release rate of the $CCSD_{pM}$ formulations may be due to the differences in their solubilities, water penetration time inside the capsule, and relative time for the alkalizer to maintain the alkaline microenvironment. Once $CCSD_{pM}$ formulations were in contact with water, the alkalizer modulates the solution surrounding the $CCSD_{pM}$ to enable CC's transformation into an unprotonated state [44]. Besides the alkalizer, another contributing factor may be the wetting ability of the polymer along with the transformation of the crystallinity state into the amorphous state (from results of solid-state characterization).

The amount of moisture can directly affect a drug's physical stability as well as the recrystallization phenomenon. Here, the water content of all the formulations (F1–F5) was also measured. About 10.9% moisture was observed in the F4 formulation, the highest among the ASDs. On the other hand, F1 had the lowest moisture content at about 5.96%, which was correlated to its smallest amount of hydrophilic polymer among the formulations (Figure 4C). The differences in the moisture content might be due to incomplete drying after spray drying and a varying amount of PVPK30 that attribute to different hygroscopicity in the formulations. After reviewing the results from the dissolution, solubility, and moisture content studies, F1 was selected for further characterization and assessment as it had the highest solubility, a better drug release rate, and lower moisture content.

3.3. Assessment of Selected $CCSD_{pM}$ Formulations

The in vitro dissolution profile of the selected $CCSD_{pM}$, F1, was investigated at various solutions including distilled water and solutions at pH 1.2, 4.0 and 6.8, and then compared with the dissolution profile of the PM and the free CC (Figure 5). It was observed that F1 had a substantially higher drug release rate at all conditions than the PM or the free CC. At pH 1.2 and 4.0, the drug release of F1 was above 60% within 60 min; at higher pH, F1's drug release was above 90%. On the other hand, no significant changes were observed in the release characteristics of the free CC under different conditions. However, significant variations of drug release were observed in the case of PM. There was a difference of approximately 30% in drug release at pH 4.0 solution and distilled water whereas more than a difference of 60% in drug release at pH 1.2 and 6.8 between PM and F1. The low drug release rate of PM further confirmed the superiority of $CCSD_{pM}$ F1. The variation in drug release from F1 at different pH media solution suggest that there is an influence of pre-existing pH conditons of media (diffusion layer) in the microenvironmental pH modulation capacity of alkalizer. It was also seen that the pH of the dissolution solution was not altered drastically during the experiment, and all the dissolution profiles were correlated to the solution's pH.

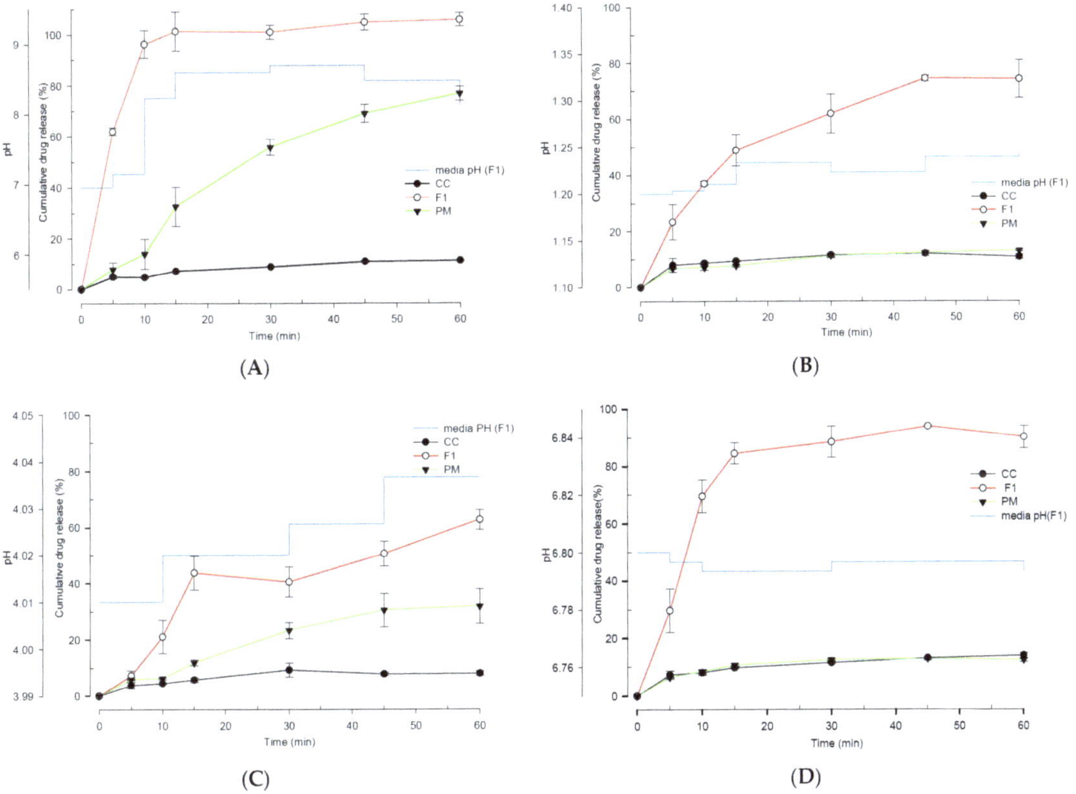

Figure 5. The in vitro dissolution study of CC from capsules filled with optimized formulation (F1), physical mixture (PM), and pure drug in (**A**) distilled water, (**B**) a solution at pH 1.2, (**C**) a solution at pH 4.0 and (**D**) a solution at pH 6.8. Each value represents the mean of three experiments (n = 3), and the error bar represents the standard deviation.

In addition, the saturated solubility of F1, PM, and free CC was studied at pH 1.2, 4.0, and 6.8 and in water (Table 2). The optimized $CCSD_{PM}$, F1, displayed notable improvement in the saturated solubility over free CC and the PM. F1's saturated solubility was more than 30,000-fold of that of free CC and at least 3-fold of that of PM. F1's improvements in dissolution and solubility over the PM are due to ASDs that transform crystalline materials into amorphous forms and the solubilization, stabilization, and wetting effects of the polymers and alkalizers [44]. Further, a drug loading study showed that F1 had the highest drug content at about 99%, which could be correlated with its excellent dissolution profile.

Table 2. The solubility of the free CC, physical mixture (PM), and F1 in solutions with different pH.

Medium	CC (μg/mL)	PM (μg/mL)	F1 (μg/mL)
Water	1.03 ± 0.06	7613.11 ± 6480.31	31,156.05 ± 4552.69
pH 1.2	0.89 ± 0.13	10,462.60 ± 6492.75	32,212.37± 4785.75
pH 4.0	0.48 ± 0.03	103.78 ± 76.71	31,095.11 ± 5395.98
pH 6.8	2.30 ± 0.37	822.71 ± 171.25	38,424.75 ± 7539.25

Each value represents the mean of three experiments (n = 3) ± standard deviation.

3.4. Physiochemical Characterization

The solid-state properties of free CC, PM, and F1 were investigated using characterization tools, such as SEM, DSC, and XRD. The external morphological view of CC,

PVPK30, SC, PM, and F1 was imaged with SEM (Figure 6). The CC powder appeared as irregularly shaped crystalline structures (Figure 6A), whereas PVPK30 and SC had spherical particles with a smooth surface and fine particles with no distinctive shape, respectively (Figure 6B,C). The PM (Figure 6D) in the same ratio as F1 had the alkalizer and drug particles adhering to the carrier's surface. Surprisingly, F1 appeared to have spherical and some dented particles without the presence of drug particles on its outer surface (Figure 6E).

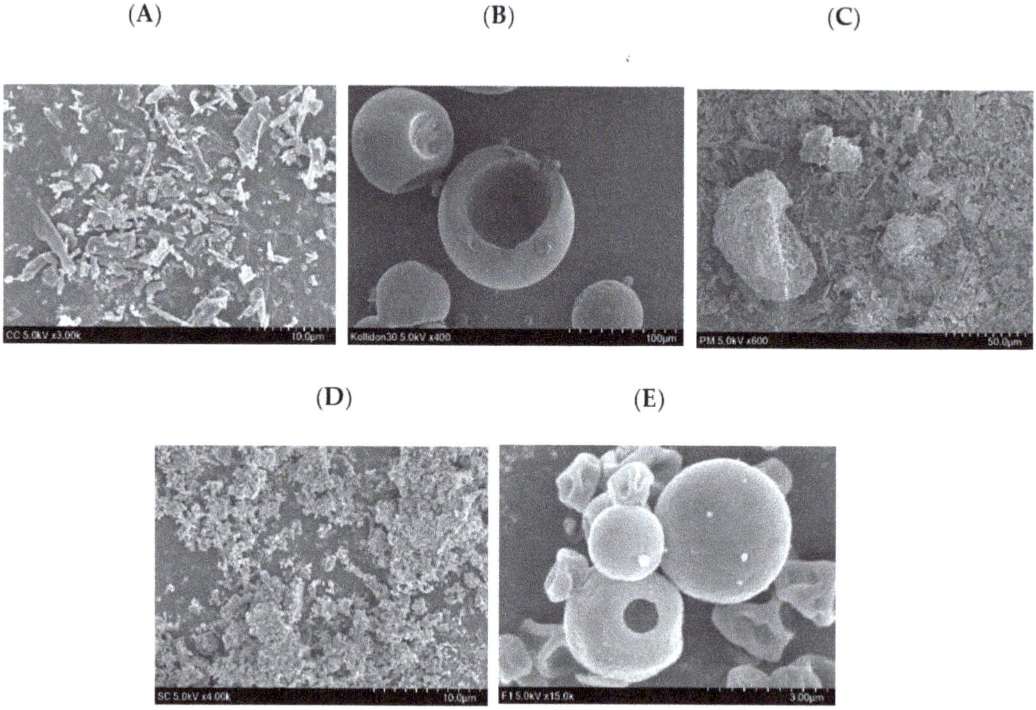

Figure 6. SEM image of (**A**) CC powder, (**B**) PVPK30, (**C**) SC (Na_2CO_3), (**D**) physical mixture (PM), and (**E**) F1.

On the other hand, DSC analysis revealed the thermal characteristics of pure drug CC, PVPK30, SC, and F1 (Figure 7A). The DSC curve of CC showed an endothermic peak around 170 °C, consistent with the previous finding that CC was thermally stable at below 162 °C [45,46]. The sharp endothermic peak also confirms that CC's structure is crystalline. Moreover, PVPK30 and SC had not shown any characteristic sharp endothermic peak except the broad endothermic peak at 50–130 °C for PVPK30 and 70–85 °C and 110–112 °C for SC. In addition, DSC of PM revealed a reduced endothermic peak of CC, suggesting weak interaction with the carriers. However, CC's characteristic endothermic peak is absent in the F1 DSC curve, suggesting inhibited crystallinity.

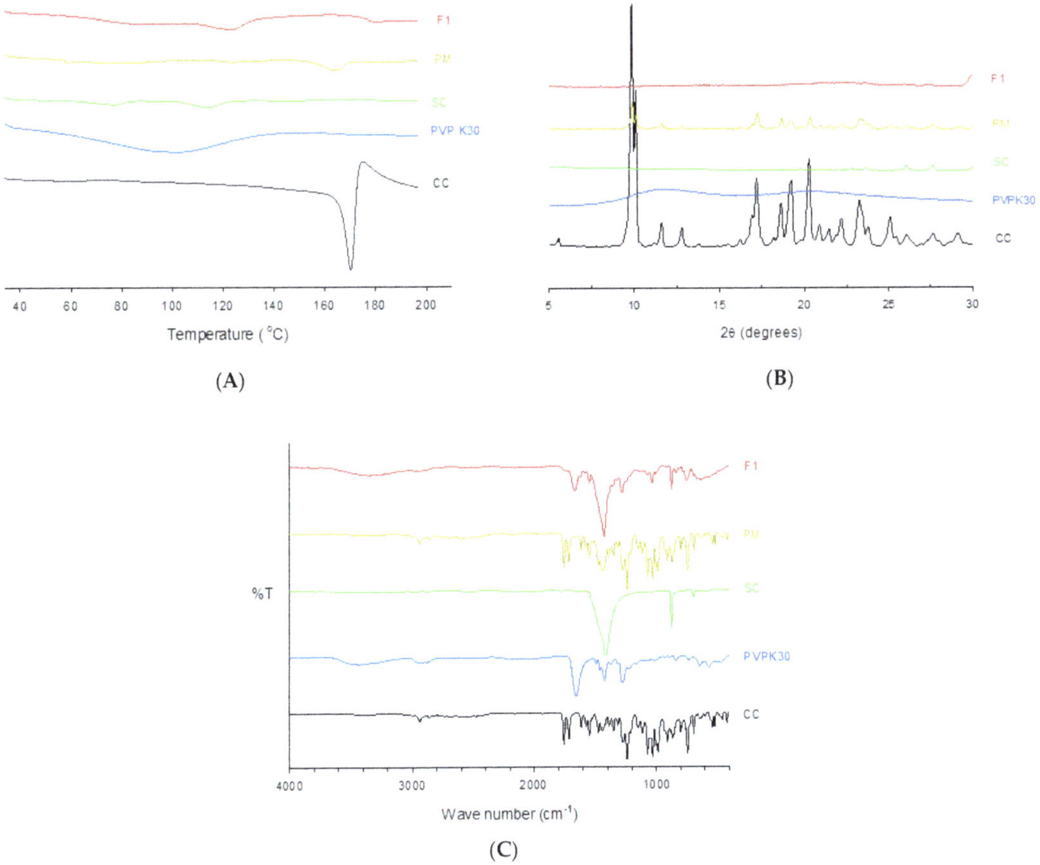

Figure 7. The differential scanning calorimetry (DSC) (**A**), powder X-ray diffraction (PXRD) (**B**), and FTIR (**C**) analysis of CC, PVPK30, SC, PM, and F1.

The powder X-ray diffraction (PXRD) of CC, PVPK30, SC, PM and F1 were performed (Figure 7B). The diffraction pattern of CC shows numerous distinctive peaks up to 30°, corroborating with its highly crystalline nature [46]. In contrast, PVPK30 had no peaks due to its amorphous nature. Additionally, SC's PXRD pattern showed smaller and fewer peaks, consistent with its reduced crystalline form. In addition, the PM retained intrinsic peaks of the respective ingredients with a reduced crystalline form. Lastly, the characteristic peaks of CC and SC were absent in the F1 sample, again consistent with F1's amorphous nature.

The FTIR analysis was used to investigate the drug-polymer interaction in ASDs as it will unveil the mechanism of stabilization of ASD. The FTIR spectrum of CC, PVPK30, SC, PM, and F1 was compared (Figure 7C). The CC spectra revealed prominent peaks bands characteristic of the polymeric form I of CC [47]; the aromatic and aliphatic CH stretching in 3070–2855 cm^{-1} range with peaks at 3068, 3000, 2940, and 2860 cm^{-1}; the C=O group stretching from the asymmetric organic carbonate -OC(=O)O- moiety with an intense band at 1753 cm^{-1}; an ester carbonyl group at 1713 cm^{-1}; the -NH bending at 1622 cm^{-1}; and the aromatic C-N stretching at 1348 cm^{-1} and C-O ether stretch at 1032 cm^{-1}. PVPK-30 showed distinct -C=O stretching at 1651 cm^{-1} and broad absorption bands at 3434 cm^{-1} from -OH stretching vibrations, correlating to the broad endotherm peak in the DSC study. SC's spectrum also exhibited a broad band peaking at 1420 cm^{-1} and sharp peaks at 872 and 702 cm^{-1}. Further, the PM exhibited a characteristic peak of CC and other excipients along with some superimposition. $CCSD_{pM}$ F1's spectra retained the characteristic peaks of CC with some enclosure suggesting weak inter-molecular H-bonding. Further examination in conjunction with other techniques, such as Raman spectroscopy and ^1H NMR, will provide more insights into the phenomena, such as the masking and shifting in spectra.

3.5. Stability Studies

The stability study of a formulation uncovers the changes in the quality parameters under normal and stress conditions within a time frame. Different variables, such as the manufacturing process, quality of drug, excipient, and packaging material, may impact a product's quality over time. However, the impact of heat and moisture has been identified as the principal factor determining product quality [48]. The in vitro drug release studies confirm that $CCSD_{pM}$(F1) under real-time and accelerated stability conditions have comparable release characteristics (Figure 8). All the samples had more than 90% cumulative drug release in 30 min, indicating a consistent release profile with the 0-week sample. In addition, the drug content of F1 after 12 weeks in RTS and 4 weeks in ACC conditions was 96.38 ± 1.040 and 95.75 ± 3.53%, respectively, indicating an absence of potential degradations (Table 3).

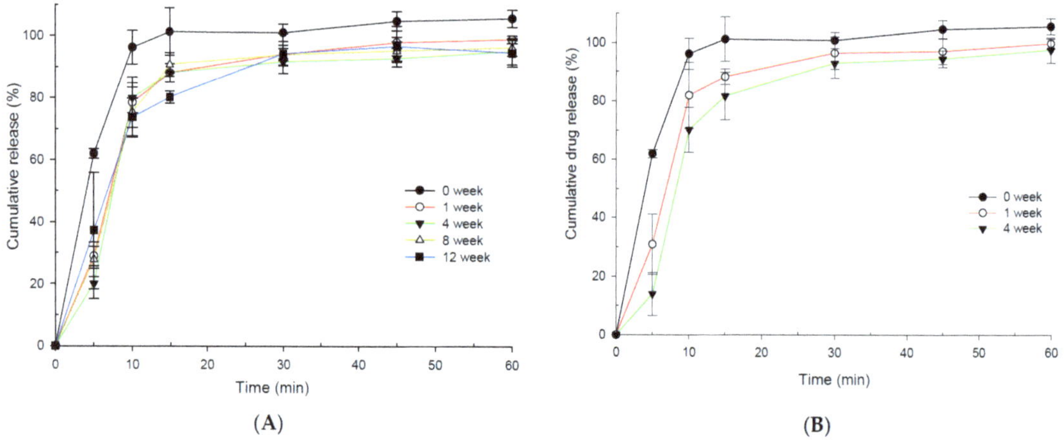

Figure 8. The stability study of $CCSD_{pM}$ (F1). (**A**) The dissolution study after 1, 4, 8 or 12 weeks under real-time stability condition at 25 ± 2 °C and RH 60 ± 5%. (**B**) The dissolution study after 1 or 4 weeks under accelerated stability condition at 40 ± 2 °C and RH 75 ± 5%.

Table 3. Drug content study.

Weeks	Drug Content (µg/mL)	
	Real-Time Stability Condition	**Accelerated Stability Condition**
0	99.99 ± 2.55	
1	96.45 ± 2.98	96.08 ± 6.75
4	94.90 ± 1.75	95.75 ± 3.54
8	95.61 ± 3.06	-
12	96.38 ± 1.04	-

Each value represents the mean of three experiments (n = 3) ± standard deviation.

Usually, a stability study of at least six months is required to demonstrate a product's stability. However, in our study, the 4-week accelerated conditions and 12-real-time conditions provide a level of understanding of the effect of temperature and moisture on $CCSD_{pM}$ formulations. Further, a formulation's stability can be correlated with a smaller alkalizer-to-drug ratio, as high alkalizer content can give rise to instability. Though the study was of a limited time frame with only in vitro and drug content analysis, these results validate pH modulation approach to enhance absorption. Additionally, extending the study time and quantifying the impurities will further strengthen the feasibility of this approach.

3.6. Pharmacokinetic Studies

Candesartan is the major metabolite of CC that induces an antihypertensive effect. CC, the prodrug, is rapidly hydrolyzed to candesartan by the esterase in the gastrointestinal tract. As a result, only candesartan can be quantified in the plasma. Here the plasma concentration of candesartan at the 10 mg/kg dose for $CCSD_{pM}$ F1 and the pure CC was successfully quantified in rats (n = 6) using a reverse UHPLC system.

The mean plasma concentration-time plots and pharmacokinetic parameters of $CCSD_{pM}$ and pure drug are summed up in Figure 9 and Table 4, respectively. As shown in Figure 9, the mean plasma concentration of candesartan from $CCSD_{pM}$ F1 was higher than pure CC at all the time points, suggesting increased bioavailability. The maximum plasma concentration (C_{max}) in rats administered with $CCSD_{pM}$ was 188.75 ± 41.06 ng/mL, considerably higher, by 7.42-fold, than that of the pure CC at 25.44 ± 6.28 ng/mL. In addition, the *AUC* of candesartan from the rats administered with $CCSD_{pM}$, at 771.87 ± 227.63 h·ng/mL, was significantly higher than that from the pure CC administration at 173.29 ± 30.27 h·ng/mL. Other pharmacokinetic parameters, such as t half ($t_{1/2}$) was shorter in F1, while k elimination (K_{el}) and T_{max} of $CCSD_{pM}$ were similar in F1 and pure CC.

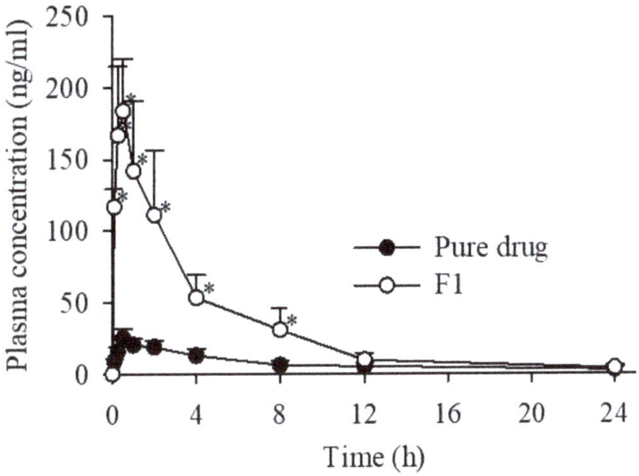

Figure 9. Plasma concentration-time profiles of candesartan after oral administration of pure drug (CC) or $CCSD_{pM}$ (F1) in rats. Each value represents the mean of six experiments (n = 6), and the error bar represents the standard deviation. * $p < 0.05$ compared to free CC.

Table 4. Pharmacokinetic parameters of pure drug (CC) powder, and $CCSD_{pM}$ formulation (F1).

Formulations	CC	F1
AUC (h·ng/mL)	173.29 ± 30.27	771.87 ± 227.63 *
C_{max} (ng/mL)	25.44 ± 6.28	188.75 ± 41.06 *
T_{max} (h)	0.83 ± 0.60	0.50 ± 0.27
$t_{1/2}$ (h)	7.47 ± 2.81	4.93 ± 1.42
K_{el} (h^{-1})	0.10 ± 0.03	0.15 ± 0.05

Each value represents the mean of six experiments (n = 6), and the error bar represents the standard deviation. * $p < 0.05$ compared to free CC.

Altogether, these data indicate that better solubility and dissolution rate at the physiological pH range increases bioavailability, resulting in a significant enhancement in oral absorption. The rapid absorption of $CCSD_{pM}$ can be due to its amorphous nature, increased solubility, and super-saturable state in the physiological environment. The use of polymers alone has also been accounted for increased absorption [31] but addition of pH modifiers was found to improve the overall performances significantly without any stability issues. However, the optimization of the use of alkalizers needs to be thoroughly examined with a better correlation between the in vitro and in vivo parameters. This study has taken a step to address the low bioavailability issues of weakly acidic drugs, such as CC, using polymers, alkalizers, and a spray drying technique to achieve notable improvement in the in vitro-in vivo, stability study. Furthermore, this strategy can help reduce the therapeutic dose due to the increase in bioavailability, excipients amount due to the lower carrier-to-drug ratio, and cost-effectiveness compared to the conventional methods.

4. Conclusions

A novel CC-loaded spray-dried ASD with pH modifiers was successfully designed and formulated to enhance candesartan's bioavailability. The optimized formulation exhibited increased solubility, enhanced dissolution with good stability. The enhanced properties could be due to the solubilization of CC by the added polymer matrix as well as the modulation of the microenvironment pH with alkalizers. In addition, polymer PVPK30 and pH modulator sodium carbonate contributed to the maintenance of a supersaturable state, increasing the absorption potential at GI lumen. The physicochemical characterization also confirmed that CC was amorphous in the dispersed state with the polymer matrix. The pharmacokinetics of optimized $CCSD_{pM}$ were remarkably increased compared to the pure CC, indicating better absorption and bioavailability. Although $CCSD_{pM}$ had good stability, long-term studies are needed to reinforce and support the pragmatic shift of formulation technology. Overall, a spray-dried ASD system based on the use of a pH modifier could be a potential approach to enhance the limited bioavailability of poorly soluble drugs.

Author Contributions: Conceptualization, investigation, methodology, writing—original draft, writing—review and editing, S.P. and D.W.K.; supervision, project administration, funding acquisition, D.W.K. All authors have read and agreed to the published version of the manuscript.

Funding: This work was supported by National Research Foundation of Korea (NRF) grants funded by the Korea government (No. 2018R1D1A1B07050598 and No. 2020R1A5A2017323).

Institutional Review Board Statement: The study was conducted according to the guidelines of the Declaration of Helsinki and approved by the Institutional Animal Care and Use Committee at Kyungpook National University (License Number: 2019-0054, Authorization date: 1 March 2019).

Informed Consent Statement: Not applicable.

Data Availability Statement: The data presented in this study are available in the paper here.

Conflicts of Interest: The authors declare no conflict of interest.

References

1. Wells, J.A.; McClendon, C.L. Reaching for high-hanging fruit in drug discovery at protein-protein interfaces. *Nature* **2007**, *450*, 1001–1009. [CrossRef] [PubMed]
2. Hauss, D.J. Oral lipid-based formulations. *Adv. Drug Deliv. Rev.* **2007**, *59*, 667–676. [CrossRef] [PubMed]
3. Lindenberg, M.; Kopp, S.; Dressman, J.B. Classification of orally administered drugs on the World Health Organization Model list of Essential Medicines according to the biopharmaceutics classification system. *Eur. J. Pharm. Biopharm.* **2004**, *58*, 265–278. [CrossRef]
4. Dokoumetzidis, A.; Macheras, P. A century of dissolution research: From Noyes and Whitney to the Biopharmaceutics Classification System. *Int. J. Pharm.* **2006**, *321*, 1–11. [CrossRef] [PubMed]
5. Sheth, P.; Sandhu, H.; Singhal, D.; Malick, W.; Shah, N.; Serpil Kislalioglu, M. Nanoparticles in the Pharmaceutical Industry and the Use of Supercritical Fluid Technologies for Nanoparticle Production. *Curr. Drug Deliv.* **2012**, *9*, 269–284. [CrossRef]
6. Ali, H.H.; Hussein, A.A. Oral solid self-nanoemulsifying drug delivery systems of candesartan citexetil: Formulation, characterization and in vitro drug release studies. *AAPS Open* **2017**, *3*, 6. [CrossRef]

7. Park, J.H.; Cho, J.H.; Kim, D.S.; Kim, J.S.; Din, F.U.; Kim, J.O.; Yong, C.S.; Youn, Y.S.; Oh, K.T.; Kim, D.W.; et al. Revaprazan-loaded surface-modified solid dispersion: Physicochemical characterization and in vivo evaluation. *Pharm. Dev. Technol.* **2019**, *24*, 788–793. [CrossRef]
8. Kwon, J.; Giri, B.R.; Song, E.S.; Bae, J.; Lee, J.; Kim, D.W. Spray-dried amorphous solid dispersions of atorvastatin calcium for improved supersaturation and oral bioavailability. *Pharmaceutics* **2019**, *11*, 461. [CrossRef] [PubMed]
9. Craig, D.Q.M. The mechanisms of drug release from solid dispersions in water-soluble polymers. *Int. J. Pharm.* **2002**, *231*, 131–144. [CrossRef]
10. Weuts, I.; Kempen, D.; Verreck, G.; Decorte, A.; Heymans, K.; Peeters, J.; Brewster, M.; Mooter, G. Van Den Study of the physicochemical properties and stability of solid dispersions of loperamide and PEG6000 prepared by spray drying. *Eur. J. Pharm. Biopharm.* **2005**, *59*, 119–126. [CrossRef]
11. Ali, H.H.; Hussein, A.A. Oral nanoemulsions of candesartan cilexetil: Formulation, characterization and in vitro drug release studies. *AAPS Open* **2017**, *3*, 4. [CrossRef]
12. Loftsson, T. Drug solubilization by complexation. *Int. J. Pharm.* **2017**, *531*, 276–280. [CrossRef] [PubMed]
13. Stella, V.J.; Nti-Addae, K.W. Prodrug strategies to overcome poor water solubility. *Adv. Drug Deliv. Rev.* **2007**, *59*, 677–694. [CrossRef] [PubMed]
14. Yan, Y.-D.; Kim, H.-K.; Seo, K.-H.; Lee, W.S.; Lee, G.-S.; Woo, J.-S.; Yong, C.-S.; Choi, H.-G. The Physicochemical Properties, in Vitro Metabolism and Pharmacokinetics of a Novel Ester Prodrug of EXP3174. *Mol. Pharm.* **2010**, *7*, 2132–2140. [CrossRef] [PubMed]
15. Bikiaris, D.N. Solid dispersions, Part I: Recent evolutions and future opportunities in manufacturing methods for dissolution rate enhancement of poorly water-soluble drugs. *Expert Opin. Drug Deliv.* **2011**, *8*, 1501–1519. [CrossRef]
16. Vasconcelos, T.; Sarmento, B.; Costa, P. Solid dispersions as strategy to improve oral bioavailability of poor water soluble drugs. *Drug Discov. Today* **2007**, *12*, 1068–1075. [CrossRef]
17. He, Y.; Ho, C. Amorphous Solid Dispersions: Utilization and Challenges in Drug Discovery and Development. *J. Pharm. Sci.* **2015**, *104*, 3237–3258. [CrossRef] [PubMed]
18. Singh, A.; Van den Mooter, G. Spray drying formulation of amorphous solid dispersions. *Adv. Drug Deliv. Rev.* **2016**, *100*, 27–50. [CrossRef] [PubMed]
19. Vasconcelos, T.; Marques, S.; das Neves, J.; Sarmento, B. Amorphous solid dispersions: Rational selection of a manufacturing process. *Adv. Drug Deliv. Rev.* **2016**, *100*, 85–101. [CrossRef]
20. Laitinen, R.; Löbmann, K.; Strachan, C.J.; Grohganz, H.; Rades, T. Emerging trends in the stabilization of amorphous drugs. *Int. J. Pharm.* **2013**, *453*, 65–79. [CrossRef]
21. Marsac, P.J.; Li, T.; Taylor, L.S. Estimation of drug-polymer miscibility and solubility in amorphous solid dispersions using experimentally determined interaction parameters. *Pharm. Res.* **2009**, *26*, 139–151. [CrossRef]
22. Kanaujia, P.; Poovizhi, P.; Ng, W.K.; Tan, R.B.H. Amorphous formulations for dissolution and bioavailability enhancement of poorly soluble APIs. *Powder Technol.* **2015**, *285*, 2–15. [CrossRef]
23. Gordon, M.; Taylor, J.S. Ideal copolymers and the second-order transitions of synthetic rubbers. i. non-crystalline copolymers. *J. Appl. Chem.* **2007**, *2*, 493–500. [CrossRef]
24. Hancock, B.C.; Shamblin, S.L.; Zografi, G. Molecular Mobility of Amorphous Pharmaceutical Solids Below Their Glass Transition Temperatures. *Pharm. Res. An Off. J. Am. Assoc. Pharm. Sci.* **1995**, *12*, 799–806.
25. BASF Kollidon. *Polyvinylpyrrolidone Excipients*; BASF: Ludwigshafen, Germany, 2008; pp. 1–331.
26. Taniguchi, C.; Kawabata, Y.; Wada, K.; Yamada, S.; Onoue, S. Microenvironmental pH-modification to improve dissolution behavior and oral absorption for drugs with pH-dependent solubility. *Expert Opin. Drug Deliv.* **2014**, *11*, 505–516. [CrossRef]
27. Farag Badawy, S.I.; Hussain, M.A. Microenvironmental pH modulation in solid dosage forms. *J. Pharm. Sci.* **2007**, *96*, 948–959. [CrossRef]
28. McClellan, K.J.; Goa, K.L. Candesartan cilexetil. A review of its use in essential hypertension. *Drugs* **1998**, *56*, 847–869. [CrossRef]
29. Sharma, G.; Beg, S.; Thanki, K.; Katare, O.P.; Jain, S.; Kohli, K.; Singh, B. Systematic development of novel cationic self-nanoemulsifying drug delivery systems of candesartan cilexetil with enhanced biopharmaceutical performance. *RSC Adv.* **2015**, *5*, 71500–71513. [CrossRef]
30. Zhang, Z.; Gao, F.; Bu, H.; Xiao, J.; Li, Y. Solid lipid nanoparticles loading candesartan cilexetil enhance oral bioavailability: In vitro characteristics and absorption mechanism in rats. *Nanomed. Nanotechnol. Biol. Med.* **2012**, *8*, 740–747. [CrossRef]
31. Surampalli, G.; Nanjwade, B.K.; Patil, P.A.; Chilla, R. Novel tablet formulation of amorphous candesartan cilexetil solid dispersions involving P-gp inhibition for optimal drug delivery: In vitro and in vivo evaluation. *Drug Deliv.* **2014**, *23*, 1–15.
32. AboulFotouh, K.; Allam, A.A.; El-Badry, M.; El-Sayed, A.M. A Self-Nanoemulsifying Drug Delivery System for Enhancing the Oral Bioavailability of Candesartan Cilexetil: Ex Vivo and In Vivo Evaluation. *J. Pharm. Sci.* **2019**, *108*, 3599–3608. [CrossRef] [PubMed]
33. Gao, F.; Zhang, Z.; Bu, H.; Huang, Y.; Gao, Z.; Shen, J.; Zhao, C.; Li, Y. Nanoemulsion improves the oral absorption of candesartan cilexetil in rats: Performance and mechanism. *J. Control. Release* **2011**, *149*, 168–174. [CrossRef]
34. Ilevbare, G.A.; Liu, H.; Edgar, K.J.; Taylor, L.S. Maintaining supersaturation in aqueous drug solutions: Impact of different polymers on induction times. *Cryst. Growth Des.* **2013**, *13*, 740–751. [CrossRef]

35. Trasi, N.S.; Taylor, L.S. Effect of polymers on nucleation and crystal growth of amorphous acetaminophen. *CrystEngComm* **2012**, *14*, 5188–5197. [CrossRef]
36. Vandecruys, R.; Peeters, J.; Verreck, G.; Brewster, M.E. Use of a screening method to determine excipients which optimize the extent and stability of supersaturated drug solutions and application of this system to solid formulation design. *Int. J. Pharm.* **2007**, *342*, 168–175. [CrossRef]
37. Blaabjerg, L.I.; Grohganz, H.; Lindenberg, E.; Löbmann, K.; Müllertz, A.; Rades, T. The influence of polymers on the supersaturation potential of poor and good glass formers. *Pharmaceutics* **2018**, *10*, 164. [CrossRef]
38. International Conference on Harmonisation of Technical Requirements for Registration of Pharmaceuticals for Human Use (ICH). Available online: https://www.ncbi.nlm.nih.gov/pmc/articles/PMC4544148/ (accessed on 4 March 2021).
39. Figueroa-Campos, A.; Sánchez-Dengra, B.; Merino, V.; Dahan, A.; González-Álvarez, I.; García-Arieta, A.; González-Álvarez, M.; Bermejo, M. Candesartan Cilexetil In Vitro–In Vivo Correlation: Predictive Dissolution as a Development Tool. *Pharmaceutics* **2020**, *12*, 633. [CrossRef]
40. Li, N.; Taylor, L.S. Tailoring supersaturation from amorphous solid dispersions. *J. Control. Release* **2018**, *279*, 114–125. [CrossRef]
41. Brouwers, J.; Brewster, M.E.; Augustijns, P. Supersaturating Drug Delivery Systems: The Answer to Solubility-Limited Oral Bioavailability? *J. Pharm. Sci.* **2009**, *98*, 2549–2572. [CrossRef]
42. Chavan, R.B.; Thipparaboina, R.; Kumar, D.; Shastri, N.R. Evaluation of the inhibitory potential of HPMC, PVP and HPC polymers on nucleation and crystal growth. *RSC Adv.* **2016**, *6*, 77569–77576. [CrossRef]
43. Kim, D.W.; Kwon, M.S.; Yousaf, A.M.; Balakrishnan, P.; Park, J.H.; Kim, D.S.; Lee, B.J.; Park, Y.J.; Yong, C.S.; Kim, J.O.; et al. Comparison of a solid SMEDDS and solid dispersion for enhanced stability and bioavailability of clopidogrel napadisilate. *Carbohydr. Polym.* **2014**, *114*, 365–374. [CrossRef] [PubMed]
44. Tran, P.H.L.; Tran, T.T.D.; Lee, K.H.; Kim, D.J.; Lee, B.J. Dissolution-modulating mechanism of pH modifiers in solid dispersion containing weakly acidic or basic drugs with poor water solubility. *Expert Opin. Drug Deliv.* **2010**, *7*, 647–661. [CrossRef] [PubMed]
45. Buda, V.; Baul, B.; Andor, M.; Man, D.E.; Ledeţi, A.; Vlase, G.; Vlase, T.; Danciu, C.; Matusz, P.; Peter, F.; et al. Solid state stability and kinetics of degradation for candesartan—Pure compound and pharmaceutical formulation. *Pharmaceutics* **2020**, *12*, 86. [CrossRef]
46. Chi, Y.; Xu, W.; Yang, Y.; Yang, Z.; Lv, H.; Yang, S.; Lin, Z.; Li, J.; Gu, J.; Hill, C.L.; et al. Three Candesartan Salts with Enhanced Oral Bioavailability. *Cryst. Growth Des.* **2015**, *15*, 3707–3714. [CrossRef]
47. Matsunaga, H.; Eguchi, T.; Nishijima, K.; Enomoto, T.; Sasaoki, K.; Nakamura, N. Solid-State Characterization of Candesartan Cilexetil (TCV-116): Crystal Structure and Molecular Mobility. *Chem. Pharm. Bull. (Tokyo)* **1999**, *47*, 182–186. [CrossRef]
48. Cha, J.; Gilmor, T.; Lane, P.; Ranweiler, J.S. 12-Stability Studies. In *Handbook of Modern Pharmaceutical Analysis*; Ahuja, S., Scypinski, S.B.T.S., Eds.; Academic Press: Cambridge, MA, USA, 2011; Volume 10, pp. 459–505, ISBN 1877-1718.

pharmaceutics

MDPI

Article

Development of Lipid–Polymer Hybrid Nanoparticles for Improving Oral Absorption of Enoxaparin

Bo Tang [1,2,3], Yu Qian [1] and Guihua Fang [1,*]

[1] School of Pharmacy, Nantong University, 19 Qixiu Road, Nantong 226001, China; tangbo@ntu.edu.cn (B.T.); syfsxyhh18@163.com (Y.Q.)
[2] School of Pharmacy, Shenyang Pharmaceutical University, 103 Wenhua Road, Shenyang 110016, China
[3] Yabang Medical Research Institute, 66 Changhong Road, Changzhou 213145, China
* Correspondence: fangguihua@ntu.edu.cn; Tel.: +86-0513-85051726

Received: 21 May 2020; Accepted: 25 June 2020; Published: 30 June 2020

check for updates

Abstract: Enoxaparin, an anticoagulant that helps prevent the formation of blood clots, is administered parenterally. Here, we report the development and evaluation of lipid–polymer hybrid nanoparticles (LPHNs) for the oral delivery of enoxaparin. The polymer poloxamer 407 (P407) was incorporated into lipid nanoparticles to form gel cores and ensure high encapsulation efficiency and the controlled release of enoxaparin. In vitro results indicated that 30% of P407 incorporation offered higher encapsulation efficiency and sustained the release of enoxaparin. Laser confocal scanning microscopy (LCSM) images showed that LPHNs could not only significantly improve the accumulation of enoxaparin in intestinal villi but also facilitate enoxaparin transport into the underlayer of intestinal epithelial cells. In vivo pharmacokinetic study results indicated that the oral bioavailability of enoxaparin was markedly increased about 6.8-fold by LPHNs. In addition, its therapeutic efficacy against pulmonary thromboembolism was improved 2.99-fold by LPHNs. Moreover, LPHNs exhibited excellent biocompatibility in the intestine. Overall, the LPHN is a promising delivery carrier to boost the oral absorption of enoxaparin.

Keywords: enoxaparin; lipid–polymer hybrid nanoparticles; oral; intestinal absorption

1. Introduction

Heparin is an anticoagulant that prevents the formation of blood blots, and it has shown great prevention and therapeutic efficacy in terms of deep-vein thrombosis (DVT), pulmonary embolism (PE), and venous thrombosis [1] clinically. Low molecular weight heparin (LMWH) is obtained from unfractionated heparin (UFH) by chemical and enzymatic depolymerization [2]. Enoxaparin, one of the most commonly used LMWH, holds a longer half-life in vivo than UFH, which reduces the administration frequency [3]. However, its oral absorption is still low due to its large molecular weight, high anionic charges, and first-pass effect in the liver [4–6]. Therefore, it is administered via the parenteral route, which is less convenient and has lower compliance for patients. To translate the administration route from injection to oral delivery, it is quite crucial to increase the oral absorption of LMWH [7,8]. With the advances in nanotechnology, polymer- and lipid-based nanocarriers such as polymeric micelles [9], polymeric nanoparticles [10], lipid nanocapsules [11], microemulsions [12], and solid lipid nanoparticles [13] have been intensively used to facilitate the oral absorption of LMWH. Rationally designed nanocarriers are able to overcome the hurdles encountered during the absorption process through following ways, including (1) protecting drugs from acidic degradation in the stomach; (2) increasing the intestinal epithelial permeability; (3) facilitating intestinal lymphatic transport [13–18].

Solid lipid nanoparticles (SLNs) are colloidal drug delivery systems consisting of surfactant-stabilized lipids that are solid both at room and body temperature [13]. They integrate the advantages of liposomes, polymeric nanoparticles, and emulsions. In addition, SLNs possess a solid lipid core matrix, so they are used to encapsulate lipophilic drugs in most cases [19,20]. Because LMWH is hydrophilic, the encapsulation efficiency of LMWH in the SLNs is low, which leads to insufficient therapeutic concentration in vivo. This is due to hydrophilic drugs having limited loading quantity and homogeneity in the lipid cores. To improve the encapsulation efficiency of LMWH in the SLNs, conjugating lipidic molecules with LMWH via chemical synthesis was reported in a previous study [13]. Although the oral absorption of LMWH is significantly improved in this way, there may be some problems associated with the chemical modification of LMWH. Since LMWH exerts its therapeutic effects by binding to antithrombin III (AT III) via a unique pentasaccharide motif [21], chemical synthesis may increase the risk of reducing or losing the activity of LMWH. To avoid the possibility of reducing or losing drug activity, a common alternative strategy is to prepare LMWH-loaded SLNs by a double emulsion (water-in-oil-in-water, W/O/W) method. However, the encapsulation efficiency of LMWH in the SLNs is still unsatisfactory. Therefore, a new encapsulation strategy is needed to further improve the encapsulation efficiency of LMWH.

It has been reported that hydrophilic viscosity-enhancing agents such as propylene glycol (PG) and polyethylene glycol (PEG) 400 and PEG 600 are able to increase the encapsulation efficiency of insulin in the SLNs [22]. Inspired by this, hydrogels may be an alternative. Hydrogels, a network of polymer chains, are often used for the delivery of hydrophilic drugs with higher drug loading [23]. Poloxamer 407 (P407) is a triblock copolymer consisting of a central hydrophobic block and two hydrophilic blocks of polyethylene glycol at both ends. P407-based hydrogels exhibit interesting nature at certain concentration levels. That is, they are in a liquid state below gelation temperature and turn into a viscosity-enhancing gel above gelation temperature [24,25].

Encouraged by the advantage of SLNs and hydrogels, we attempted to fabricate lipid–polymer hybrid nanoparticles (LPHNs) for the oral delivery of enoxaparin. In this study, poloxamer 407 is used to improve the encapsulation efficiency and control the release of enoxaparin. The lipid–polymer hybrid nanoparticles were characterized in terms of size and zeta potential, encapsulation efficiency, and particle morphology. In vitro release behavior was also investigated. The intestinal absorption was evaluated by laser confocal scanning microscopy. In addition, in vivo absorption, in vivo efficacy, and safety tests were performed by rat experiments. In all, we attempt to investigate whether lipid–polymer hybrid nanoparticles can increase encapsulation efficiency and boost the oral absorption of enoxaparin.

2. Materials and Methods

2.1. Materials

Enoxaparin (mean MW 4251 Da, 101 IU/mg) was purchased from Hangzhou Jiuyuan Gene Engineering Co., Ltd. (Hangzhou, China). Precirol ATO 5 (glyceryl palmitostearate) was kindly donated by Gattefosse (Lyon, France). Egg yolk lecithin (E80) was obtained from Lipoid KG (Ludwigshafen, Germany), and Tween 80 was purchased from BASF (Ludwigshafen, Germany). Poloxamer 407 (BASF, Ludiwigshafen, Germany) was purchased from Xi'an Yuelai Medical Technology Co., Ltd. (Xi'an, China). Fluorescein isothiocyanate (FITC) was obtained from Shanghai Golden Wheat Biotechnology Co., Ltd. (Shanghai, China). Tissue-Tek O.C.T. compound (SAKURA, Torrance, CA, USA) was purchased from Nantong Qixiang Biotechnology Co., Ltd. (Nantong, China). Activated partial thromboplastin time (APTT) assay kits were obtained from Nanjing Caobenyuan Biotechnology Co., Ltd. (Nanjing, China). All other chemicals were of analytical grade.

2.2. Preparation of Lipid–Polymer Hybrid Nanoparticles (LPHNs)

Enoxaparin-loaded LPHNs were prepared as follows. In brief, 12.5 mg of enoxaparin was dissolved in 0.5 mL-differentiated ratios of poloxamer 407 (P407) aqueous solution at 4 °C. Then, 10 mg E 80 and 40 mg Precirol ATO 5 were dissolved in 2 mL dichloromethane (DCM). DCM was dropped into 0.2 mL of P407 aqueous solution containing enoxaparin. Then, this mixed solution was ultrasonicated using a probe sonicator (Ningbo Xinzhi Biological Technology Co. Ltd., Ningbo, China) for 2 min at 500 W to obtain primary W/O emulsion. Subsequently, 2% Tween 80 aqueous solution added to the obtained primary emulsion followed by ultrasonication for 1 min at 380 W. Finally, the obtained formulation was transferred into a flask to remove the DCM at 34 °C, using a rotary evaporator (Eyela, Tokyo, Japan). The preparation method for enoxaparin-loaded SLNs was the same as that for enoxaparin-loaded LPHNs, except that no P407 was in the aqueous solution.

2.3. *In Vitro Characteristics*

2.3.1. Size, Zeta Potential, and Encapsulation Efficiency

The particle size and size distribution of prepared nanoparticles were measured by 90 plus zeta (Brookhaven, MS, USA) at room temperature. The zeta potential of nanoparticles was tested using the 90 plus zeta by electrophoretic laser doppler anemometry at room temperature. All the samples were diluted with deionized water, and measurements were taken in triplicate.

The encapsulation efficiency of enoxaparin in nanoparticles was determined by an ultra-filtration method [26]. An appropriate amount of nanoparticle dispersion was added in a Millipore Amicon®Ultra filteration tube (MWCO: 100 kDa). Free enoxaparin was separated from the nanoparticle dispersion by centrifugation at 2000 rpm for 15 min. To determine the total amount of the drug, including the free drug in the dispersion and encapsulated drug in the nanoparticles, an appropriate amount of nanoparticle dispersion was destroyed by DCM, and the released enoxaparin was extracted by deionized water. The enoxaparin in the ultrafiltrate and nanoparticle dispersion was determined by the Azure II colorimetric method using a multimode microplate reader (Bio Tek, Winooski, VT, USA) at 606 nm [27]. The linearity range of this method was determined between 0 and 6 μg/mL, with a linear correlation coefficient of 0.9973. All samples were measured in triplicate. The encapsulation efficiency (EE) of enoxaparin was calculated using the following equation:

$$EE\% = \frac{W_{totaldrug} - W_{freedrug}}{W_{totaldrug}} \quad (1)$$

where $W_{\text{total drug}}$ is the total amount of drug in the nanoparticle dispersion, and $W_{\text{free drug}}$ is the total amount of drug in the ultrafiltrate.

In addition, the prepared nanoparticle suspension was placed at 4 °C in a refrigerator for 1 week to determine whether the encapsulation efficiency changes with time.

2.3.2. Particle Morphology

The morphology of nanoparticles was examined by transmission electron microscopy (TEM). Samples of nanoparticles were diluted with deionized water, dropped onto a copper grid, and then stained with phosphotungstic acid. The samples were subjected to TEM (JEOL, Tokyo, Japan) after drying.

2.3.3. In Vitro Drug Release

In vitro release of enoxaparin from the nanoparticles was studied using the dialysis method, and an enoxaparin solution was used as control. Briefly, 2 mL of nanoparticle suspension was transferred into dialysis bags (Biosharp Biotechnology Co. Ltd., Hefei, China, MWCO: 14 kDa) and dialysis bags were immersed into a beaker containing 25 mL pH 6.8 phosphate buffer. Then, the beaker was placed in a 37 °C water bath with a magnetic stirring speed of 150 rpm. At a predetermined time point, the medium in the beaker was withdrawn, followed by replacement with the same volume of fresh release medium. The released enoxaparin content was determined by the Azure II colorimetric method, as mentioned in the previous part.

2.4. Intestinal Absorption

To investigate the intestinal absorption of nanoparticles, in vivo experiments were conducted in rats. All animal studies were conducted according to the guidelines of the local Institute Animal Ethical Care Committee (IAEC, 20180512-003). To visualize the intestinal absorption, fluorescein isothiocyanate (FITC) was used to label enoxaparin. FITC was conjugated with enoxaparin according to the method previously described [28]. Briefly, 2 mg of FITC dissolved in dimethylsulfoxide was slowly added to 0.1 M sodium carbonate, and then added in 50 mg of enoxaparin. The reaction was performed in a ice-water bath, with a stirring speed of 150 rpm in the dark. After 8 h, the reaction was stopped by adding an ammonium chloride solution. Then, the resulting FITC-enoxaparin conjugate was introduced into a dialysis bag (MWCO: 1000 Da) to remove the byproduct. The dialyzed product was lyophilized at −50 °C to obtain FITC-labeled enoxaparin. Male SD rats (200 ± 20 g) were given FITC-enoxaparin solution and FITC-enoxaparin LPHN2 by gavage at a dosage of 505 IU/kg. After 30 min, the rats were sacrificed, and then the jejunum was removed, washed, and fixed with 4% paraformaldehyde for 4 h at room temperature, and dehydrated with 20% sucrose solution. The segments were frozen in cryo-embedding media, sectioned at 20 μm, and placed on polysine-coated slides. The sections were fixed with 4% paraformaldehyde for 30 min and rinsed three times with pH 7.4 phosphate buffer, and the intestine sections were then incubated with 20 μL of 4′,6-diamidino-2-phenylindole (DAPI) for 10 min in the dark to stain the nucleus, followed by mounting with antifluorescence quenching reagent. Finally, the sections were observed under a Leica SP8 laser confocal scanning microscope.

2.5. In Vivo Pharmacokinetic Study in Rats

In vivo absorption of nanoparticles was studied in rats. Male SD rats (200 ± 20 g) were divided randomly into three groups, with four rats per group. After fasting for 24 h, the rats were given enoxaparin solution and enoxaparin-loaded LPHN2 by gavage at a dose of 1010 IU/kg. At predetermined time intervals (0, 1, 3, 5, 8, 12 h), blood samples (about 0.5 mL) were drawn from the rats. Plasma was obtained by centrifugation (6000 rpm, 10 min) and analyzed by measuring the activated partial thromboplastin time (APTT) value according to a standard commercial kit. The absolute bioavailability (F) of orally administered formulations was calculated by comparing their AUC with that intravenous injection of enoxaparin solution (101 IU/kg).

2.6. In Vivo Efficacy in Mice

The in vivo prevention of pulmonary thromboembolism of nanoparticles was studied in mice. Male Kunming mice (18~22 g) were divided randomly into four groups, with 12 mice per group. Two groups were treated with enoxaparin solution and enoxaparin-loaded LPHN3 via intragastric administration at a single dosage of 1010 IU/kg, respectively. Two groups were given 100 μL of enoxaparin solution (101 IU/kg) and saline as control. Two hours after administration, all groups were intravenously injected with 100 μL of 1250 IU/kg thrombin to induce hind limb paralysis or death. The number of dead or paralyzed mice was recorded within 20 min; the results are shown as a percentage of protection.

2.7. Safety Evaluation

To investigate whether nanoparticles cause intestinal membrane damage or not, a histopathological examination was conducted. In this experiment, enoxaparin-loaded nanoparticles were given orally to rats at 1010 IU/kg, and physiological saline was given orally as a control. Then, the rats were sacrificed after 2 and 8 h. The jejunum was removed from rats and placed in 5% formaldehyde solution and stained with hematoxylin-erosin for histological studies.

2.8. Statistical Analysis

Statistical analysis was performed using a Student's t-test. Data were expressed as mean ± SD. Statistical significance was represented by * $p < 0.05$ and ** $p < 0.01$.

3. Results and Discussion

3.1. Preparation and Characterization of Lipid–Polymer Hybrid Nanoparticles

Double W/O/W emulsification technology was used to prepare enoxaparin-loaded lipid–polymer hybrid nanoparticles. Poloxamer 407 acted as the polymer core to load the drug. The schematic diagram of enoxaparin-loaded lipid–polymer hybrid nanoparticles is presented in Figure 1A. To screen the optimal amount of poloxamer 407, a control group (SLNs) was created with the absence of P407, and three different ratios (20%, 30%, 40%, *w/v*) of poloxamer 407 were tested. Their size and encapsulation efficiency are summarized in Table 1. The tested amount of P407 had no significant influence on particle size, polydispersity index, or zeta potential, but it led to different encapsulation efficiencies for enoxaparin. When the amount of P407 was set as 30%, the enoxaparin-loaded LPHN possessed a higher encapsulation efficiency of 65.72%. The results suggest that the addition of an appropriate concentration of P407 into the double emulsion could improve the encapsulation efficiency of enoxaparin. The higher encapsulation efficiency of LPHN2 could possibly be attributed to its appropriate viscosity. P407 is a thermo-sensitive polymer, and it can form gels when the ambient temperature is above gelation temperature. According to previous research [3,24,29], the increase in P407 concentration in the gel increases its viscosity. When the amount of P407 is 20%, its viscosity is not enough to restrain the enoxaparin in the internal gel core. Theoretically, the addition of 40% P407 could offer the highest encapsulation efficiency. However, the gel formed by 40% of P407 is too viscous to be dispersed well by ultrasonication, leading to lower encapsulation efficiency. Hence, LPHN2 was selected as the formulation in the following experiments. To investigate if the encapsulation efficiency of LPHN2 was changed with time, we tested the encapsulation efficiency after storage at 4 °C for one week. The encapsulation efficiency of LPHN2 stored at 4 °C for one week was 64.01%, which indicated that the encapsulation efficiency of LPHN2 could be kept unchanged for at least one week.

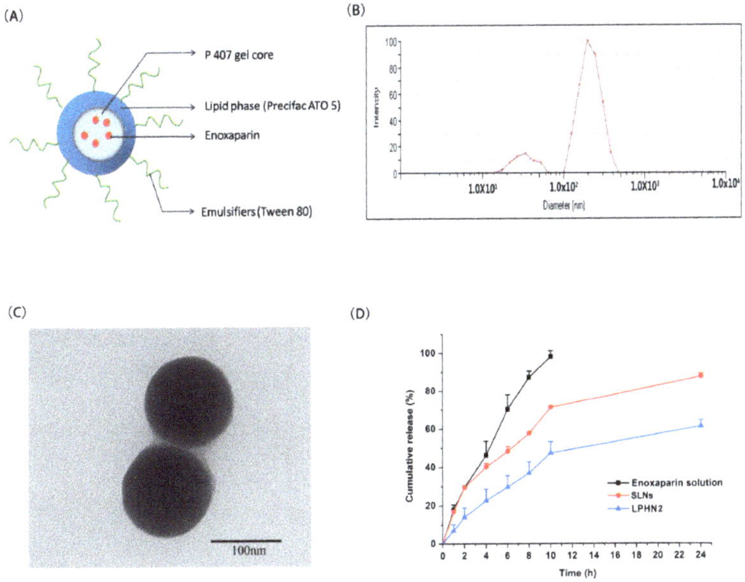

Figure 1. (**A**) Schematic representation of the structure of enoxaparin-loaded lipid hybrid nanoparticles. (**B**) The size distribution of lipid–polymer hybrid nanoparticle 2 (LPHN2). (**C**) The transmission electron microscopy (TEM) morphology of LPHN2. (**D**) In vitro release of profiles of enoxaparin from enoxaparin solution, enoxaparin-loaded solid lipid nanoparticles (SLNs), and enoxaparin-loaded LPHN2 (n = 3).

Table 1. Characterization of enoxaparin-loaded lipid-polymer hybrid nanoparticles at 3 different ratios of poloxamer 407 (n = 3).

Amount of P407	Size (nm)	PI	ζ Potential (mV)	EE (%)
0% (SLNs)	159.40 ± 1.59	0.293 ± 0.010	−21.83 ± 3.94	43.21 ± 3.79
20% (LPHN1)	149.70 ± 1.71	0.264 ± 0.030	−17.47 ± 1.20	43.14 ± 7.52
30% (LPHN2)	149.75 ± 2.45	0.293 ± 0.009	−14.71 ± 1.93	65.72 ± 14.33
40% (LPHN3)	153.19 ± 0.79	0.274 ± 0.002	−20.04 ± 1.59	59.47 ± 11.66

PI, polydispersity index; ζ potential, zeta potential; EE, encapsulation efficiency.

The average size of LPHN2 was about 150 nm, with a low PI (<0.30) (Figure 1B). In addition, there is a size distribution ranging from 10 to 100 nm in Figure 1B, which may be caused by the formation of Tween 80-based micelles in nanoparticle suspensions. The zeta potential of LPHN2 was slightly negative (−14.71 mV), which may be attributed to negatively charged egg lecithin in the surface of the LPHN.

Transmission electron microscopy (TEM) has been extensively used to observe the surface morphology of nanoparticles. The TEM image of LPHN2 is shown in Figure 1C, indicating that LPHN was spherical and about 150 nm in size, consistent with dynamic light scattering results.

The release of enoxaparin from LPHN2 was evaluated in pH 6.8 phosphate buffer and compared with the in vitro release of 0% P407-prepared SLNs and enoxaparin solution. The in vitro release profiles of enoxaparin solution, SLNs, and LPHN2 are shown in Figure 1D. Almost 98% of the drug released from the enoxaparin solution was within 10 h, which indicates that enoxaparin can diffuse freely through the dialysis bag. In contrast with the SLNs, there was a controlled and sustained release of enoxaparin from the LPHN2. Approximately 87% of the cumulative amount of enoxaparin was released from SLNs within 24 h. In the case of LPHN2, the percentage cumulative release of enoxaparin was about 61% within 24 h. The in vitro release result indicated that the incorporation of 30% P407 could control and sustain the enoxaparin release from LPHN compared with free P407 SLNs. There are two reasons to explain why LPH2 exhibited sustained release behavior in contrast with traditional lipid nanoparticles (SLNs). On the one hand, LPHN2 has higher encapsulation efficiency. For most of the drugs, they should diffuse from the nanoparticles first, and then release into the medium. Therefore, less amounts of free drugs could be released from the nanoparticles. On the other hand, the viscous gel core may delay drug diffusion from nanoparticles into the release medium.

3.2. Intestinal Absorption

The absorption of enoxaparin-loaded LPHN2 in the intestine of rats was visualized by LCSM after oral administration. Figure 2 shows the intestine fluorescence signals after the intragastric administration of FITC-labeled enoxaparin solution and LPHN2. The LCSM images suggest that a more intense fluorescence was observed in the intestine after administration of FITC-labeled enoxaparin-loaded LPHN2 in comparison with the administration of FITC-labeled enoxaparin solution. In addition, the fluorescence signal can be viewed under a layer of intestinal epithelial cells, as indicated by the red arrows. Therefore, the LCSM results indicate that the drug in LPHN2 was not only accumulated in the surface of intestinal villi but had also penetrated the underlayer of intestinal epithelial cells.

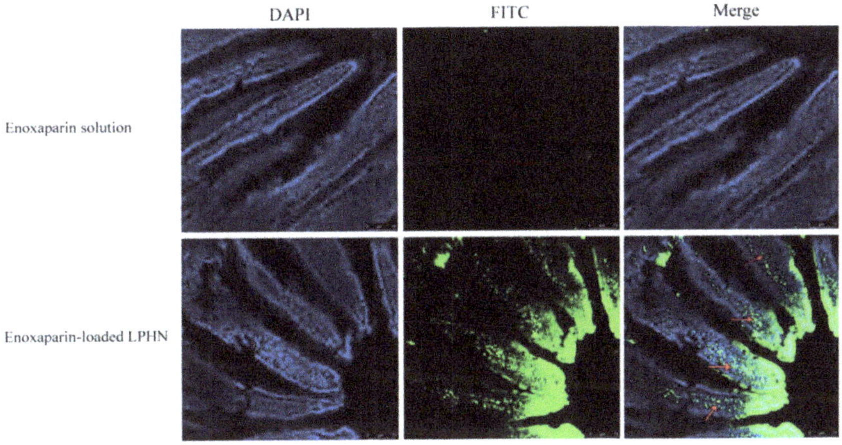

Figure 2. The LCSM images of the jejunum of rats at 0.5 h after administration of FITC-labeled (green) enoxaparin solution (the upper) and LPHN2 (the bottom). Cell nuclei of the jejunum sections were stained by DAPI (blue).

3.3. *In Vivo Pharmacokinetic Study in Rats*

In vivo pharmacokinetic behavior of enoxaparin-loaded LPHNs was investigated by measuring APTT in rats after intragastric administration, as shown in Figure 3. The main pharmacokinetic parameters are summarized in Table 2. The absolute bioavailability (F_{abs}) of enoxaparin-loaded LPHN2 was 14.2%, a 6.8-fold increase compared with enoxaparin solution. The results indicate that the oral bioavailability of enoxaparin could be improved by lipid–polymer hybrid nanoparticles. As we know, the basic mechanisms that nanoparticles could improve oral absorption of drugs are as follows [30,31]: (1) encapsulation of drug to avoid degradation in the gastrointestinal tract before reaching the absorption site; (2) improving intestinal epithelial cell uptake. For drugs that are unstable in the gastrointestinal tract, high encapsulation efficiency is the precondition of oral absorption enhancement by nanoparticles. There are several reasons that could explain why LPHNs enhance the oral absorption of enoxaparin. On the one hand, LPHNs have higher encapsulation efficiency to protect enoxaparin from degradation in the stomach. On the other hand, on the basis of the intestinal absorption of LPHNs, LPHNs could overcome the mucus layer to facilitate enoxaparin entry to under layer of intestinal epithelial cells, followed by absorption into the systemic circulation.

Table 2. Main pharmacokinetic parameters after peroral administration of enoxaparin formulations in rats at a dosage of 1010 IU/kg ($n = 4$). * $p < 0.05$ represents a significant improvement in absolute bioavailability in comparison with enoxaparin solution (p.o.).

Formulations	T_{max} (h)	$AUC_{0-12\,h}$ (s·h)	F_{abs} (%)
Enoxaparin solution (i.v.)	-	182.3 ± 44.2	100.0
Enoxaparin solution (p.o.)	0.5	37.6 ± 10.0	2.1
Enoxaparin-loaded LPHN2 (p.o.)	3	258.3 ± 93.1	14.2*

i.v. means intravenous injection; p.o. means peroral administration.

Despite the results that LPHNs can improve the oral bioavailability of enoxaparin, its absolute bioavailability is still not high enough. There are several reasons that may explain this: (1) The encapsulation efficiency of enoxaparin in the LPNH is about 65%, and almost 35% of enoxaparin is a free drug in LPHN dispersion, and free enoxaparin usually has low oral bioavailability; (2) the nanoparticles must overcome the mucus layer before they are transported across the epithelium.

Although one part of the nanoparticles can penetrate the mucus layer and be transported across the epithelium, other parts of the nanoparticle may be trapped in the mucus layer and eliminated from the gastrointestinal tract, owing to the mucus layer being renewed every 1~2 h [32]. Therefore, more rationally designed nanocarriers with higher encapsulation efficiency and stronger mucus layer permeability are needed to further improve the absolute oral bioavailability of enoxaparin.

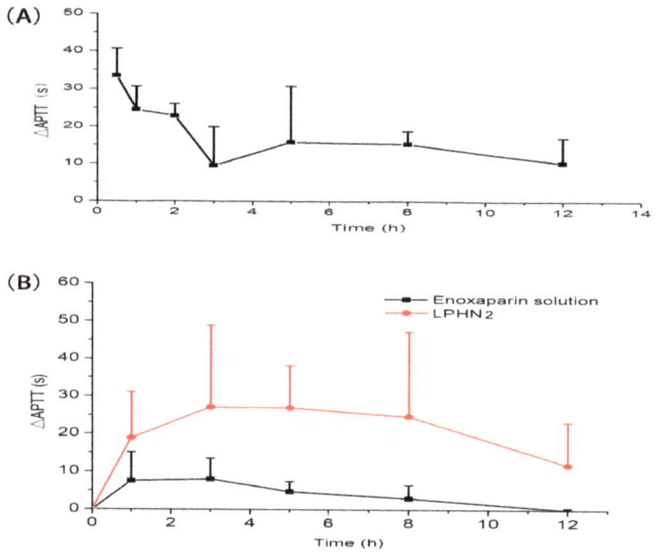

Figure 3. Mean Δ activated partial thromboplastin time (APTT) over time after a single intravenous injection of enoxaparin solution at a dosage of 101 IU/kg (**A**), and oral administration of enoxaparin solution and enoxaparin-loaded LPHN2 at a dosage of 1010 IU/kg (**B**) (n = 4).

3.4. *In Vivo Efficacy*

In vivo prevention of pulmonary thromboembolism of nanoparticles was studied in mice. As shown in Table 3, the inhibition effect was 58.3% when enoxaparin solution was intravenously administered. The inhibition effect of enoxaparin-loaded LPHN2 was 50.0%, 2.99-fold higher than that of enoxaparin solution after oral administration, which further indicated that lipid–polymer hybrid nanoparticles are effective in improving oral absorption and the inhibition effect of enoxaparin against thrombin-induced thrombosis.

Table 3. Inhibition effect of pulmonary thromboembolism by orally administered various enoxaparin formulations (n = 12).

Formulations	Inhibition Effect (% protection)
Saline (i.v.)	8.3
Enoxaparin solution (i.v.)	58.3
Enoxaparin solution (p.o.)	16.7
Enoxaparin-loaded LPHN2 (p.o.)	50.0

i.v. means intravenous injection; p.o. means peroral administration.

3.5. *Safety Evaluation*

To investigate whether nanoparticles cause intestinal membrane damage or not, a histopathological examination was conducted. The results of pathological sections are shown in Figure 4. The histological studies indicated that there were no significant changes in the morphology and structure of the intestine exposed to enoxaparin-loaded LPHN2. The mucosal erosions and disruption of the enterocytes did not appear. Hence, LPHN is biocompatible in vivo as well as safe for the oral delivery of enoxaparin.

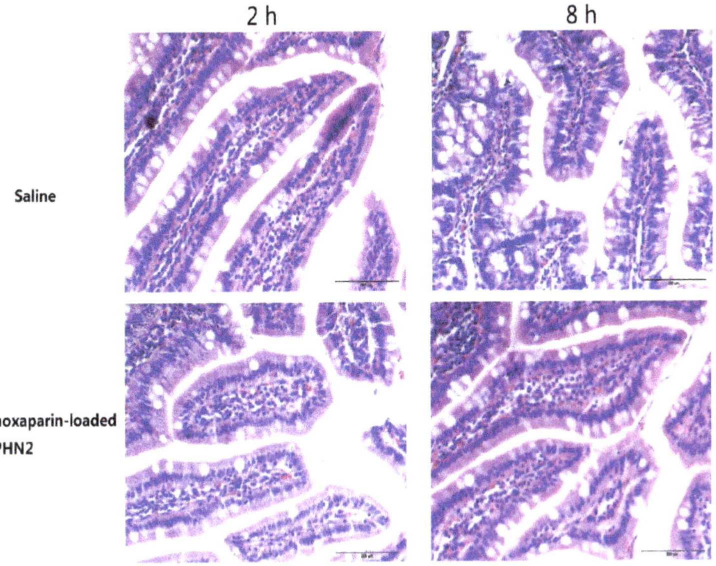

Figure 4. Morphology of intestinal mucosa of rats after oral administration of physiological saline- and enoxaparin-loaded LPHN2 after 2 and 8 h. Scale bar: 200 μm.

4. Conclusions

In summary, lipid–polymer hybrid nanoparticles (LPHNs) were prepared by double emulsification technology. The concentration of poloxamer 407 was optimized to ensure the high encapsulation efficiency of enoxaparin. Compared with traditional lipid nanoparticles, LPHNs possess not only higher encapsulation efficiency of enoxaparin, but also sustained release. In addition, optimized LPHNs could increase the concentration of enoxaparin in intestinal villi and facilitate enoxaparin penetration into the underlayer of enterocytes. Results of an in vivo pharmacokinetic study and an in vivo efficacy study further confirmed the superiority of LPHNs with regard to absorption-enhancing effects. In conclusion, rationally designed LPHNs could be excellent nanocarriers for oral delivery of enoxaparin.

Author Contributions: Conceptualization, G.F.; methodology, G.F.; software, B.T.; validation, G.F. and B.T.; formal analysis, G.F., B.T., and Y.Q.; investigation, G.F., B.T., and Y.Q.; data curation, B.T. and Y.Q.; writing—original draft preparation, G.F.; writing—review and editing, G.H.F.; funding acquisition, G.F. and B.T. All authors have read and agreed to the published version of the manuscript.

Funding: This work was supported by the Nantong Science and Technology Project (JC2019100), Natural Science Fund for Colleges and Universities in Jiangsu Province, No. 18KJB350009, and Natural Science Foundation of Jiangsu Province, No. BK20170445.

Conflicts of Interest: The authors declare no conflict of interest.

References

1. Hirsh, J.; Warkentin, T.E.; Shaughnessy, S.G.; Anand, S.S.; Halperin, J.L.; Raschke, R.; Granger, C.; Ohman, E.M.; Dalen, J.E. Heparin and Low-Molecular-Weight Heparin Mechanisms of Action, Pharmacokinetics, Dosing, Monitoring, Efficacy, and Safety. *Chest* **2001**, *119*, 64S–94S. [CrossRef] [PubMed]

2. Gray, E.; Mulloy, B.; Barrowcliffe, T.W. Heparin and low-molecular-weight heparin. *Thromb. Haemost.* **2008**, *99*, 807–818. [PubMed]
3. Fang, G.; Zhou, J.; Qian, Y.; Gou, J.; Yang, X.; Tang, B. Development and evaluation of thermo-sensitive hydrogel system with nanocomplexes for prolonged subcutaneous delivery of enoxaparin. *J. Drug Deliv. Sci. Technol.* **2018**, *48*, 118–124. [CrossRef]
4. Wang, L.; Li, L.; Sun, Y.; Tian, Y.; Li, Y.; Li, C.; Junyaprasert, V.B.; Mao, S. Exploration of hydrophobic modification degree of chitosan-based nanocomplexes on the oral delivery of enoxaparin. *Eur. J. Pharm. Sci. Off. J. Eur. Fed. Pharm. Sci.* **2013**, *50*, 263–271. [CrossRef] [PubMed]
5. Wang, L.; Li, L.; Sun, Y.; Ding, J.; Li, J.; Duan, X.; Li, Y.; Junyaprasert, V.B.; Mao, S. In vitro and in vivo evaluation of chitosan graft glyceryl monooleate as peroral delivery carrier of enoxaparin. *Int. J. Pharm.* **2014**, *471*, 391–399. [CrossRef]
6. Motlekar, N.A.; Youan, B.B. The quest for non-invasive delivery of bioactive macromolecules: A focus on heparins. *J. Control. Release Off. J. Control. Release Soc.* **2006**, *113*, 91–101. [CrossRef]
7. Neves, A.R.; Correia-da-Silva, M.; Sousa, E.; Pinto, M. Strategies to Overcome Heparins' Low Oral Bioavailability. *Pharmaceuticals* **2016**, *9*, 37. [CrossRef]
8. Fang, G.; Tang, B. Advanced delivery strategies facilitating oral absorption of heparins. *Asian J. Pharm. Sci.* **2020**. [CrossRef]
9. Valimaki, S.; Khakalo, A.; Ora, A.; Johansson, L.S.; Rojas, O.J.; Kostiainen, M.A. Effect of PEG-PDMAEMA Block Copolymer Architecture on Polyelectrolyte Complex Formation with Heparin. *Biomacromolecules* **2016**, *17*, 2891–2900. [CrossRef]
10. Ibrahim, S.S.; Osman, R.; Awad, G.A.; Mortada, N.D.; Geneidy, A.S. Low molecular weight heparins for current and future uses: Approaches for micro- and nano-particulate delivery. *Drug Deliv.* **2016**, *23*, 2661–2667. [CrossRef]
11. Ramadan, A.; Lagarce, F.; Tessier-Marteau, A.; Thomas, O.; Legras, P.; Macchi, L.; Saulnier, P.; Benoit, J.P. Oral fondaparinux: Use of lipid nanocapsules as nanocarriers and in vivo pharmacokinetic study. *Int. J. Nanomed.* **2011**, *6*, 2941–2951.
12. Kim, S.K.; Lee, E.H.; Vaishali, B.; Lee, S.; Lee, Y.K.; Kim, C.Y.; Moon, H.T.; Byun, Y. Tricaprylin microemulsion for oral delivery of low molecular weight heparin conjugates. *J. Control. Release Off. J. Control. Release Soc.* **2005**, *105*, 32–42. [CrossRef] [PubMed]
13. Paliwal, R.; Paliwal, S.R.; Agrawal, G.P.; Vyas, S.P. Biomimetic solid lipid nanoparticles for oral bioavailability enhancement of low molecular weight heparin and its lipid conjugates: In vitro and in vivo evaluation. *Mol. Pharm.* **2011**, *8*, 1314–1321. [CrossRef] [PubMed]
14. Rong, W.-T.; Lu, Y.-P.; Tao, Q.; Guo, M.; Lu, Y.; Ren, Y.; Yu, S.-Q. Hydroxypropyl-Sulfobutyl-β-Cyclodextrin Improves the Oral Bioavailability of Edaravone by Modulating Drug Efflux Pump of Enterocytes. *J. Pharm. Sci.* **2014**, *103*, 730–742. [CrossRef] [PubMed]
15. Lu, Y.; Liu, S.; Zhao, Y.; Zhu, L.; Yu, S. Complexation of Z-ligustilide with hydroxypropyl-beta-cyclodextrin to improve stability and oral bioavailability. *Acta Pharm.* **2014**, *64*, 211–222. [CrossRef]
16. Bagre, A.P.; Jain, K.; Jain, N.K. Alginate coated chitosan core shell nanoparticles for oral delivery of enoxaparin: In vitro and in vivo assessment. *Int. J. Pharm.* **2013**, *456*, 31–40. [CrossRef]
17. Meissner, Y.; Ubrich, N.; Ghazouani, F.E.; Maincent, P.; Lamprecht, A. Low molecular weight heparin loaded pH-sensitive microparticles. *Int. J. Pharm.* **2007**, *335*, 147–153. [CrossRef]
18. Fan, B.; Xing, Y.; Zheng, Y.; Sun, C.; Liang, G. pH-responsive thiolated chitosan nanoparticles for oral low-molecular weight heparin delivery: In vitro and in vivo evaluation. *Drug Deliv.* **2016**, *23*, 238–247. [CrossRef]
19. Yuan, H.; Chen, C.Y.; Chai, G.H.; Du, Y.Z.; Hu, F.Q. Improved transport and absorption through gastrointestinal tract by PEGylated solid lipid nanoparticles. *Mol. Pharm.* **2013**, *10*, 1865–1873. [CrossRef]
20. Wong, H.L.; Bendayan, R.; Rauth, A.M.; Li, Y.; Wu, X.Y. Chemotherapy with anticancer drugs encapsulated in solid lipid nanoparticles. *Adv. Drug Deliv. Rev.* **2007**, *59*, 491–504. [CrossRef]
21. Hirsh, J.; Anand Sonia, S.; Halperin Jonathan, L.; Fuster, V. Mechanism of Action and Pharmacology of Unfractionated Heparin. *Arterioscler. Thromb. Vasc. Biol.* **2001**, *21*, 1094–1096. [CrossRef] [PubMed]
22. Boushra, M.; Tous, S.; Fetih, G.; Korzekwa, K.; Lebo, D.B.; Xue, H.Y.; Wong, H.L. Development and evaluation of viscosity-enhanced nanocarrier (VEN) for oral insulin delivery. *Int. J. Pharm.* **2016**, *511*, 462–472. [CrossRef] [PubMed]

23. Lin, Z.; Gao, W.; Hu, H.; Ma, K.; He, B.; Dai, W.; Wang, X.; Wang, J.; Zhang, X.; Zhang, Q. Novel thermo-sensitive hydrogel system with paclitaxel nanocrystals: High drug-loading, sustained drug release and extended local retention guaranteeing better efficacy and lower toxicity. *J. Control. Release Off. J. Control. Release Soc.* **2014**, *174*, 161–170. [CrossRef] [PubMed]
24. Tang, X.; Huang, K.; Gui, H.; Wang, J.; Lu, J.; Dai, L.; Zhang, L.; Wang, G. Pluronic-based micelle encapsulation potentiates myricetin-induced cytotoxicity in human glioblastoma cells. *Int. J. Nanomed.* **2016**, *11*, 4991–5002. [CrossRef]
25. Wang, P.; Li, Y.; Jiang, M. Effects of the multilayer structures on Exenatide release and bioactivity in microsphere/thermosensitive hydrogel system. *Colloids Surf. B Biointerfaces* **2018**, *171*, 85–93. [CrossRef]
26. Fang, G.; Tang, B.; Chao, Y.; Xu, H.; Gou, J.; Zhang, Y.; Tang, X. Cysteine-Functionalized Nanostructured Lipid Carriers for Oral Delivery of Docetaxel: A Permeability and Pharmacokinetic Study. *Mol. Pharm.* **2015**, *12*, 2384–2395. [CrossRef]
27. Jiao, Y.; Ubrich, N.; Marchand-Arvier, M.; Vigneron, C.; Hoffman, M.; Lecompte, T.; Maincent, P. In Vitro and In Vivo Evaluation of Oral Heparin–Loaded Polymeric Nanoparticles in Rabbits. *Circulation* **2002**, *105*, 230–235. [CrossRef]
28. Hoffart, V.; Ubrich, N.; Lamprecht, A.; Bachelier, K.; Vigneron, C.; Lecompte, T.; Hoffman, M.; Maincent, P. Microencapsulation of Low Molecular Weight Heparin into Polymeric Particles Designed with Biodegradable and Nonbiodegradable Polycationic Polymers. *Drug Deliv.* **2003**, *10*, 1–7. [CrossRef]
29. Sherif, S.; Bendas, E.R.; Badawy, S. The clinical efficacy of cosmeceutical application of liquid crystalline nanostructured dispersions of alpha lipoic acid as anti-wrinkle. *Eur. J. Pharm. Biopharm. Off. J. Arb. Fur Pharm. Verfahr. e.V* **2014**, *86*, 251–259. [CrossRef]
30. Lakkireddy, H.R.; Urmann, M.; Besenius, M.; Werner, U.; Haack, T.; Brun, P.; Alie, J.; Illel, B.; Hortala, L.; Vogel, R.; et al. Oral delivery of diabetes peptides—Comparing standard formulations incorporating functional excipients and nanotechnologies in the translational context. *Adv. Drug Deliv. Rev.* **2016**, *106*, 196–222. [CrossRef]
31. Malhaire, H.; Gimel, J.-C.; Roger, E.; Benoît, J.-P.; Lagarce, F. How to design the surface of peptide-loaded nanoparticles for efficient oral bioavailability? *Adv. Drug Deliv. Rev.* **2016**, *106*, 320–336. [CrossRef] [PubMed]
32. Hansson, G.C. Mucus and mucins in diseases of the intestinal and respiratory tracts. *J. Intern. Med.* **2019**, *285*, 479–490. [CrossRef] [PubMed]

pharmaceutics

MDPI

Article

Hydrogel Formulations Incorporating Drug Nanocrystals Enhance the Therapeutic Effect of Rebamipide in a Hamster Model for Oral Mucositis

Noriaki Nagai [1,*], Ryotaro Seiriki [1], Saori Deguchi [1], Hiroko Otake [1], Noriko Hiramatsu [2], Hiroshi Sasaki [3] and Naoki Yamamoto [3]

[1] Faculty of Pharmacy, Kindai University, 3-4-1 Kowakae, Higashi-Osaka, Osaka 577-8502, Japan; 1611610157u@kindai.ac.jp (R.S.); 2045110002h@kindai.ac.jp (S.D.); hotake@phar.kindai.ac.jp (H.O.)

[2] Laboratory of Molecularbiology and Histochemistry, Fujita Health University Institute of Joint Research, 1-98 Dengakugakubo, Kutsukake, Toyoake, Aichi 470-1192, Japan; norikoh@fujita-hu.ac.jp

[3] Department of Ophthalmology, Kanazawa Medical University, 1-1 Daigaku, Uchinada, Kahoku, Ishikawa 920-0293, Japan; sasaki-h@k5.dion.ne.jp (H.S.); naokiy@kanazawa-med.ac.jp (N.Y.)

* Correspondence: nagai_n@phar.kindai.ac.jp; Tel.: +81-6-4307-3638

check for updates

Received: 21 May 2020; Accepted: 8 June 2020; Published: 9 June 2020

Abstract: A mouthwash formulation of rebamipide (REB) is commonly used to treat oral mucositis; however, this formulation does not provide sufficient treatment or prevention in cases of serious oral mucositis. To improve treatment, we attempted to design a hydrogel incorporating REB nanocrystals (R-NPs gel). The R-NPs gel was prepared by a bead mill method using carbopol hydrogel, methylcellulose and 2-hydroxypropyl-β-cyclodextrin, and another hydrogel incorporating REB microcrystals (R-MPs gel) was prepared following the same protocol but without the bead mill treatment. The REB particle size in the R-MPs gel was 0.15–25 μm, and while the REB particle size was 50–180 nm in the R-NPs gel. Next, we investigated the therapeutic effect of REB nanocrystals on oral mucositis using a hamster model. Almost all of the REB was released as drug nanocrystals from the R-NPs gel, and the REB content in the cheek pouch of hamsters treated with R-NPs gel was significantly higher than that of hamsters treated with R-MPs gel. Further, treatment with REB hydrogels enhanced the healing of oral wounds in the hamsters. REB accumulation in the cheek pouch of hamsters treated with the R-NPs gel was prevented by an inhibitor of clathrin-dependent endocytosis (CME) (40 μM dynasore). In conclusion, we designed an R-NPs gel and found that REB nanocrystals are taken up by tissues through CME, where they provide a persistent effect resulting in an enhancement of oral wound healing.

Keywords: rebamipide; nanocrystals; oral mucositis; hydrogel; endocytosis

1. Introduction

Pain caused by serious oral mucositis affects food intake, nutrition, speaking, and swallowing, can cause life-threatening bacteremia, and ultimately leads to poor quality of life for patients [1,2]. Chemoradiotherapy for patients with head and neck cancer often causes serious oral mucositis, and the severe pain interferes with subsequent treatment and quality of life [3–5]. Previous studies have shown that reactive oxygen species cause cell apoptosis, DNA damage, and enhanced production of proinflammatory cytokines [6], and that these factors greatly impact mucositis. Therefore, topical granulocyte macrophage colony stimulating factors, anti-inflammatory agents and mucosal coating agents are widely used as medical therapies for oral mucositis [7]. In addition, Caphosol®, MuGard®, Mucotrol™, Gelclair®, Episil® and Palifermin have surfaced on the market. Caphosol® is a supersaturated calcium phosphate, electrolyte mouth rinse used as artificial saliva, and MuGard® (oral mucoadhesive) causes the formation of a protective coating over oral mucosa. Mucotrol™ is a mixture of herbal agents that is used as an oral gel wafer and includes sorbitol, *Cyamopsis tetragonolobus*, stearic acid, magnesium stearate and aloe. Gelclair® is a viscous gel that is used as a mouthwash and forms a protective film by adhering to the mucosa of the oropharyngeal cavity, helping to provide pain relief in mouth lesions. Episil® is a lipid-based fluid developed for the management and relief of pain associated with oral lesions of various aetiologies such as oral mucositis, a painful side effect of cancer therapies. Palifermin is a truncated human recombinant keratinocyte growth factor produced in *Escherichia coli*. The keratinocyte growth factor stimulates the growth of cells that line the surface of the mouth and intestinal tract. However, serious oral mucositis remains a frequent and critical complication of head and neck cancers [8–10].

Rebamipide (REB), 2-(4-chlorobenzoylamino)-3-[2(1H)-quinolinone-4-yl]-propionic acid, was developed by Otsuka Pharmaceutical Co., Ltd. (Tokyo, Japan) for the treatment of gastric ulcers, gastritis, and dry eye syndrome. It was reported that REB scavenges free radicals, exhibits an anti-inflammatory action and improves blood flow [11,12]. In addition, REB increases endogenous prostaglandins E2 and I2, leading to antibacterial effects, mucin secretagogue activity and anti-inflammatory action [13,14]. The efficacy of REB for the treatment of oral mucositis was first reported by Matsuda et al. in 1994, and a resulting mouthwash containing REB has been used as a therapy for mucositis caused by radiotherapy [15], chemotherapy [16] and Behcet's disease [7]. Furthermore, a pilot randomized controlled trial (RCT) reported that mouthwash containing REB reduces the onset of oral mucositis caused by chemoradiotherapy and radiotherapy [15,17,18]. The various pharmacological effects of REB include suppression of the induction of mucus secretion [19], promotion of endogenous prostaglandin production in the gastric mucosa [20,21], anti-free radical action [12], neutrophil activation [22,23], inhibition of inflammatory reactions [24–26] and up-regulation of epidermal growth factor and its receptor [27]. Pharmacokinetic studies using experimental animals have shown that REB acts directly on peptic ulcers and gastritis [28], and that a 4% REB liquid preparation is the optimal concentration for a mouthwash in terms of safety and efficacy profiles [18]. However, sufficient drug efficacy is difficult to obtain since the mouth-washing agent has a short residence time in the oral cavity, and a local concentration of REB on the oral mucosa cannot be maintained via a mouthwash containing liquid REB. We aimed to prepare mucoadhesive formulations, and focused to design the formulations incorporating drug nanocrystals into a hydrogel net. Moreover, we investigated the mucoadhesive properties, drug release and the uptake of REB into the cheek pouch tissue in the REB hydrogel.

It is important to consider the structure of the three-dimensional network in sputum to efficiently deliver REB particles to the oral mucosa. It has been reported that gastrointestinal mucus and cystic fibrosis sputum almost completely block the delivery of particles larger than 500 nm [29–31]. In addition, the mucoadhesive properties of a formulation are enhanced by decreasing their particle size, since this increases the relative surface area [32]. Therefore, we hypothesized that nanocrystals with a particle diameter smaller than 200 nm would be a suitable carrier of REB for the treatment of oral mucositis. We previously found that drug nanocrystals were taken up by cells, provided high efficiency, and showed that a hydrogel is suitable as a base for gel formulations, since the drug nanocrystals were easily released from the hydrogel base [33–35]. In this study, we attempted to design a hydrogel formulation containing REB nanocrystals smaller than 200 nm by incorporating the drug nanocrystals into a hydrogel net, and to demonstrate the usefulness of these REB nanocrystals as a therapy for oral mucositis.

2. Materials and Methods

2.1. Animals

Male golden or Syrian hamsters (*Mesocricetus auratus*, weight 98 ± 2.6 g) were purchased from Shimizu Laboratory Supplies Co., Ltd. (Kyoto, Japan). All animal experiments were approved by the animal experimental committee in Kindai University on 1 April 2019 (approval number KAPS-31-016).

2.2. Preparation of REB Hydrogel

Hydrogel formulations incorporating REB nanocrystals were prepared according to previous reports [33,34]. REB powder (0.4%; Wako Pure Chemical Industries, Ltd., Osaka, Japan), 0.5% methylcellulose (MC; Shin-Etsu Chemical Co., Ltd., Tokyo, Japan) and 5% 2-hydroxypropyl-β-cyclodextrin (HPβCD; Nihon Shokuhin Kako Co., Ltd., Tokyo, Japan) were added to distilled water containing 0.1 mm zirconia beads, and crushed at 5500 rpm for 1 min by a Micro Smash MS-100R (TOMY SEIKO Co. Ltd., Tokyo, Japan). The mill treatment was repeated 30 times, after which the dispersions were milled at 1500 rpm for 3 h with a Shake Master NEO (Bio-Medical Science Co., Ltd., Tokyo, Japan). The milled dispersions were incorporated into a Carbopol® 934 hydrogel net (Serva, Heidelberg, Germany) and used as hydrogel formulations incorporating REB nanocrystals (R-NPs gel) in this study. Hydrogel formulations incorporating REB microcrystals (R-MPs gel) were prepared by mixing the 0.4% REB powder, 0.5% MC and 5% HPβCD in the distilled water, and incorporated the REB microcrystals into Carbopol® 934 hydrogel net.

2.3. Characteristics of REB Hydrogels

The characteristics of the REB hydrogels were analyzed according to previous studies [33,34]. Briefly, the particle size distributions of the R-MPs gels were measured by a SALD-7100 (refractive index, 1.60-0.10i; Shimadzu Corp., Kyoto, Japan), and the particle size distribution and particle number of the R-NPs gel were determined using NANOSIGHT LM10 (viscosity, 1.27 mPa·s; QuantumDesign Japan, Tokyo, Japan). The atomic force microscopy (AFM) image of the REB nanocrystals was obtained using a SPM-9700 (Shimadzu Corp., Kyoto, Japan), and the crystal form was determined by a powder X-ray diffraction (XRD) Mini Flex II (Rigaku Co., Tokyo, Japan). The zeta potential of REB was analyzed by a model 502 zeta potential analyzer (Nihon Rufuto Co., Ltd., Tokyo, Japan). REB concentrations were measured on a HPLC LC-20AT system (Shimadzu Corp. Kyoto, Japan) with an Inertsil® ODS-3 column (GL Science Co., Inc., Tokyo, Japan) with detection at 287 nm. Methyl p-hydroxybenzoate was used as an internal standard, and the mobile phase was 50 mM phosphate buffer/acetonitrile (75/25 *v*/*v*) at a flow rate of 0.25 mL/min. The uniformity of the REB in the gels was determined as follows: 0.3 g of REB hydrogel was divided into 10 parts (0.03 g) and dissolved in *N*,*N*-dimethylformamide. The REB contents in the dissolved samples were measured by the HPLC method described above. In this study, the standard deviation (SD) of the REB levels in the 10 hydrogel divisions represents the non-uniformity of REB in the hydrogel.

2.4. Permeation Study from REB Hydrogels

Drug release from the REB hydrogels was analyzed according to the previous study using a Franz diffusion cell set on an MF™-MEMBRANE FILTER with a pore size of 220 nm (Merck Millipore, Tokyo, Japan) [33–35]. The reservoir chamber of the cell was filled with 12.2 mL of 10 mM phosphate buffer consist of sodium phosphate and potassium phosphate according to the Japanese Pharmacopoeia, 17th Edition (JP XVII), and the pH was adjusted by NaOH (pH 7.4). A total of 0.3 g of 0.4% REB hydrogels was added to the donor side. We collected 50 μL samples of phosphate from the reservoir chamber over time and replaced them with the same volume of 10 mM phosphate buffer. The nanoparticle size distribution, number, and released REB levels in the samples were measured by the NANOSIGHT and HPLC methods described in Section 2.3.

2.5. REB Contents in Hamsters Treated with REB Hydrogels

In this study, 10 μM cytochalasin D (phagocytosis inhibitor) [36], 2 μM rottlerin (MP—macropinocytosis inhibitor) [37], 40 μM dynasore (CME—clathrin-dependent endocytosis inhibitor) [38] and 54 μM nystatin (CavME—caveolae-dependent endocytosis inhibitor) [36] were used as inhibitors for each type of endocytosis. A total of 0.1 g of 0.4% REB hydrogel with or without endocytosis inhibitors was applied to the cheek pouch of hamsters and maintained for 2 or 8 h.

After that, the hamsters were euthanized under deep isoflurane anesthesia, and the cheek pouches were carefully collected. The collected cheek pouches were homogenized in *N,N*-dimethylformamide to extract the REB. Blood was collected from the vena cava, centrifuged at 20,400 g and a temperature of 4 °C for 20 min, and the supernatants were used as samples. REB levels in both the cheek pouch and blood samples were measured by HPLC, as described above.

2.6. Measurement of Wound Area in the Hamster Model for Oral Mucositis

Hamsters were anesthetized with isoflurane (3%, rate of flow 1 L/min), and 25 μL of 10% acetic acid was injected into the cheek pouch. After 2 days, the hamsters were used in experiments as a model for oral mucositis. A total of 0.1 g of REB hydrogel was applied once a day (10:00 a.m.) and the wound images were monitored by a digital camera. The wound size was measured daily with an image. The initial areas of the wound (0 days) were as follows: non-treated hamsters (None), 10.8 ± 0.76; vehicle-treated hamsters (Vehicle), 10.2 ± 3.3; R-MPs-treated hamsters, 10.3 ± 3.3; R-NPs-treated hamsters, 10.7 ± 1.9 (mm^2; means ± standard error of mean (SEM), n = 5–8). The values (%) were calculated as the ratio to the initial area of the respective wound.

2.7. Measurement of Wound Area in the Hamster Model for Oral Mucositis

The cheek pouches of euthanized hamsters were removed and fixed at room temperature using a tissue quick fixation solution (SUPER FIX, Kurabo Industries, Osaka, Japan). The fixed tissues were prepared in paraffin blocks by the general protocol, and serial sections with a thickness of 4 μm were prepared using a microtome. Hematoxylin and eosin (H&E) staining was performed for morphological observation, and immunostaining was performed with a multi-cytokeratin antibody to identify the oral mucosal epithelium; endogenous peroxidase treatment was performed with 0.3% hydrogen peroxide methanol; and microwave treatment was performed (90 °C, 20 min) in citric acid buffer (pH 6.0) for antigen activation. Samples were incubated with anti-multi-cytokeratin mouse monoclonal antibody (1:200, Clone: AE1/AE3, Leica Biosystems Nussloch GmbH) for 30 min at 37 °C. After three washes with phosphate buffer solution, samples were incubated with universal immune-peroxidase polymer (anti-mouse antibody, Histofine® Simple Stain MAX PO (M), Nichirei Biosciences, Tokyo, Japan) for 30 min at 37 °C. Samples were again washed three times with phosphate buffer solution, color washed with 3,3′-diaminobenzidine tetrahydrochloride (DAB) solution for 30 s, washed with water, and nuclear stained with Meyer's hematoxylin solution (Muto Chemical Co., Ltd., Tokyo, Japan) for 5 min. Specimens were observed using a biological upright microscope (Power BX-51, Olympus, Tokyo, Japan) with a digital camera (4× and 10× object lenses, DP-71, Olympus), and photographed at the central area of the oral wound.

2.8. Statistical Analysis

Data are shown as the mean ± SEM, and ANOVA, Student's t-test and Dunnett's multiple comparisons were used to analyze statistical differences.

3. Results

3.1. Design and Characteristics of the R-NPs Gel

Bead mill is a known method to prepare drug nanocrystals. We attempted to prepare REB nanocrystals using the bead mill method and investigated the characteristics of the hydrogel with REB nanocrystals. Figure 1 shows the particle size distribution of REB in the hydrogel. The aggregates of REB particles were observable in the R-MPs gel (Figure 1A,B) with the naked eye; however, bead mill treatment caused a decrease in REB particle size, after which aggregates were no longer visible in the R-NPs gel (Figure 1A,C). The particle size distribution was 50–180 nm after mill treatment (Figure 1C), and the AFM image also showed the REB particles crushed to nano-size (Figure 1D). In addition, we demonstrated the characteristics of the REB in the R-NPs gel (Figure 2). The REB content in R-NPs gel was uniform in comparison with the R-MPs gel (Figure 2A), and the REB solubility in the R-NPs gel was higher than that in the R-MPs gel (Figure 2B). On the other hand, the crystal form of REB was maintained in the R-NPs gel (Figure 2C), and the crystal structure of REB nanocrystals in the hydrogel was similar to that in the REB microcrystals. These results showed that the form did not affect the difference on its solubility. Moreover, we evaluated the stability of R-NPs gel. In this study, the zeta potential of the REB nanocrystals was −11.9 mV, and no differences were observed in the size, content or form of the REB nanocrystals in hydrogel for one month.

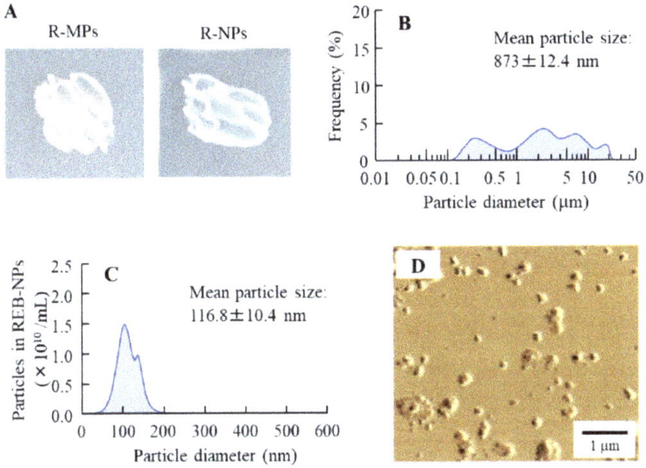

Figure 1. Condition of rebamipide (REB) in REB hydrogels. (**A**) Photographs of the R-MPs gel (hydrogel with incorporated rebamipide microcyrstals) and R-NPs gel (hydrogel with incorporated rebamipide nanocrystals). (**B**,**C**) Particle size in the R-MPs (**B**) and R-NPs (**C**) gels. (**D**) AFM image of the R-NPs gel. Bead mill treatment decreased the particle size of REB to the range of 50–180 nm.

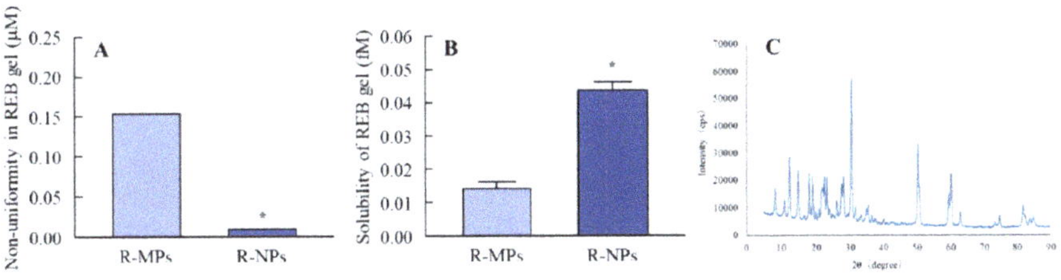

Figure 2. Characteristics of REB in the R-MPs and R-NPs gels. (**A**) Non-uniformity in REB particle distribution in the R-MPs and R-NPs gels. (**B**) Solubility of REB in the R-MPs and R-NPs gels. (**C**) XRD pattern of REB particles after bead mill treatment. $N = 7$. * $p < 0.05$ vs. R-MPs for each category. The mill-treated REB retained its crystal structure, but the uniformity of REB distribution in the R-NPs gel was higher than the non-milled REB in the R-MPs gel. Moreover, solubility of REB was increased by bead mill treatment.

3.2. Endocytic Uptake of REB Nanocrystals into Cheek Pouch Tissue

In the investigation of the mechanism for drug permeation in tissues, an evaluation of drug release from the hydrogel is necessary. Figure 3 shows the REB released from the hydrogel. The release of REB was observed for both the R-MPs and R-NPs gels, but the levels released from the R-NPs gel were significantly higher (Figure 3A). Almost all of the REB released from R-MPs gel was of the solution type, while drug nanocrystals were detected in the reservoir chamber after treatment with the R-NPs gel (Figure 3B,C). Next, we examined REB levels in the cheek pouch of hamsters treated with the R-MPs and R-NPs gels (Figure 4A). Eight hours after treatment, the REB levels in hamsters treated with the R-NPs gel were 25-fold higher than in hamsters treated with the R-MPs gel. We then investigated whether endocytosis is related to the uptake of REB into the cheek pouch tissue (Figure 4B,C). Co-treatment with nystatin, rottlerin or cytochalasin D did not affect REB levels in the cheek pouch of hamsters treated with the R-NPs gel. In contrast, co-treatment with dynasore resulted in a significant decrease in tissue REB levels, indicating that CME is related to the uptake of REB into the cheek pouch tissue. We also examined the REB levels in the blood of hamsters 0–8 h after treatment with REB hydrogels. No REB was detected in the plasma of hamsters treated with either the R-MPs or R-NPs gels.

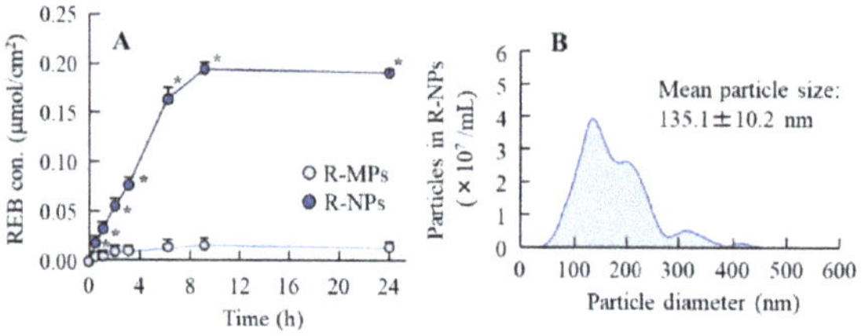

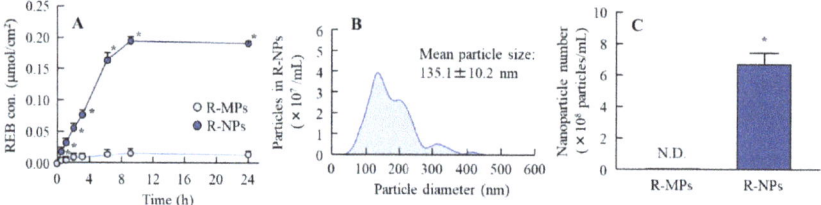

Figure 3. Drug release from R-MPs and R-NPs gels through a 220-nm pore membrane. (**A**) Release behavior of REB from R-MPs and R-NPs gels through a membrane. (**B**) and (**C**) Size distribution (**B**) and number (**C**) of REB nanocrystals in the reservoir chamber 24 h after R-NPs application. $n = 7$. N.D., not detectable. * $p < 0.05$ vs. R-MPs gel for each category. REB was released from the R-NPs gel in the form of nanocrystals.

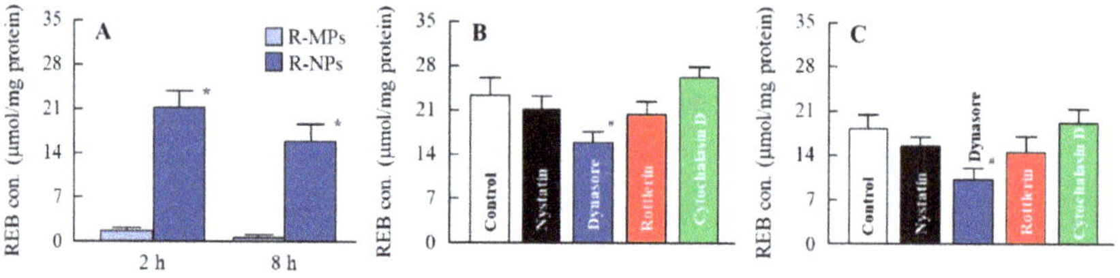

Figure 4. Changes in REB content in the cheek pouch of hamsters treated with REB hydrogels for oral mucositis. (**A**) REB contents in the cheek pouch of hamsters 2 and 8 h after treatment with R-MPs and R-NPs gels. (**B**,**C**) REB contents in the cheek pouch of hamsters treated with endocytosis inhibitors 2 h (**B**) and 8 h (**C**) after the application of R-MPs and R-NPs gels. Control—R-NPs-treated hamster. Nystatin—nystatin-treated hamster treated with R-NPs. Dynasore—dynasore-treated hamster treated with R-NPs. Rottlerin—rottlerin-treated hamster treated with R-NPs. Cytochalasin D—cytochalasin D-treated hamster treated with R-NPs. $n = 5–7$. * $p < 0.05$, vs. R-MPs for each category. # $p < 0.05$ vs. Control for each category. REB content in hamsters treated with R-NPs gel was higher than in those treated with R-MPs gel; the CME pathway appears to be related to the penetration of REB into the cheek pouch tissues from the hydrogel formulations.

3.3. *Effect of REB Hydrogel on Oral Wound Healing in the Hamster Model*

Figure 5 shows the therapeutic potential of the REB hydrogels for oral mucositis. The wounds in the hamsters injected with acetic acid remained uncured after three days with an area of 8.1 ± 0.5 mm^2. Although the oral wound in hamsters treated with vehicle also remained uncured after three days (8.0 ± 0.3 mm^2), hamsters treated with R-MPs gel showed a decrease in the oral wound area to 6.3 ± 0.4 mm^2. However, treatment with the R-NPs gel significantly enhanced healing of the wound, with the area reduced to 2.3 ± 0.3 mm^2 three days after the injection of acetic acid. Further, we examined wounds histologically by H&E staining and multi-cytokeratin immunostaining (Figure 6). The None and Vehicle group hamsters showed a degeneration and thickening of the oral mucosal epithelium, migration of inflammatory cells, (♠) and dilated blood vessels (black arrowheads) in the mucosal lamina propria. A regenerated oral mucosal epithelium (white arrowhead) was partially observed in the wounds of hamsters treated with the R-MPs or R-NPs gels, and inflammatory cell levels were reduced in the mucosal lamina propria (Figure 6A). A proliferation of basal cells in the regenerated oral mucosal epithelium was present in hamsters treated with the R-MPs and R-NPs gels (yellow arrowheads, Figure 6B). Oral mucosal epithelial cells containing multi-cytokeratin were stained brown by DAB. The multi-cytokeratin-positive cells in the None group were degenerated and necrotic, and the mucosal lamina propria underlying the mucosal epithelium was thickened (♣1). In the Vehicle group, the degenerated and necrotic mucosal epithelium was almost shedding, and the mucosal lamina propria was thickened as in the None group, with further migration of inflammatory cells (♣2). Regenerated oral mucosal epithelium was observed in the wounds of some of the hamsters treated with the R-MPs or R-NPs gels. The regenerated oral mucosal epithelium included basal cells (white arrowheads) and layers of multi-cytokeratin-positive cells (*) toward the surface of the mucosa (Figure 6C,D).

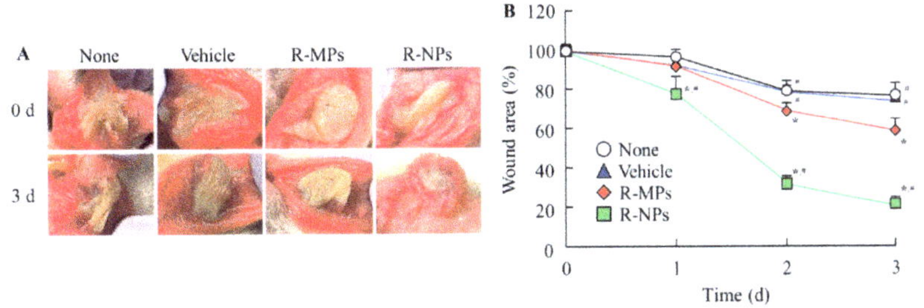

Figure 5. Therapeutic effect of R-NPs gel on wounds in the cheek pouch of hamsters. (**A**) Representative images of the cheek pouch of the hamster model for oral mucositis 0 and 3 d after treatment with REB hydrogels. (**B**), Wound area in the cheek pouch of the hamster model 0–3 d after treatment with REB hydrogels. n = 5–8. * $p < 0.05$, vs. Vehicle for each category. # $p < 0.05$ vs. R-MPs gel for each category. Treatment with REB hydrogel enhanced the therapeutic effect on oral mucositis. The wound areas in hamsters treated with R-NPs gel were significantly smaller than in hamsters treated with R-MPs gel.

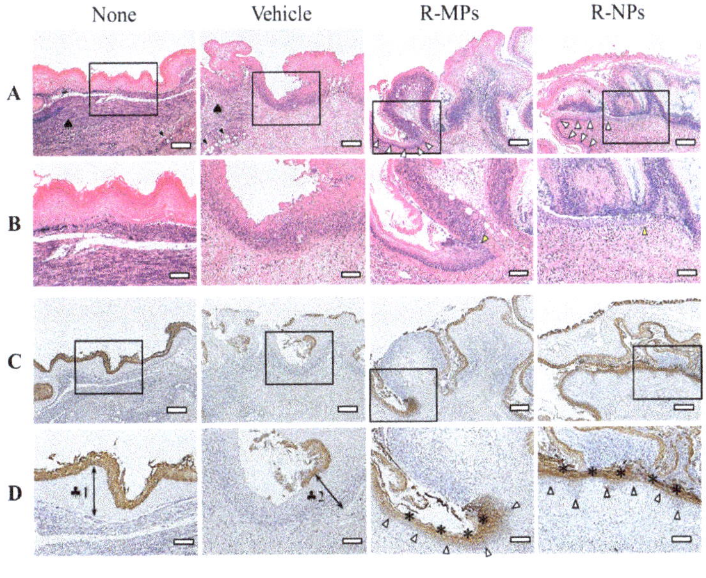

Figure 6. Microscopic effects of the R-NPs gel on oral mucositis. (**A**) Images of H&E-stained cheek

pouch tissue specimens from a hamster with oral mucositis three days after treatment with REB hydrogels (4× objective lens; bars indicate 200 μm). (**B**) High magnification images in the areas delineated by the squares in Figure A (10× objective lens; bars indicate 100 μm). (**C**) Images of immunostaining for multi-cytokeratin in the serial sections shown in Figure A (4× objective lens; bars indicate 200 μm). (**D**) High magnification images of the areas delineated by the squares in Figure C (10× objective lens; bars indicate 100 μm).

4. Discussion

Oral mucositis is the most common painful mucosal lesion, but traditional treatments, such as a mouthwash containing REB, do not provide sufficient treatment or prevention of this condition in serious cases [6,8,39]. Therefore, it is essential to look for effective treatments with few or no adverse effects. In this study, we developed a hydrogel formulation incorporating REB nanocrystals (R-NPs gel) and showed that CME is related to the uptake of REB nanocrystals into the cheek pouch tissue of hamsters. In addition, we found that R-NPs gel releases high levels of REB into tissues and provides a useful therapy for oral mucositis in the hamster model (Figure 7).

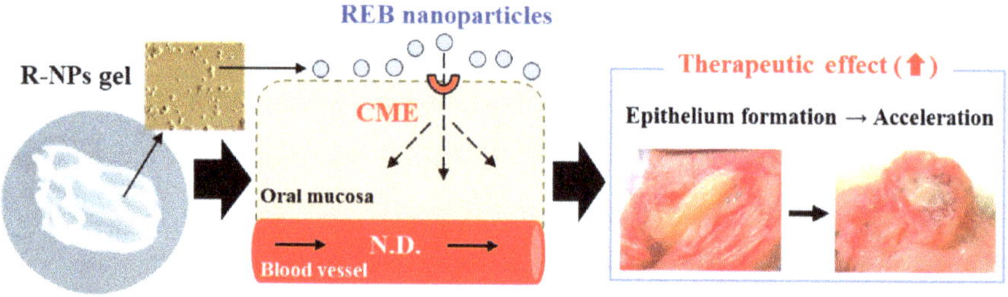

Figure 7. Drug delivery pathway and therapeutic effect of R-NPs gel in the cheek pouch of the hamster model for oral mucositis. N.D., not detectable.

Daniel et al. reported limited diffusion of particles larger than 0.5 μm through the mucin layer [31]. Szentkuti [30] showed that particles larger than 1 μm (1.09 μm diameter) do not accumulate on the surface of cell membranes and are undetectable 30 min after application, but the mucoadhesive properties of particles that are 415 nm in diameter are higher and they do accumulate on the apical membranes of surface epithelium cells and remain there for more than 30 min after treatment [30]. These reports suggest that the mucoadhesive properties of a drug increase as particle size decreases, and that the preparation of particles smaller than 400 nm in diameter is needed for application as a drug delivery system (DDS) for therapy of oral mucositis. Break down and build up methods have been used to prepare drug nanocrystals, and we previously succeeded in preparing drug nanocrystals of indomethachin and tranilast with an average particle diameter smaller than 100 nm by applying the bead mill method in the presence of various excipients, such as a cellulose compound and cyclodextrin [40,41]. Moreover, we showed that these drug nanocrystals show high mucoadhesive properties and bioavailability in the small intestine of rats [42,43]. Therefore, we tried to prepare nanocrystals of REB according to our previous protocol [40,41]. The particle size of the REB in the R-NPs gel was in the range of 50–180 nm (Figure 1C,D), so even the largest particle was smaller than 200 nm. Moreover, REB nanocrystals were dispersed uniformly in the hydrogel (Figure 1A) and were released from the R-NPs gel to a significantly greater extent than the R-MPs gel. In addition, REB was released from the hydrogel as drug nanocrystals, since REB nanocrystals were detected in the reservoir chamber of the Franz diffusion cell after passage through a 220 nm pore membrane (Figure 3).

The cheek pouches of a hamster represent a stable environment and drugs that are taken into them do not get washed away. Therefore, wounds in a hamster's cheek pouch are widely used as an animal model for the study of drug accumulation and the therapeutic effect on oral mucositis. We used this model in our study and found that the accumulation and persistence of REB in the cheek pouch of hamsters treated with the R-NPs gel were remarkably higher in comparison with treatment using the R-MPs gel (Figure 4A). This showed that the cellular uptake of REB nanocrystals was higher than microcrystals in the oral mucosa. In addition, R-NPs gel provided a significant increase in wound healing (Figure 5). The mucosal epithelium of acetic acid-denatured cheek pouch tissues underwent regeneration following treatment with R-MPs and R-NPs, and the number of inflammatory cells observed in the mucosal lamina propria were reduced in comparison with the None and Vehicle treatment groups. Treatment with both the R-MPs and R-NPs gels produced regeneration of the layered structure of the mucosal epithelium, but regeneration was greater in hamsters treated with the R-NPs gel (Figure 6). These results suggest that the REB particle size is suitable for use in a DDS to the oral mucosa, and show that treatment with the R-NPs gel can provide effective therapy for oral wound healing. On the other hand, no REB was detected in the plasma of hamsters treated with either hydrogel. The levels of blood flow and blood volume in the hamster cheek pouch may relate to the non-systemic distribution of REB. These results suggest that the therapeutic effect on oral wound healing by REB is local and not a systemic side effect in the hamster model.

It is important to clarify the mechanism for the enhancement of accumulation, persistence and therapeutic effect of REB in the cheek pouch of hamsters treated with R-NPs gel. In general, solubility is related to tissue penetration and cell uptake, and the solubility of REB in the R-NPs gel was increased by bead mill treatment. Cyclodextrin shows an inclusion ability for drugs, and inclusion enhances the solubility of poorly soluble drugs such as REB. In fact, the solubility of REB in an R-MPs gel without HPβCD is 0.0043 ± 0.0004 fM (n = 5), and the liquid REB levels in the hydrogel are lower than in the R-MPs gel containing 5% HPβCD. We also measured REB solubility in the R-NPs gel without 5% HPβCD and found it to be 0.016 ± 0.003 fM (n = 5). Thus, the amount of liquid REB is decreased when HPβCD is removed from the R-MPs gel formulation. However, the liquid REB level in the hydrogel formulation incorporating REB nanocrystals and 5% HPβCD was similar to that of the R-MPs gel. These results suggest that the inclusion ability of the drug by HPβCD is enhanced with a decrease in particle size and is related to the increase in REB solubility. Both the liquid (solution) and crystalline types are mixed in the hydrogel formulations incorporating REB nanocrystals, and this enhancement of REB solubility may affect REB release from the hydrogel and uptake into the tissue. Otherwise, the amount of liquid REB in the hydrogel was small, with almost all REB existing as nanocrystals. Therefore, we also investigated the mechanism for the accumulation of drug nanocrystals in the cheek pouch tissue.

The rate of mucosal absorption and retention of drug nanocrystals with a particle diameter smaller than 200 nm is high [29–32,43], and energy-dependent endocytosis is related to drug uptake in the cells and tissues of the small intestine [42]. Considering this, we investigated whether energy-dependent endocytosis is related to the uptake of REB nanocrystals into cheek pouch tissue by using various inhibitors of energy-dependent endocytosis. Energy-dependent endocytosis is classified into four pathways: Phagocytosis, MP, CME and CavME [44,45]. Large particles (0.5–5 μm) are taken up by phagocytosis, and somewhat smaller particles (100 nm–5 μm) are taken up by MP. CME and CavME relate to the uptake of particles smaller than those taken up by MP: <120 nm for CME and <80 nm for CavME [46]. Each of these energy-dependent endocytosis pathways can be specifically inhibited by different inhibitors: 10 μM cytochalasin D inhibits phagocytosis [36], 2 μM rottlerin inhibits MP [37], 40 μM dynasore inhibits CME [38] and 54 μM nystatin inhibits CavME [36]. Co-treatment of R-NPs gel and either cytochalasin D, rottlerin or nystatin had no effect of the amount of REB taken up by cheek pouch tissue. REB content in the cheek pouch of hamsters co-treated with R-NPs gel and dynasore were significantly decreased (Figure 4B,C). These results suggest that the REB nanocrystals are taken up into cheek pouch tissue by the CME pathway, resulting in the enhancement of wound healing (Figures 5 and 6).

5. Conclusions

We designed a hydrogel formulation incorporating REB nanocrystals (R-NPs gel) and found that most of the REB is released from the hydrogel as drug nanocrystals, which are taken up into the tissue through the CME pathway. REB provides a persistent effect, resulting in an enhancement of oral wound healing. It is possible that the R-NPs gel can provide useful therapy for serious oral mucositis. The development of formulations incorporating drug nanocrystals, such as hydrogels and mouthwashes, may be helpful when designing oral DDS for poorly soluble drugs.

Author Contributions: Conceptualization, N.N.; Data curation, R.S., S.D., H.O. and N.Y.; Formal analysis, R.S., S.D., H.O., N.H. and N.Y.; Funding acquisition, N.N.; Investigation, R.S., S.D., H.O., N.H. and N.Y.; Methodology, N.N., R.S., H.S. and N.Y.; Supervision, N.N.; Visualization, N.N.; Writing—original draft, N.N., H.S. and N.Y.; Writing—review & editing, N.N. All authors have read and agreed to the published version of the manuscript.

Funding: This work was supported in part by a grant, 18K06769, from the Ministry of Education, Culture, Sports, Science, and Technology of Japan.

Conflicts of Interest: The authors declare that the research was conducted in the absence of any commercial or financial relationships that could be construed as a potential conflicts of interest.

References

1. Sciubba, J.J.; Goldenberg, D. Oral complications of radiotherapy. *Lancet Oncol.* **2006**, *7*, 175–183. [CrossRef]
2. Rodríguez-Caballero, A.; Torres-Lagares, D.; Robles-García, M.; Pachón-Ibáñez, J.; González-Padilla, D.; Gutiérrez-Pérez, J.L. Cancer treatment-induced oral mucositis: A critical review. *Int. J. Oral Maxillofac. Surg.* **2012**, *41*, 225–238. [CrossRef]
3. Donnelly, J.P.; Blijlevens, N.M.; Verhagen, C.A. Can anything be done about oral mucositis? *Ann. Oncol.* **2003**, *14*, 505–507. [CrossRef]
4. Sonis, S.T. Oral mucositis in cancer therapy. *J. Support. Oncol.* **2004**, *2*, 3–8.
5. Trotti, A.; Bellm, L.A.; Epstein, J.B.; Frame, D.; Fuchs, H.J.; Gwede, C.K.; Komaroff, E.; Nalysnyk, L.; Zilberberg, M.D. Mucositis incidence, severity and associated outcomes in patients with head and neck cancer receiving radiotherapy with or without chemotherapy: A systematic literature review. *Radiother. Oncol.* **2003**, *66*, 253–262. [CrossRef]
6. Sonis, S.T.; Elting, L.S.; Keefe, D.; Peterson, D.E.; Schubert, M.; Hauer-Jensen, M.; Bekele, B.N.; Raber-Durlacher, J.; Donnelly, J.P.; Rubenstein, E.B. Perspectives on cancer therapy-induced mucosal injury: Pathogenesis, measurement, epidemiology, and consequences for patients. *Cancer* **2004**, *100*, 1995–2025. [CrossRef] [PubMed]
7. Prescribing Information: Mucosta®Tablets 100 mg, Ohtsuka Japan Inc. 2017. Available online: https://www.pmda.go.jp/PmdaSearch/iyakuDetail/GeneralList/2329021 (accessed on 20 May 2020). (In Japanese).
8. Lalla, R.V.; Bowen, J.; Barasch, A.; Elting, L.; Epstein, J.; Keefe, D.M.; McGuire, D.B.; Migliorati, C.; Nicolatou-Galitis, O.; Peterson, D.E.; et al. MASCC/ISOO clinical practice guidelines for the management of mucositis secondary to cancer therapy. *Cancer* **2014**, *120*, 1453–1461. [CrossRef] [PubMed]
9. Bensinger, W.; Schubert, M.; Ang, K.K.; Brizel, D.; Brown, E.; Eilers, J.G.; Elting, L.; Mittal, B.B.; Schattner, M.A.; Spielberger, R.; et al. NCCN Task Force Report. prevention and management of mucositis in cancer care. *J. Natl. Compr. Cancer Netw.* **2008**, *6*, S1–S21; quiz S22–S24.
10. Peterson, D.E.; Boers-Doets, C.B.; Bensadoun, R.J.; Herrstedt, J. ESMO Guidelines Committee Management of oral and gastrointestinal mucosal injury: ESMO Clinical Practice Guidelines for diagnosis, treatment, and follow-up. *Ann. Oncol.* **2015**, *26*, v139–v151. [CrossRef] [PubMed]
11. Murakami, K.; Okajima, K.; Uchiba, M.; Harada, N.; Johno, M.; Okabe, H.; Takatsuki, K. Rebamipide attenuates indomethacin-induced gastric mucosal lesion formation by inhibiting activation of leukocytes in rats. *Dig. Dis. Sci.* **1997**, *42*, 319–325. [CrossRef] [PubMed]
12. Yoshikawa, T.; Naito, Y.; Tanigawa, T.; Kondo, M. Free radical scavenging activity of the novel anti-ulcer agent rebsamipide studied by electron spin resonance. *Arzneimittelforschung* **1993**, *43*, 363–366. [PubMed]
13. Nanke, Y.; Kobashigawa, T.; Yago, T.; Kawamoto, M.; Yamanaka, H.; Kotake, S. Rebamipide, an Amino Acid Analog of 2(1H)-Quinolinone, Inhibits the Formation of Human Osteoclasts. *BioMed Res. Int.* **2016**, *2016*, 6824719. [CrossRef] [PubMed]

14. Tanaka, H.; Fukuda, K.; Ishida, W.; Harada, Y.; Sumi, T.; Fukushima, A. Rebamipide increases barrier function and attenuates TNFalpha-induced barrier disruption and cytokine expression in human corneal epithelial cells. *Br. J. Ophthalmol.* **2013**, *97*, 912–916. [CrossRef] [PubMed]
15. Yasuda, T.; Chiba, H.; Satomi, T.; Matsuo, A.; Kaneko, T.; Chikazu, D.; Miyamatsu, H. Preventive effect of rebamipide gargle on chemoradiotherpy-induced oral mucositis in patients with oral cancer: A pilot study. *J. Oral Maxillofac. Res.* **2011**, *2*, e3. [CrossRef] [PubMed]
16. Nabeta, I.; Nakamura, K.; Kimura, M.; Kaya, M.; Tsuneizumi, M.; Nakagami, K.; Kawarasaki, T.; Honma, M. The effect of rebamipide for prevention of mucositis associated with anthracycline chemotherapy for breast cancer. *J. Jpn. Soc. Hosp. Pharm.* **2010**, *46*, 1629–1634. (In Japanese)
17. Chaitanya, B.; Pai, K.M.; Yathiraj, P.H.; Fernandes, D.; Chhaparwal, Y. Rebamipide gargle in preventive management of chemo-radiotherapy induced oral mucositis. *Oral Oncol.* **2017**, *72*, 179–182. [CrossRef]
18. Yokota, T.; Ogawa, T.; Takahashi, S.; Okami, K.; Fujii, T.; Tanaka, K.; Iwae, S.; Ota, I.; Ueda, T.; Monden, N.; et al. Efficacy and safety of rebamipide liquid for chemoradiotherapy-induced oral mucositis in patients with head and neck cancer: A multicenter, randomized, double-blind, placebo-controlled, parallel-group phase II study. *BMC Cancer* **2017**, *17*, 314. [CrossRef]
19. Ishihara, K.; Komuro, Y.; Nishiyama, N.; Yamasaki, K.; Hotta, K. Effect of rebamipide on mucus secretion by endogenous prostaglandin-independent mechanism in rat gastric mucosa. *Arzneimittelforschung* **1992**, *42*, 1462–1466.
20. Yamasaki, K.; Kanbe, T.; Chijiwa, T.; Ishiyama, H.; Morita, S. Gastric mucosal protection by OPC-12759, a novel antiulcer compound, in the rat. *Eur. J. Pharmacol.* **1987**, *142*, 23–29. [CrossRef]
21. Kleine, A.; Kluge, S.; Peskar, B.M. Stimulation of prostaglandin biosynthesis mediates gastroprotective effect of rebamipide in rats. *Dig. Dis. Sci.* **1993**, *38*, 1441–1449. [CrossRef]
22. Nagano, C.; Azuma, A.; Ishiyama, H.; Sekiguchi, K.; Imagawa, K.; Kikuchi, M. Rebamipide suppresses formyl-methionyl-leucylphenylalanine (fMLP)-induced superoxide production by inhibiting fMLP-receptor binding in human neutrophils. *J. Pharmacol. Exp. Ther.* **2001**, *297*, 388–394.
23. Kobayashi, T.; Zinchuk, V.S.; del Saz, E.G.; Jiang, F.; Yamasaki, Y.; Kataoka, S.; Okada, T.; Tsunawaki, S.; Seguchi, H. Suppressive effect of rebamipide, an antiulcer agent, against activation of human neutrophils exposed to formyl-methionyl-leucyl-phenylalanine. *Histol. Histopathol.* **2000**, *15*, 1067–1076.
24. Masamune, A.; Yoshida, M.; Sakai, Y.; Shimosegawa, T. Rebamipide inhibits ceramide-induced interleukin-8 production in Kato III human gastric cancer cells. *J. Pharmacol. Exp. Ther.* **2001**, *298*, 485–492.
25. Kim, C.D.; Kim, H.H.; Hong, K.W. Inhibitory effect of rebamipide on the neutrophil adherence stimulated by conditioned media from helicobacter pylori-infected gastric epithelial cells. *J. Pharmacol. Exp. Ther.* **1999**, *288*, 133–138.
26. Arakawa, T.; Kobayashi, K.; Yoshikawa, T.; Tarnawski, A. Rebamipide: Overview of its mechanisms of action and efficacy in mucosal protection and ulcer healing. *Dig. Dis. Sci.* **1998**, *43*, 5S–13S.
27. Tarnawski, A.; Arakawa, T.; Kobayashi, K. Rebamipide treatment activates epidermal growth factor and its receptor expression in normal and ulcerated gastric mucosa in rats: One mechanism for its ulcer healing action? *Dig. Dis. Sci.* **1998**, *43*, 90S–98S.
28. Shioya, Y.; Kashiyama, E.; Okada, K.; Kusumoto, N.; Abe, Y. Metabolic fate of the anti-ulcer agent, (±)-2-(4-chlorobenzoylamino)-3-[2(1H)-quinolinon-4-yl]propionic acid (OPC-12759): Absorption, distribution, and excretion in rats and dogs. *Iyakuhin Kenkyu* **1989**, *20*, 522–533.
29. Sanders, N.N.; De Smedt, S.C.; Van Rompaey, E.; Simoens, P.; De Baets, F.; Demeester, J. Cystic fibrosis sputum: A barrier to the transport of nanospheres. *Am. J. Respir. Crit. Care Med.* **2000**, *162*, 1905–1911. [CrossRef]
30. Szentkuti, L. Light microscopical observations on luminally administered dyes, dextrans, nanospheres and microspheres in the pre-epithelial mucus gel layer of the rat distal colon. *J. Control. Release* **1997**, *46*, 233–242. [CrossRef]
31. Norris, D.A.; Sinko, P.J. Effect of size, surface charge and hydrophobicity on the translocation of polyestyrene microspheres through gastrointestinal mucin. *J. Appl. Polym. Sci.* **1997**, *63*, 1481–1492. [CrossRef]
32. Bravo-Osuna, I.; Vauthier, C.; Farabollini, A.; Palmieri, G.F.; Ponchel, G. Mucoadhesion mechanism of chitosan and thiolated chitosan-poly(isobutyl cyanoacrylate) core-shell nanoparticles. *Biomaterials* **2007**, *28*, 2233–2243. [CrossRef]

33. Nagai, N.; Ishii, M.; Seiriki, R.; Ogata, F.; Otake, H.; Nakazawa, Y.; Okamoto, N.; Kanai, K.; Kawasaki, N. Novel Sustained-Release Drug Delivery System for Dry Eye Therapy by Rebamipide Nanoparticles. *Pharmaceutics* **2020**, *12*, 155. [CrossRef]
34. Nagai, N.; Iwamae, A.; Tanimoto, S.; Yoshioka, C.; Ito, Y. Pharmacokinetics and Antiinflammatory Effect of a Novel Gel System Containing Ketoprofen Solid Nanoparticles. *Biol. Pharm. Bull.* **2015**, *38*, 1918–1924. [CrossRef]
35. Nagai, N.; Ogata, F.; Otake, H.; Nakazawa, Y.; Kawasaki, N. Design of a transdermal formulation containing raloxifene nanoparticles for osteoporosis treatment. *Int. J. Nanomed.* **2018**, *13*, 5215–5229. [CrossRef]
36. Mäger, I.; Langel, K.; Lehto, T.; Eiríksdóttir, E.; Langel, U. The role of endocytosis on the uptake kinetics of luciferin-conjugated cell-penetrating peptides. *Biochim. Biophys. Acta Biomembr.* **2012**, *1818*, 502–511. [CrossRef]
37. Hufnagel, H.; Hakim, P.; Lima, A.; Hollfelder, F. Fluid phase endocytosis contributes to transfection of DNA by PEI-25. *Mol. Ther.* **2009**, *17*, 1411–1417. [CrossRef]
38. Malomouzh, A.I.; Mukhitov, A.R.; Proskurina, S.E.; Vyskocil, F.; Nikolsky, E.E. The effect of dynasore, a blocker of dynamin-dependent endocytosis, on spontaneous quantal and non-quantal release of acetylcholine in murine neuromuscular junctions. *Dokl. Biol. Sci.* **2014**, *459*, 330–333. [CrossRef]
39. Nicolatou-Galitis, O.; Sarri, T.; Bowen, J.; Di Palma, M.; Kouloulias, V.E.; Niscola, P.; Riesenbeck, D.; Stokman, M.; Tissing, W.; Yeoh, E.; et al. Systematic review of anti-inflammatory agents for the management of oral mucositis in cancer patients. *Support. Care Cancer* **2013**, *21*, 3179–3189. [CrossRef]
40. Nagai, N.; Ito, Y.; Okamoto, N.; Shimomura, Y. A nanoparticle formulation reduces the corneal toxicity of indomethacin eye drops and enhances its corneal permeability. *Toxicology* **2014**, *319*, 53–62. [CrossRef]
41. Nagai, N.; Ito, Y. Therapeutic Effects of Gel Ointments containing Tranilast Nanoparticles on Paw Edema in Adjuvant-Induced Arthritis Rats. *Biol. Pharm. Bull.* **2014**, *37*, 96–104. [CrossRef]
42. Ishii, M.; Fukuoka, Y.; Deguchi, S.; Otake, H.; Tanino, T.; Nagai, N. Energy-Dependent Endocytosis is Involved in the Absorption of Indomethacin Nanoparticles in the Small Intestine. *Int. J. Mol. Sci.* **2019**, *20*, 476. [CrossRef] [PubMed]
43. Nagai, N.; Ito, Y. Effect of Solid Nanoparticle of Indomethacin on Therapy for Rheumatoid Arthritis in Adjuvant-Induced Arthritis Rat. *Biol. Pharm. Bull.* **2014**, *37*, 1109–1118. [CrossRef] [PubMed]
44. Wang, J.; Byrne, J.D.; Napier, M.E.; DeSimone, J.M. More effective nanomedicines through particle design. *Small* **2011**, *7*, 1919–1931. [CrossRef] [PubMed]
45. Rappoport, J.Z. Focusing on clathrin-mediated endocytosis. *Biochem. J.* **2008**, *412*, 415–423. [CrossRef]
46. Zhang, S.; Li, J.; Lykotrafitis, G.; Bao, G.; Suresh, S. Size-dependent endocytosis of nanoparticles. *Adv. Mater.* **2009**, *21*, 419–424. [CrossRef]

MDPI
St. Alban-Anlage 66
4052 Basel
Switzerland
Tel. +41 61 683 77 34
Fax +41 61 302 89 18
www.mdpi.com

Pharmaceutics Editorial Office
E-mail: pharmaceutics@mdpi.com
www.mdpi.com/journal/pharmaceutics

www.ingramcontent.com/pod-product-compliance
Lightning Source LLC
LaVergne TN
LVHW070707100526
838202LV00013B/1046